Arthritis Sourcebook

Basic Consumer Health Information about Specific Forms of Arthritis and Related Disorders, Including Rheumatoid Arthritis, Osteoarthritis, Gout, Polymyalgia Rheumatica, Psoriatic Arthritis, Spondyloarthropathies, Juvenile Rheumatoid Arthritis, and Juvenile Ankylosing Spondylitis; Along with Information about Medical, Surgical, and Alternative Treatment Options, and Including Strategies for Coping with Pain, Fatigue, and Stress

Edited by Allan R. Cook. 575 pages. 1998. 0-7808-0201-2. $78.

Back & Neck Disorders Sourcebook

Basic Information about Disorders and Injuries of the Spinal Cord and Vertebrae, Including Facts on Chiropractic Treatment, Surgical Interventions, Paralysis, and Rehabilitation, Along with Advice for Preventing Back Trouble

Edited by Karen Bellenir. 548 pages. 1997. 0-7808-0202-0. $78.

"The strength of this work is its basic, easy-to-read format. Recommended."
— Reference and User Services Quarterly, Winter '97

Blood & Circulatory Disorders Sourcebook

Basic Information about Blood and Its Components, Anemias, Leukemias, Bleeding Disorders, and Circulatory Disorders, Including Aplastic Anemia, Thalassemia, Sickle-Cell Disease, Hemochromatosis, Hemophilia, Von Willebrand Disease, and Vascular Diseases; Along with a Special Section on Blood Transfusions and Blood Supply Safety, a Glossary, and Source Listings for Further Help and Information

Edited by Karen Bellenir and Linda M. Shin. 575 pages. 1998. 0-7808-0203-9. $78.

Brain Disorders Sourcebook

Basic Consumer Health Information about Strokes, Epilepsy, Amyotrophic Lateral Sclerosis (ALS/Lou Gehrig's Disease), Parkinson's Disease, Brain Tumors, Cerebral Palsy, Headache, Tourette Syndrome, and More; Along with Statistical Data, Treatment and Rehabilitation Options, Coping Strategies, Reports on Current Research Initiatives, a Glossary, and Resource Listings for Additional Help and Information

Edited by Karen Bellenir. 600 pages. 1999. 0-7808-0229-2. $78.

Burns Sourcebook

Basic Information about Various Types of Burns and Scalds, Including Flame, Heat, Electrical, Chemical, and Sun; Along with Short- and Long-Term Treatments, Tissue Reconstruction, Plastic Surgery, Prevention Suggestions, and First Aid

Edited by Allan R. Cook. 600 pages. 1999. 0-7808-0204-7. $78.

Cancer Sourcebook, 1st Edition

Basic Information on Cancer Types, Symptoms, Diagnostic Methods, and Treatments, Including Statistics on Cancer Occurrences Worldwide and the Risks Associated with Known Carcinogens and Activities

Edited by Frank E. Bair. 932 pages. 1990. 1-55888-888-8. $78.

"Written in nontechnical language. Useful for patients, their families, medical professionals, and librarians."
— Guide to Reference Books, '96

"Designed with the non-medical professional in mind. Libraries and medical facilities interested in patient education should certainly consider adding the Cancer Sourcebook to their holdings. This compact collection of reliable information . . . is an invaluable tool for helping patients and patients' families and friends to take the first steps in coping with the many difficulties of cancer."
— Medical Reference Services Quarterly, Winter '91

"Specifically created for the nontechnical reader . . . an important resource for the general reader trying to understand the complexities of cancer."
— American Reference Books Annual, '91

"This publication's nontechnical nature and very comprehensive format make it useful for both the general public and undergraduate students." — Choice, Oct '90

New Cancer Sourcebook, 2nd Edition

Basic Information about Major Forms and Stages of Cancer, Featuring Facts about Primary and Secondary Tumors of the Respiratory, Nervous, Lymphatic, Circulatory, Skeletal, and Gastrointestinal Systems, and Specific Organs; Statistical and Demographic Data; Treatment Options; and Strategies for Coping

Edited by Allan R. Cook. 1,313 pages. 1996. 0-7808-0041-9. $78.

"This book is an excellent resource for patients with newly diagnosed cancer and their famil... The dia...
...ghly rec-
...in their

...Oct '97

...n is ex-
...ral read-
..., Jan '97

Continues next page

Cancer Sourcebook, 3rd Edition

Basic Information about Major Forms and Stages of Cancer, Featuring Facts about Primary and Secondary Tumors of the Respiratory, Nervous, Lymphatic, Circulatory, Skeletal, and Gastrointestinal Systems, and Specific Organs, Statistical and Demographic Data, Treatment Options, and Strategies for Coping

Edited by Edward J. Prucha. 800 pages. 1999. 0-7808-0227-6. $78.

Cancer Sourcebook for Women

Basic Information about Specific Forms of Cancer That Affect Women, Featuring Facts about Breast Cancer, Cervical Cancer, Ovarian Cancer, Cancer of the Uterus and Uterine Sarcoma, Cancer of the Vagina, and Cancer of the Vulva; Statistical and Demographic Data; Treatments, Self-Help Management Suggestions, and Current Research Initiatives

Edited by Allan R. Cook and Peter D. Dresser. 524 pages. 1996. 0-7808-0076-1. $78.

". . . written in easily understandable, non-technical language. Recommended for public libraries or hospital and academic libraries that collect patient education or consumer health materials."
— *Medical Reference Services Quarterly, Spring '97*

"Would be of value in a consumer health library. . . . written with the health care consumer in mind. Medical jargon is at a minimum, and medical terms are explained in clear, understandable sentences."
— *Bulletin of the MLA, Oct '96*

"The availability under one cover of all these pertinent publications, grouped under cohesive headings, makes this certainly a most useful sourcebook."
— *Choice, Jun '96*

"Presents a comprehensive knowledge base for general readers. Men and women both benefit from the gold mine of information nestled between the two covers of this book. Recommended."
— *Academic Library Book Review, Summer '96*

"This timely book is highly recommended for consumer health and patient education collections in all libraries."
— *Library Journal, Apr '96*

Cancer Sourcebook for Women, 2nd Edition

Basic Information about Specific Forms of Cancer That Affect Women, Featuring Facts about Breast Cancer, Cervical Cancer, Ovarian Cancer, Cancer of the Uterus and Uterine Sarcoma, Cancer of the Vagina, and Cancer of the Vulva, Statistical and Demographic Data, Treatments, Self-Help Management Suggestions, and Current Research Initiatives

Edited by Edward J. Prucha. 600 pages. 1999. 0-7808-0226-8. $78.

Cardiovascular Diseases & Disorders Sourcebook

Basic Information about Cardiovascular Diseases and Disorders, Featuring Facts about the Cardiovascular System, Demographic and Statistical Data, Descriptions of Pharmacological and Surgical Interventions, Lifestyle Modifications, and a Special Section Focusing on Heart Disorders in Children

Edited by Karen Bellenir and Peter D. Dresser. 683 pages. 1995. 0-7808-0032-X. $78.

". . . comprehensive format provides an extensive overview on this subject."
— *Choice, Jun '96*

". . . an easily understood, complete, up-to-date resource. This well executed public health tool will make valuable information available to those that need it most, patients and their families. The typeface, sturdy non-reflective paper, and library binding add a feel of quality found wanting in other publications. Highly recommended for academic and general libraries. "
— *Academic Library Book Review, Summer '96*

Communication Disorders Sourcebook

Basic Information about Deafness and Hearing Loss, Speech and Language Disorders, Voice Disorders, Balance and Vestibular Disorders, and Disorders of Smell, Taste, and Touch

Edited by Linda M. Ross. 533 pages. 1996. 0-7808-0077-X. $78.

"This is skillfully edited and is a welcome resource for the layperson. It should be found in every public and medical library."
— *Booklist Health Sciences Supplement, Oct '97*

Congenital Disorders Sourcebook

Basic Information about Disorders Acquired during Gestation, Including Spina Bifida, Hydrocephalus, Cerebral Palsy, Heart Defects, Craniofacial Abnormalities, Fetal Alcohol Syndrome, and More, Along with Current Treatment Options and Statistical Data

Edited by Karen Bellenir. 607 pages. 1997. 0-7808-0205-5. $78.

"Recommended reference source." — *Booklist, Oct '97*

Consumer Issues in Health Care Sourcebook

Basic Information about Health Care Fundamentals and Related Consumer Issues, Including Exams and Screening Tests, Physician Specialties, Choosing a Doctor, Using Prescription and Over-the-Counter Medications Safely, Avoiding Health Scams, Managing Common Health Risks in the Home, Care Options for Chronically or Terminally Ill Patients, and a List of Resources for Obtaining Help and Further Information

Edited by Karen Bellenir. 592 pages. 1998. 0-7808-0221-7. $78.

Continues in back end sheets

Forensic Medicine
SOURCEBOOK

Health Reference Series

Health Reference Series

First Edition

Forensic Medicine
SOURCEBOOK

*Basic Consumer Information for the
Layperson about Forensic Medicine, Including
Crime Scene Investigation, Evidence Collection and
Analysis, Expert Testimony, Computer-Aided
Criminal Identification, Digital Imaging in
the Courtroom, DNA Profiling, Accident
Reconstruction, Autopsies, Ballistics, Drugs and
Explosives Detection, Latent Fingerprints, Product
Tampering, and Questioned Document
Examination; Along with Statistical Data,
a Glossary of Forensics Terminology, and Listings
of Sources for Further Help and Information*

Edited by
Annemarie S. Muth

Omnigraphics, Inc.

Penobscot Building / Detroit, MI 48226

Bibliographic Note

Because this page cannot legibly accommodate all the copyright notices, the Bibliographic Note portion of the Preface constitutes an extension of the copyright notice.

Beginning with books published in 1999, each new volume of the *Health Reference Series* will be individually titled and called a "First Edition." Subsequent updates will carry sequential edition numbers. To help avoid confusion and to provide maximum flexibility in our ability to respond to informational needs, the practice of consecutively numbering each volume will be discontinued.

Edited by Annemarie S. Muth

Health Reference Series

Karen Bellenir, *Series Editor*
Peter D. Dresser, *Managing Editor*
Joan Margeson, *Research Associate*
Dawn Matthews, *Verification Assistant*
Margaret Mary Missar, *Research Coordinator*
Jenifer Swanson, *Research Associate*

Omnigraphics, Inc.

Matthew P. Barbour, *Vice President, Operations*
Laurie Lanzen Harris, *Vice President, Editorial Director*
Thomas J. Murphy, *Vice President, Finance and Comptroller*
Peter E. Ruffner, *Senior Vice President*
Jane J. Steele, *Marketing Consultant*

Frederick G. Ruffner, Jr., Publisher

Library of Congress Cataloging-in-Publication Data

Forensic medicine sourcebook : basic consumer information for the layperson about Forensic medicine . . . / edited by Annemarie S. Muth.
    p. cm.
Includes bibliographical references and index.
ISBN 0-7808-0232-2 (Lib. bdg.)
1. Medical jurisprudence Popular works. I. Muth, Annemarie.
RA1053.F67 1999   99-26967
614'.1—dc21   CIP

∞

Printed in the United States

Table of Contents

Part III: Forensic Medicine/Science Subspecialties

Part IV: Emerging Forensic Subspecialties

Part V: Advances in Crime Investigation

Part VI: The Courtroom

Part VII: Additional Help and Information

Preface

About This Book

Forensic medicine explores the legal aspects of medicine. From its beginnings, the task of forensic practitioners has been to preserve, quantify, and interpret physical evidence pertinent to a legal case. In the past, this might have involved a rudimentary examination of a corpse to determine the cause of death. As medical science advanced, scientists could analyze more minute, even microscopic, forms of physical evidence, such as the chemical composition of hair and blood samples, to better determine the cause of death, or to identify the victim or perpetrator of a crime. Today, in many cases, such scientific assessment has invalidated the testimony of witnesses and overturned legal decisions; DNA testing results have exonerated previously convicted prisoners.

There is a keen interest among the general public about the advancements in forensic medicine. This book takes a layperson's look at this topic. It briefly explores the history of forensic medicine and how related sciences assist our justice system today. It includes statistics on the frequency of homicides and autopsies in the United States, a glossary of pertinent terminology, and a chapter of resource listings for further information. It features articles from both government and private sector organizations on how new forensic practices and technologies may further the precise analysis of evidence taken from a crime scene or the scene of a natural disaster. It also demonstrates how and why the justice system consults forensic specialists and explains their changing role in the legal process.

How to Use This Book

This book is divided into parts and chapters. Parts focus on broad areas of interest. Chapters are devoted to single topics within a part.

Part I: Overview briefly defines the forensic sciences, provides a forensic science timeline, and features statistics on suspicious deaths, autopsies, and death investigation jurisdictions in the United States and Canada,

Part II: Crime Scene and Laboratory Investigation describes the collection and preservation of evidence at crime scenes, evidence photography, handling domestic violence cases, examining the corpse at the scene of the crime, determining the age of the victim from skeletal remains, examining the corpse for signs of rapid anoxial death (asphyxia), and describing the analytical tools of the forensic chemist.

Part III: Forensic Medicine / Science Subspecialties features articles describing in some depth the work of each of the forensic subspecialists: the forensic pathologist, psychiatrist, nurse, anthropologist, toxicologist, odontologist, entomologist, palynologist, geologist, engineer, firearms identification specialist, and questioned documents examiner.

Part IV: Emerging Forensic Subspecialties provides information about new forensic subspecialties that either use a new technology or method to detect or analyze evidence. These include automated DNA typing, criminal profiling, computer-aided victim and criminal identification, bite mark evidence, latent fingerprint technology, language-based author identification, diatom testing for drowning victims, and drugs and explosives detection.

Part V: Advances in Crime Investigation includes chapters describing new forensic laboratories, new laboratory regulations and prescribed tests, and new investigative organizations. This section covers a wide range of topics including child fatality review teams, hair and urinalysis in drug detection, gunshot residue analysis, condom trace evidence, and product tampering.

Part VI: The Courtroom discusses how evidence is admitted in a case, the role of the expert medical witness, how DNA has overturned previous court decisions, and the use of computer-aided graphics to reconstruct a crime or accident.

Part VII: Additional Help and Information provides a glossary of forensics terminology and a list of forensics-related organizations and online sites that may be contacted for further information.

Bibliographic Note

This volume contains documents and excerpts from publications issued by the following U.S. government agencies: Centers for Disease Control and Prevention (CDC), Federal Bureau of Investigation (FBI), Food and Drug Administration (FDA), National Center for Environmental Health (NCEH), National Criminal Justice Reference Service (NCJRS), National Institute of Justice (NIJ), National Law Enforcement and Corrections Technology Center (NLECTC), and National Library of Medicine (NLM).

In addition, this volume contains copyrighted documents from the following organizations and individuals: The Art Engineering Company; Herbert L. Blitzer, Institute for Forensic Imaging; Harold J. Bursztajn, M.D., Harvard Medical School; Jason A. Byrd, Ph.D., University of Florida; Jeffrey Scott Doyle, Kentucky State Police, Jefferson Regional Forensic Laboratory; Forensic Sciences Foundation, Inc. (FSF); John A. Giacobbe, Eastern New Mexico University, Portales; William J. Graves, Centre of Forensic Sciences, University of Toronto; Indiana University and Purdue University, Indianapolis (IUPUI); Knowledge Solutions LLC; Karen L. Kwek, University of Toronto; Virginia A. Lynch, M.S.N, R.N., F.A.A.F.S.; John Mustard, Centre of Forensic Sciences, University of Toronto; National Association of Medical Examiners (NAME); National Forensic Center (NFC); James O. Pex, Oregon State Police, Coos Bay Forensic Laboratory; Michael S. Pollanen, Ph.D., Office of the Chief Coroner of Ontario, Canada; George Schiro, Louisiana State Police Crime Laboratory; T. C. Forensic Pty Ltd.; TH Geological Services, Inc.; Carrie M. Weiler, B.A., King County Medical Examiner's Office, Seattle; and Emily J. Will, Certified Document Examiner. Copyrighted articles from *Chemical & Engineering News, Clinical Infectious Diseases, Forensic Sourcebook99 / CD-ROM, International Journal of Legal Medicine, Journal of Psychosocial Nursing and Mental Health Services, Journal of the American Dental Association, The Police Chief, The Scientist,* and *Today's Chemist at Work* are also included.

Full citation information is provided on the first page of each chapter. Every effort has been made to secure all necessary rights to reprint the copyrighted material. If any omissions have been made, please contact Omnigraphics to make corrections for future editions.

Acknowledgements

In addition to the many organizations and agencies who contributed the material that is included in this book, thanks go to Margaret Mary Missar for her tireless efforts in tracking down documents, Jenifer Swanson for her researching and internet expertise, and Dawn Matthews for her verification assistance.

Note from the Editor

This book is part of Omnigraphics' *Health Reference Series*. The series provides basic information about a broad range of medical concerns. It is not intended to serve as a tool for diagnosing illness, in prescribing treatments, or as a substitute for the physician/patient relationship. All persons concerned about medical symptoms or the possibility of disease are encouraged to seek professional care from an appropriate health care provider.

Our Advisory Board

The *Health Reference Series* is reviewed by an Advisory Board comprised of librarians from public, academic, and medical libraries. We would like to thank the following board members for providing guidance to the development of this series:

Nancy Bulgarelli,
William Beaumont Hospital Library, Royal Oak, MI

Karen Morgan,
Mardigian Library, University of Michigan, Dearborn, MI

Rosemary Orlando,
St. Clair Shores Public Library, St. Clair Shores, MI

Health Reference Series *Update Policy*

The inaugural book in the *Health Reference Series* was the first edition of *Cancer Sourcebook* published in 1992. Since then, the *Series* has been enthusiastically received by librarians and in the medical community. In order to maintain the standard of providing high-quality health information for the lay person, the editorial staff at Omnigraphics felt it was necessary to implement a policy of updating volumes when warranted.

Medical researchers have been making tremendous strides, and the challenge to stay current with the most recent advances is one our editors take seriously. Each decision to update a volume will be made on an individual basis. Some of the considerations will include how much new information is available and the feedback we receive from people who use the books. If there's a topic you would like to see added to the update list, or an area of medical concern you feel has not been adequately addressed, please write to:

Editor
Health Reference Series
Omnigraphics, Inc.
2500 Penobscot Bldg.
Detroit, MI 48226

The commitment to providing on-going coverage of important medical developments has also led to some technical changes in the *Health Reference Series*. Beginning with books published in 1999, each new volume will be individually titled and called a "First Edition." Subsequent updates will carry sequential edition numbers. To help avoid confusion and to provide maximum flexibility in our ability to respond to informational needs, the practice of consecutively numbering each volume will be discontinued.

Part One

Overview

Chapter 1

Forensic Science

The Role of the Forensic Scientist

The forensic sciences form a vital part of the entire justice and regulatory system. Still, some of its disciplines have become identified primarily with law enforcement, an image enhanced by television and movies. This is misleading because forensic scientists may be involved in all aspects of a criminal case, and the results of their work may serve either the defense or the prosecution. The forensic scientist's skill is to use all the information available to determine facts.

Though closely identified with the criminal justice system, the forensic scientist plays an increasingly active role in the civil justice arena. Issues of law and/or fact which may require forensic science expertise range from questions of the validity of a signature on a will, to a claim of products liability, to questions of whether a corporation is complying with environmental laws.

The work of the forensic scientist reduces the number of cases entering the overloaded court system by assisting the decision-makers before a case reaches the court. The facts developed by forensic scientists often show either the prosecuting or defense attorneys that an issue does not merit a court hearing. This decision is based on scientific

Excerpted from "The Forensic Sciences Foundation, Inc., Career Brochure," [Online] undated. Available: http://www.aafs.org/career/CareerBroch.html. Produced by The Forensic Sciences Foundation, Inc., P.O. Box 669, Colorado Springs, CO 80901-0669. For complete contact information, please refer to Chapter 56, "Resources." Reprinted with permission.

investigation, not circumstantial evidence or the sometimes unreliable testimony of witnesses.

The legal system is based on the belief that the legal process results in justice. This has come under some question in recent years. Of course, the forensic scientist cannot change skepticism and mistrust singlehandedly. He or she can, however, contribute to restoring faith in judicial processes by using science and technology in the search for facts in civil, criminal, and regulatory matters.

Criminalistics

Criminalistics is the analysis, comparison, identification, and interpretation of physical evidence. The main role of the criminalist is to objectively apply the techniques of the physical and natural sciences to examine physical evidence, and thereby prove the existence of a crime or make connections. The criminalist provides information to investigators, attorneys, judges, or juries. This information is helpful in determining the innocence or guilt of the suspect.

Because of the variety of human activity which may surround a crime, the range of material which may be physical evidence is almost limitless. Evidence may be so small that a microscope is needed to see it, or it may be as large as a truck. It may be as subtle as a whiff of a flammable gas at an arson scene or as obvious as a pool of blood at a homicide scene. The enormous range of material challenges the ingenuity of the criminalist. He or she examines and identifies hair, fibers, blood and seminal stains, alcohol, drugs, paint, glass, botanicals, soil, flammable gases, and safe insulating material; restores smeared or smudged markings; and identifies firearms and compares bullets, tool markings, and foot prints.

Using analytical skill and practical experience, the criminalist separates significant evidence from that having little or no probative value. Next, the criminalist sorts, compares, or identifies the evidence, developing useful information for an investigation or trial. It may be established, for example, that a bullet has been fired from a particular gun or that a fragment of plastic from the scene of a hit-and-run accident has broken off a particular car. This type of analysis is difficult; it requires an eye for detail, a broad practical scientific background, and the ability to apply these skills in court with full knowledge of the ethical responsibilities involved.

Perhaps the most important task of the criminalist lies in interpreting the results of findings to determine the circumstances at the time a crime occurred, or perhaps to support a witness's statement.

4

Reconstructing the events of a crime is often very difficult. It requires an understanding of human behavior, of the physical laws and processes involved, and the recognition of how they interact.

Finally, any findings must be conveyed to the other elements of the criminal justice system. This is usually done by written reports or expert testimony. The criminalist must express conclusions so that technical details are understood by the court and the jury. The criminalist undertakes a serious challenge on behalf of society and, by fulfilling this responsibility, derives great personal satisfaction.

Engineering Sciences

Overview/Definition

An engineer applies the principles of mathematics and science for the benefit of mankind. Innovation and problem-solving are key traits of an engineer. The forensic engineer, more specifically, applies the art and science of engineering to the purpose of the law. Most requests for services involve civil suits; however, the forensic engineer may also assist in the prosecution or defense of criminal or regulatory matters.

Education and Training

Forensic engineering is a specialized practice of the engineering sciences, not a separate discipline. Few universities offer courses in forensic engineering, therefore, the forensic engineer must develop his own credentials. The minimum education required is a bachelor's degree in engineering or an allied science. It is recommended that the forensic engineer have advanced degrees, when appropriate, and be a registered Professional Engineer. The forensic engineer must be highly competent, ethical, credible, and should have extensive professional experience in the subject matter under consideration. Other essential capabilities include writing and speaking skills as well as evidence handling techniques. Knowledge and understanding of legal procedures and standards of proof are definite advantages. Active participation in professional organizations and continuing education are highly recommended.

Role of the Forensic Engineer

Questions posed to forensic engineers are in subjects as varied as the specialties of the engineers themselves. Typical subjects include: failure analysis, accident reconstruction, causes and origins of fires or explosions, design review, quality evaluation of construction or manufacturing, maintenance procedures, and environment definition. The scopes may range from entire communication networks or transportation systems to the molecular composition or grain structure of a specific component. Structures examined may range from skyscrapers or bridges to surgical implants or bones. Conclusions are applied in personal injury litigation, construction claims, contract or warranty disputes, patent or copyright infringements, and criminal and regulatory matters.

In most legal disputes involving engineering issues, each party will hire its own engineer(s) or consultation and to testify on its behalf. In other words, the forensic engineer's work is subject to the scrutiny of other highly qualified professionals.

Employment Opportunities

Forensic engineers may be employees of large corporations or government agencies. However, most forensic engineers are employed by small firms or are self-employed. Some perform their services on a part-time basis or in addition to their other work (e.g., a college professor providing forensic engineering consultations). The competent, ethical, credible, and professional forensic engineer is in high demand, now and in the foreseeable future.

Forensic Pathology

Pathology is the study of disease. This is done by the examination of the body at autopsy, of tissues removed during surgery, and by analysis of fluids from the body, such as blood or urine, in the clinical pathology laboratory.

Forensic pathology is a specialization in pathology requiring additional training. Forensic pathology is the application of the principles of pathology, and of medicine in general, to the legal needs of society. Forensic pathologists perform autopsies to determine what caused a person's death and the manner of death (natural, accident, suicide, homicide, or undetermined). The autopsies are ordered under the law. There is much emphasis on violent deaths (deaths due to homicide, accident, or suicide) in the forensic pathologist's work. Autopsies also are performed in cases of the sudden death of an apparently healthy individual, someone who had never seen a doctor (unattended death), a person who dies in police custody, suspicious or unusual deaths, deaths that may be the result of a surgical or diagnostic procedure which could be a therapeutic misadventure, or on one who dies while being an inmate of a public institution. The laws of each jurisdiction specify which types of death must be reported to the medical examiner or coroner. Many of these deaths are due to natural causes.

The forensic pathologist's involvement and investigation includes visiting the scene of death (where the subject died). Gathering information about what happened at the time and place of the subject's death, what he or she was doing, and the health of the subject are of vital importance. The forensic examination of a body includes examining the clothing on the body, the body itself, and the internal examination of the organs in the body which is the autopsy. The autopsy may include microscopic and x-ray examinations of the tissues of the body.

The forensic pathologist works in coordination with other branches of the forensic sciences. Various types of evidence may be collected, including fingernail clippings and scrapings in an assault case, swabs for examination for sperm and seminal fluid, hair samples, and fibers on the deceased's clothing and body. These specimens are evidence in a case and are sent to the crime laboratory for examination by a criminalist. Other specimens obtained at autopsy are for toxicology study. These could be blood, urine, stomach contents, bile, liver, kidney, lungs, brains, nail clippings, and hair. These specimens are sent to the toxicologist for analysis for the presence of alcohol, drugs, and other chemicals. Bullets, shotgun pellets, and wadding may be recovered at the autopsy. These are sent to the crime laboratory for examination by a firearms examiner for matching to a specific gun.

The forensic pathologist must record all the information obtained in a written report and, when indicated, in photographic records. The report must be without bias. This work may lead to the conviction of an assailant, or it may protect an innocent person. The forensic pathologist must give depositions and testify in court about the autopsy findings and toxicologic results in criminal and civil law suits. Testimony given must be neutral, presenting the scientific facts accurately and clearly for the jury and the court's deliberations.

The work of the forensic pathologist reaches out to the family of the person who died, to that person's physician, to law enforcement officers, to attorneys who are settling the estate or who are prosecuting or defending a criminal or civil suit, and to public health workers. The forensic pathologist's work will touch those who are left to deal with the loss and trauma caused by a death in a very personal way.

Jurisprudence

Law is the center of forensic sciences. To expand the definition stated earlier, forensic science is the application of scientific principles and technological practices to the purposes of justice in the study and resolution of criminal, civil, and regulatory issues. This includes presentation of testimony in courts of law and administrative tribunals. To be fully effective, one not only must be an expert in the skills of one's discipline, but also must be an expert in communicating findings in legal proceedings, while conforming with the laws governing collection, preservation, and admissibility of evidence.

The lawyer who uses expert testimony in cases involving family, criminal, personal injury, environmental, and administrative law must have a basic knowledge of all the forensic sciences and must be articulate in presenting the findings of the expert witness. However qualified one may be as an expert witness, and however accurate the analysis of the evidence, these tests and analyses will have diminished in value if the lawyer is untrained in the basic knowledge of that field and is unprepared to present the evidence effectively. The lawyer plays a critical role in advancing the search for truth?the ultimate goal of this system of justice.

Forensic Psychiatry and Behavioral Science

Forensic psychiatry is a subspecialty of psychiatry in which scientific and clinical expertise is applied to legal issues in legal contexts embracing civil, criminal, correctional, or legislative matters. Forensic psychiatry should be practiced in accordance with the professional guidelines and ethical principles of psychiatry. The difference between forensic psychiatry and clinical psychiatry is that the former deals with legal issues, while the latter deals with individual therapies.

A broad range of legal issues is addressed by forensic psychiatry and behavioral science. In family and domestic relations laws, one must consider such issues as juvenile delinquency, child custody, parental fitness, children in need of supervision, abrogation of parental rights, spouse abuse, child neglect, abandonment of children, adoption and foster care. In criminal law, one must be mindful of the patient's competence to stand trial, competence to waive legal representation, competence to be sentenced, competence to be executed, guilt by reason of mental illness or diminished responsibility, and innocence by reason of mental disease or mental defect. Involuntary psychiatric hospitalization, rights to refuse treatment, informed consent, competence to participate in do-not-resuscitate decisions, capacity to testify, competence to become engaged, married, or divorced, contractual capacity, disability compensation, and medical malpractice are issues included within civil law.

For every one of these psychiatric-legal issues, there are a variety of different legal criteria. Those criteria may be found in legislated statutes, in case law decisions, in government administrative codes, or in private contractors' documents (e.g., insurance policies). Each of the fifty states and the federal government has its own set of laws, cases, codes, and valid contracts. Even though a single issue may be under consideration, the criteria used to decide that issue depends on whether it is a federal or state legal case and which court has jurisdiction over the case.

Education and Training

Psychiatrists are medical doctors who have completed twelve years of education between college, medical school, and residency training in psychiatry. Forensic psychiatrists also will have additional education and experience in areas relevant for the law.

Some forensic psychiatrists take an additional one or two years of post-residency training in psychiatry-and-the-law. Others pursue a career of independent study and on-the-job training. The American Board of Forensic Psychiatry (ABFP) certifies competence of those specialists who have passed its series of examinations. The two principal sponsors of the ABFP are the American Academy of Forensic Sciences (AAFS) and the American Academy of Psychiatry and the Law (AAPL). There is also an Accreditation Council on Fellowships in Forensic Psychiatry that certifies the quality of post-residency subspecialty fellowship training programs; AAFS and AAPL have both endorsed the Accreditation Council's work.

Psychologists major in behavioral science during their four years of college, have completed an additional one to two years of training for a masters degree, and have spent an additional four to six years in graduate school to obtain a Ph.D. in psychology. Some psychologists take postdoctoral fellowship training in forensic psychology. Some psychologists have independently studied and obtained on-the-job training in forensic psychology. These specialists then apply to the American Board of Forensic Psychology for certification through examination.

Physical Anthropology

The next time you read in the newspaper or hear on the radio and TV that a body or skeleton has been found, it is likely that a forensic anthropologist will be contacted to identify it. Forensic anthropologists are also called to identify individuals killed in disasters such as plane crashes, explosions, fires and other tragedies resulting in the loss of life and mutilation of bodies. In this society, identification of the dead is important for many reasons. The initial step in homicide investigations is usually determining the identity of the victim. This not only concerns relatives of the deceased, but also judicial authorities who need to know whether someone is alive or dead so that wills can be read, estates settled, second marriages can be contracted, and so forth. Law enforcement agencies need to know if recovered bones are human or nonhuman. If they are human and of recent origin, the individual must be identified, and the cause of death and time elapsed since death need to be determined.

The person performing this task is usually a physical anthropologist who has specialized in the study of human skeletal biology. Physical anthropologists have a long tradition of the study of human skeletal remains from ancient societies. The techniques they have developed to determine sex, age, ancestral background (race), health status, markers of trauma and occupational stress and stature in life also have proven extremely useful in forensic sciences.

Education and Training

Forensic anthropologists usually earn a Ph.D. in anthropology with an emphasis on the study of human osteology and anatomy. It is necessary to gain practical experience in forensic anthropology before court systems will accept an individual as an expert witness in the field.

Forensic anthropology obtained professional recognition in the American Academy of Forensic Sciences (AAFS) in 1972 when the AAFS established a Physical Anthropology Section at its annual meeting. Five years later, the American Board of Forensic Anthropology was created for the purpose of certifying experts in the field of forensic anthropology as well as establishing a forum for all members of the section who perform forensic anthropology services. For membership in the AAFS and for Board certification, it is necessary to demonstrate practical experience, as judged by case reports that are submitted for review. For Board certification, a Ph.D. is required and a written and practical examination must be passed.

Employment Opportunities

Forensic anthropologists are employed at many of the major universities and colleges. They teach courses, conduct research in forensic anthropology, and work as consultants on cases submitted by law enforcement authorities. Others are employed by museums, conducting much of the same work as their academic colleagues. A number of forensic anthropologists are hired by medical examiners' offices, as knowledge of the capabilities of forensic anthropologists has become widely known among forensic scientists. Another employer is the military which utilizes anthropological expertise in identifying victims of war, atrocities, and major military accidents.

Forensic anthropologists are skilled in the identification of skeletal materials. In addition to their efforts to document age, sex, stature, race, and other characteristics of the specimens under investigation, they are familiar with various types of injuries and can work with forensic pathologists to establish cause of death. Many forensic anthropologists have training in archaeological methods and assist law enforcement agencies in the initial investigations of crime scenes. Anthropologists, with their naturalistic approach to recovery of skeletons, examination of animal remains, and analysis of soil and vegetation patterns, can successfully recover human remains from different kinds of terrain, e.g., deserts, forests, riverine systems, etc.

Some forensic anthropologists are skilled in the art of facial reproduction which involves the modeling of how a face may have appeared in the living subject for which the only surviving evidence is a skull. Other forensic anthropologists have developed skills in the determination of time elapsed since death by examining insect remains and states of body decomposition.

Questioned Documents

The document examiner discovers and proves the facts regarding documents. The bulk of the examiner's caseload rests upon answering questions regarding authorship, authenticity, alterations, additions, and erasures. However, a document examiner may be called upon to determine the significance of inks, paper, writing instruments, business machines, and other features of documents. A report is then prepared regarding examination findings, and the examiner stands ready to demonstrate these findings as an expert witness.

Education and Training

Questioned document or related courses are offered by colleges and universities as part of criminal justice, police science, or criminalistics programs. There is no degree with a major in questioned documents presently available in the United States. A trainee should possess a bachelor's degree, preferably in one of the sciences, and serve approximately a two-year apprenticeship under the supervision of a court qualified examiner. A trainee studies the leading texts pertaining to questioned documents, performs supervised case work, prepares court exhibits, and conducts independent research.

Employment Opportunities

Document examiners are employed in both the public and private sectors. Private examiners can be found in most major cities, whereas public examiners are employed by many large police departments as well as most state and federal law enforcement agencies. Many qualified examiners are members of the American Academy of Forensic Sciences, the American Society of Questioned Document Examiners, or are certified by the American Board of Forensic Document Examiners.

Wildlife Forensics

Wildlife forensics is a relatively new field of forensic science. Poaching violations, the development of state and federal hunting regulations, the Endangered Species Act of 1973, and the United Nations Convention on International Trade in Endangered Species (CITES) are some of the factors which helped create this new field.

Wildlife forensic labs have two primary functions: the identifying of evidence, and the linking of suspect, victim, and crime scene through physical evidence. The major difference between criminal science and wildlife forensics is that the victim (and occasionally the suspect) is an animal.

The identification of wildlife evidence, however, is more complicated than police science in that wildlife enforcement officers rarely seize whole animals (which can be readily identified by a museum or zoo expert with established taxonomic keys), but will more typically confiscate parts and products of these animals as evidence. The problem then is that the characteristics which define an animal species are rarely present in those parts or products. Wildlife forensic scientists are often required to develop new species-defining characteristics, through research with carefully documented known specimens, before they can examine evidence in a case and testify in court.

An additional complication is that, while police forensics deals with only a single species (homo sapiens), wildlife forensic scientists must be prepared to identify evidence from any species in the world that is illegally killed, smuggled, poached, or sold in an illicit market. Examples of wildlife evidence items might include blood on an illegal hunter's clothing; fresh, frozen, or smoked meats; loose hair; fur coats; reptile leather products, such as purses, belts, and shoes; loose feathers and down; carved ivory objects; sea turtle oil (suntan lotion); sea turtle shell jewelry; and powdered rhinoceros horn.

While it might seem that wildlife forensic scientists face an overwhelming task in developing new and reliable ID techniques, they do have one advantage over police-related workers: sample size is rarely a problem. Example seizures of wildlife evidence have included 20,000 pounds of suspected sea turtle meat, 10,000 pounds of ivory, and 300,000 suspected rhinoceros horn pills.

Emerging Forensic Disciplines

In addition to the established specialties discussed previously, there are many emerging areas of forensic study that are of importance to the profession. Many of these disciplines, while relatively new, are of great importance to the Forensic Sciences Foundation.

Forensic accountants, for example, often study potential white collar crime. Using accounting techniques they attempt to determine the patterns of persons who might have committed frauds. Artists and sculptors use their talents to create reconstructions which may help identify remains that are found, or to identify assailants. Computers are playing an ever increasing role in the forensic sciences and there are people who specialize as forensic computer-related crime investigators. As well, computers are often used by forensic image enhancement specialists. Enhancement specialists attempt to gather vital evidence such as fingerprints from exhibits using highly technical methods.

Forensic nurses work in both crime scene investigations and in areas such as rape crisis centers. In such settings they will work with forensic social workers. The gathering of evidence and the conducting of investigations may be done by forensic coroners, forensic crime scene investigators or forensic death (medical legal) investigators. Useful information may be provided by a forensic photographer, forensic polygraph examiner, forensic radiologist, or a forensic speech scientist who will aid in speech identification enhancement of recordings and the authenticity of transcripts and recordings.

The Forensic Sciences Foundation, Inc.

The Forensic Sciences Foundation, Inc., founded in 1969, is a nonprofit organization studying the application of science to the resolution of social and legal issues.

In 1973, the Foundation became affiliated with the American Academy of Forensic Sciences, a professional membership organization of forensic scientists. The Foundation is the educational, scientific, and research arm of the Academy.

The overall objectives of the Foundation are:

- To develop and conduct education and training programs;
- To develop new ways to improve the forensic sciences;
- To promote public education concerning all disciplines in the forensic sciences;
- To support research in fields relating to the forensic sciences.

The Specific Goals of the Foundation

Education

The Foundation develops, produces, and directs educational programs in all fields of the forensic sciences. Specifically the Foundation:

- Sponsors seminars and courses for physicians, including ACCME Accreditation;
- Publishes books on forensic science subjects.

Research

The Foundation conducts programs to:

- Assess manpower requirements;
- Assess the qualification of professionals in the field;
- Determine the state-of-the-art of the forensic sciences;
- Study the education and training requirements of the various disciplines;
- Assess the education and training opportunities in the forensic sciences;
- Evaluate the uses of forensic sciences by the justice system.

Chapter 2

Medical Examiner and Coroner Information Sharing

Introduction

Medical examiners and coroners (ME/Cs) are responsible for investigating sudden or violent deaths and for providing accurate, legally defensible determinations of the causes of these deaths. The information provided by ME/Cs plays a critical role in the judicial system and in decisions made by public safety and public health agencies.

The records of ME/Cs, which provide vital information about patterns and trends of mortality in the United States, are also an excellent source of data for public health studies and surveillance.

Until recently, however, death investigation information was not readily available to the public health community or to other human resource programs. Making this information more available is one of the goals of the Medical Examiner and Coroner Information Sharing Program (MECISP).

Excerpted from "The Medical Examiner and Coroner Information Sharing Program," [Online] 1994. Available: http://www.cdc.gov/nceh/ pubcatns/1994/cdc/brosures/me-cbro.htm. Produced by the CDC's National Center for Environmental Health. And from "So You Want to Be a Medical Detective?" [Online]. Available: http://www.thename.org/career/ career.htm. © 1996 by the National Association of Medical Examiners, 1402 S. Grand Blvd, St. Louis, MO 63104. For complete contact information, please refer to Chapter 56, "Resources." All rights reserved. Reprinted with permission.

Death Investigation Practices

Death investigation practices often vary considerably between jurisdictions (whether state, county, district, or city). Perhaps the most noticeable difference is that some jurisdictions use the coroner system and others use the medical examiner system. The type of system used may be uniform throughout a state or may vary from county to county within a state.

Coroners

A coroner is a public official, appointed or elected, in a particular geographic jurisdiction, whose official duty is to make inquiry into deaths in certain categories. The office of the coroner or "crowner" dates back to medieval days when the crowner was responsible for looking into deaths to be sure death duties were paid to the King. The coroner's primary duty in contemporary times is to make inquiry into the death and complete the certificate of death. The coroner assigns a cause and manner of death and lists them on the certificate of death. The cause of death refers to the disease, injury, or poison that caused the death. The coroner assigns a cause and manner of death and lists them on the certificate of death. The cause of death refers to the disease, injury, or poison that caused the death. The coroner also decides if a death occurred under natural circumstances or was due to accident, homicide, suicide, or undetermined means or circumstances.

Coroners are called upon to decide if a death was due to foul play. Depending upon the jurisdiction and the law defining the coroner's duties, the coroner may or may not be trained in the medical sciences. The coroner may employ physicians, pathologists, or forensic pathologists to perform autopsies when there appears to be a question or manner of death that autopsy can elucidate. In some jurisdictions, the coroner is a physician, but in may localities, the coroner is not required to be a physician nor be trained in medicine. In the absence of medical expertise, the non-physician coroner may have difficulty in sorting out subtle nonviolent and violent causes of death.

Medical Examiners

A medical examiner is a physician, hence, the title medical examiner. When acting in an official capacity, the physician medical examiner is charged, within a particular jurisdiction, with the investigation and examination of persons dying a sudden, unexpected or violent

16

death. The role of a medical examiner differs from that of the non-physician coroner in that the medical examiner is expected to bring medical expertise to the evaluation of the medical history and physical examination of the deceased. The physician medical examiner usually is not required to be a specialist in death investigation or pathology and may practice any branch of medicine. Most systems employing physicians as part-time medical examiners encourage them to take advantage of medical training for medical examiners to increase their level of medical expertise as applied to death investigation. The National Association of Medical Examiners and the American Academy Forensic Sciences are two organizations that offer specialized training.

Although ME/C information plays a critical role in decisions made by public safety and public health agencies, until recently, death investigation data was not readily available to the public health community.

A second variation in death investigation practices involves what deaths are actually to be investigated. About 20% of deaths in the United States are investigated by medical examiners or coroners, although the percentage varies from state to state. And although the guidelines for which deaths to investigate also vary widely from jurisdiction to jurisdiction, most jurisdictions require that these deaths be investigated:

- Deaths due to homicide, suicide, or accidental causes such as motor vehicle crashes, falls, burns, or the ingestion of drugs or other chemical agents.

- Sudden or suspicious deaths, deaths from sudden infant death syndrome (SIDS), and unattended deaths.

- Deaths caused by an agent or disease constituting a threat to public health. Deaths that occur while the decedents were at work.

- Deaths of people who were in custody or confinement. Deaths of other people institutionalized for reasons other than organic disease.

- Deaths of people to be cremated.

The thoroughness of death investigations (and as a result the completeness of death investigation records) also varies from case to case. Sometimes a postmortem examination may consist of only an external

examination of the body. The record of a complete death investigation, however, would include the following:

- The initial report of the death made to the ME/C office (e.g., by a family member, police officer, or attending physician).

- A determination of circumstances surrounding the death; findings of a scene investigation.

- Findings of a postmortem exam or autopsy.

- Results of laboratory tests to determine the presence of drugs, toxins, or infectious agents.

- Certification of the cause and manner of death.

MECISP Goal

In 1986, because of the lack of uniformity in death investigation policies, the frequent lack of communication between jurisdictions, and the need for more widespread distribution of death investigation data, the Centers for Disease Control and Prevention (CDC) established the MECISP. These are the primary goals of the MECISP:

- To improve the quality of death investigations in the United States and to promote the use of more standardized policies for when and how to conduct these investigations.

- To facilitate communication among death investigators, the public health community, federal agencies, and other interested groups.

- To improve the quality, completeness, management, and dissemination of information on investigated deaths.

- To promote the sharing and use of ME/C death investigation data.

MECISP Activities

Through financial and technical support, the MECISP helps ME/C offices to collect, manage, and disseminate data. The MECISP also:

- Publishes a directory that describes death investigation laws and lists the contact persons for all ME/C jurisdictions in the United States and Canada.

- Develops model death investigation forms and file structures.

- Develops model formats for annual and statistical death investigation reports. These reports are then distributed to and used by ME/C offices.

- Collaborates with medical examiners, coroners, public health researchers, and others in epidemiologic studies of deaths routinely investigated by ME/C offices.

- Conducts studies to identify problems associated with current methods of collecting death investigation and mortality data.

- Consults with ME/C offices to help them establish computerized data systems.

Chapter 3

Timeline of Forensic Medicine

Egypt and Babylonia

2000 B.C.—The Egyptians and Babylonians possessed considerable knowledge of practical anatomy, unknown for many centuries to the physicians of other nations because of religious and social prejudices against dissection of the dead (Chien, 1996).

1850 B.C.—The earliest record of a murder trial was found in Mesopotamia on a clay table dating back to about 1850 B.C. (Chien, 1996).

Greece and Rome

380 B.C.—The Greek civilization is responsible for placing medicine on a more rational basis, largely due to the scientific outlook and methods of Hippocrates (Chien, 1996).

44 B.C.—After Julius Caesar was assassinated, a Roman physician named Antistius examined the corpse, counted twenty-three wounds, and announced that only one stab wound to the chest had been fatal (Chien, 1996).

From "Forensic Medicine: Historical Timeline," in *Forensic Sourcebook99/CD-ROM,* Calgary, Alberta: Author, 1999. Available only with forensic educational course packages for distance delivery. For complete contact information, please refer to Chapter 56, "Resources." Reprinted with permission.

China

1247—The value of the autopsy was first recorded in a Chinese handbook written by Hsi Yuan Lu in 1247. So complete was this initial text that it was published with amendments up to the nineteenth century (Spitz and Fisher, 1980, cited in Schramm, 1991, p. 670).

England

900—Suicide officially became a crime under common law in tenth-century England (Spitz and Fisher, 1980, cited in Schramm, 1991, p. 670).

926—A grant of the coroner's office was recorded in historical sources (Spitz and Fisher, 1980, cited in Schramm, 1991, p. 670).

1066—"Murder" as a word originated after the Norman conquest of England in 1066 (Mant, 1987, cited in Schramm, 1991, p. 670-1).

1066—Les Murdrorum Law imposed fines if the death of a Norman nobleman occurred (Mant, 1987, cited in Schramm, 1991, p. 670-1).

1100s—Forensic medicine evolved in England from the medicolegal need to determine cause of death, so that the decision to impose a suicide penalty could be rendered (Spitz and Fisher, 1980, cited in Schramm, 1991, p. 670).

1184—The condemnation of suicide was made a part of canon law by the Roman Catholic Church in England. This law prohibited the burial of suicide victims in hallowed ground (Spitz and Fisher, 1980, cited in Schramm, 1991, p. 670).

1192—Richard the Lion-Hearted was kidnapped by Leopold of Austria and held for an enormous ransom. The English treasury wasn't large enough to cover the ransom demand, so a plan was devised to utilize corpses as a novel source of revenue. The title of "Coroner" was given to each knight who took custody of a deceased felon's property, thereby enriching the royal treasury. The title derives from the Latin "Custom placitorum coronae" or "Supervisor of the Crown's pleas" (Chien, 1996).

1194—The office of coroner in England was formally described along with the mechanism whereby appointment was to be made (Schramm, 1991, p. 670).

1100s (late)—Coroners were relieved of collecting monies due to the Crown (Mant, 1987, cited in Schramm, 1991, p. 670).

1340—Les Murdrorum Law repealed but the word "murder" had entered into the English language as a term for homicide (Mant, 1987, cited in Schramm, 1991, p. 670).

1888—Jack the Ripper, one of the best-known serial killers, terrorized London from August to November, 1888. He is thought to have murdered six or seven drunken prostitutes in the slums of the White Chapel district, each time slitting his victim's throat and eviscerating her. The killer vanished, after spreading panic throughout London (Chien, 1996).

1800s (late)—Fingerprint identification was pioneered when it was established conclusively that the ridge arrangement on every finger of every person is different and that the ridge pattern remains constant throughout life, the two basic facts on which fingerprint identification results. It was suggested that prints found at a crime scene possibly identify the perpetrator (Chien, 1996).

1975—Nearly a century after Jack the Ripper, a copycat killer began a murder spree in Leeds, England, in October, 1975. Dubbed the Yorkshire Ripper, the killer continued as a massive police manhunt escalated into the largest criminal investigation in England's history. Unlike Jack the Ripper, whose age, nationality, and true identity were never discovered, a footprint left at a murder scene finally led to the killer's arrest in 1981 (Chien, 1996).

France

1800s—The science of experimental toxicology was founded when numerous experiments were conducted with arsenic on animals, tracing the course of the poison as it travels through the body (Chien, 1996).

1800s (late)—Anthropometry or "Bertillonage," a method later replaced by fingerprint, incorporated a series of body measurements, physical descriptions, and photographs which aided police in the identification of criminals (Chien, 1996).

1900s—The development of ballistic study was pioneered by the examination and identification of spent bullets. Previously, analysis of bullet fragments could only generally identify the type of gun and ammunition used, thereby establishing the unique nature of each weapon, much like human fingerprinting (Chien, 1996).

New World (Haiti)

1533—First recorded autopsy in the New World was performed in Haiti for the purpose of determining whether Siamese twins had two souls or one (Chavarria and Shipley, 1924, cited in Schramm, 1991, p. 672).

America

1600s—First autopsy in the United States: Talbot County, Maryland (Spitz and Fisher, 1980, cited in Schramm, 1991, p. 672).

1635—First colonial coroner ruling was recorded in New England (Spitz and Fisher, 1980, cited in Schramm, 1991, p. 672).

1637—English coroner system began in the United States on January 29, 1637 (Fisher, 1973, cited in Henson, 1987, p. 76).

1647—Autopsies were performed on the bodies of criminals in Massachusetts for the purpose of teaching medical students (Spitz and Fisher, 1980, cited in Schramm, 1991, p. 672).

1700s—Paul Revere and other coroners in the New England settlements were popularly elected and had no medical training. Later, the office of the coroner was entwined in the political system and became politically powerful. Corruption of the coroner system in some areas arose from consideration and accommodation given to powerful friends of the coroner (Chien, 1996).

1800s—Little change in the United States coroner system in last 200 years (Henson, 1987, p. 76).

1800s (mid)—Autopsies were used to validate the accuracy of a diagnosis or cause of death (Hill, 1988, cited in Schramm, 1991, p. 672).

1860—Maryland ordered the coroner or his jury to require the attendance of a physician in cases of violent death (Spitz and Fisher, 1980, cited in Schramm, 1991, p. 672).

1860—Medical expertise became a formal aspect of the coroner's job (Fisher, 1973, cited in Henson, 1987, p. 76).

1868—Baltimore became the first city to have a physician as sole coroner (Spitz and Fisher, 1980, cited in Schramm, 1991, p. 672).

1868—Coroner replaced by medical examiner. Massachusetts authorized a statewide system which required that a Coroner be replaced by a physician known as a medical examiner, but restricted examinations to bodies that were presumed to have met a violent death (Schramm, 1991, p. 672).

1915—New York State abolished the coroner system and established a system of medical examiners (Spitz and Fisher, 1980, cited in Schramm, 1991, p. 673).

1915—The title of Medical Examiner was created. At this time, the office of Coroner was retained, while the head pathologist who directed investigations was given the new title (Chien, 1996).

1932—A Chair of Legal Medicine was established at Harvard University (Chien, 1996).

1950s (early)—The American Board of Pathology recognized Forensic Pathology as a sub-specialty. Currently, there are approximately 700 board-certified forensic pathologists in the United States (Chien, 1996).

1966—The National Association of Medical Examiners (NAME) was established and is responsible for establishing the standards of inspection and accreditation of medical examiner's offices in use today (Chien, 1996).

Today—Old system of electing a lay person to be coroner is gradually being replaced with medical examiners' offices (Henson, 1987, p. 76)

References

Chien, H. C. "History of Forensic Medicine." [Online] 1996. Available: http://140.116.5.4/~chungho/history.htm.

Henson, T. K. "Medicolegal Role in Detection and Prevention of Human Abuse." *Holistic Nursing Practice* 1 (2): 75-83 (1987).

Schramm, C. A. "Forensic Medicine: What the Perioperative Nurse Needs to Know." *AORN American Operating Nurses Journal* 53 (3): 669-92 (1991).

—by Arlene Kent-Wilkinson R.N., M.N.

Arlene Kent-Wilkinson is a forensic nurse educator/consultant who designs, writes, and instructs forensic multidisciplinary courses for Internet, lecture, and paper-based distance delivery. Her current forensic courses at The University of Calgary, Mount Royal College, and Athabasca University, are accessed by students globally.

Chapter 4

Death Investigation in the United States and Canada

History

In 1987, [the Centers for Disease Control and Prevention (CDC)] compiled the first death investigation manual in an effort to (1) facilitate communication between death investigators; (2) provide an up-to-date description of death investigation laws and practices; and (3) increase public awareness about death investigation systems and the importance and complexity of death investigation. Because so many individuals, government agencies, and private groups informed the CDC staff that this manual was a useful resource, CDC published revised editions in 1990, 1992, and 1995.

Methods

The original source document and format for the death investigation system description was taken from a May 1981 report, *A Study of State Laws, Death Investigation Systems, Practices and Their Impact on Those Affected by Sudden Infant Death Syndrome* (hereafter known as the 1981 Report). The 1981 Report was prepared for the Office for Maternal and Child Health, U.S. Department of Health and Human Services (DHHS), by Lawrence Johnson & Associates. In 1987,

From "Death Investigation in the United States and Canada," [Online] 1998. Available: http://www.cdc.gov/nceh/programs/mec/medir/1998. Produced by the CDC's National Center for Environmental Health. For complete contact information, please refer to Chapter 56, "Resources."

the CDC staff updated the information on death investigation laws for the 50 states and the District of Columbia, as given in the 1981 Report, on the basis of information received from either the state medical examiner, vital registrar, or medical examiner or coroner association. The American Academy of Forensic Sciences published the first manual in March 1988.

In October 1989, the CDC staff contacted the chief medical examiner, the medical examiner or coroner association, vital registrar, and attorney general for each state and the District of Columbia, and asked them to review and correct the information for their respective jurisdictions. In addition, we contacted the territorial vital registrars, attorneys general, and medical examiners to obtain information about their death investigation systems. In December 1989, we invited medical examiners and coroners in Canadian provinces to share information about their death investigation systems for inclusion in the directory. In August 1990, CDC published the 1990 revision, which was revised and published in August 1992. In August 1996, the CDC staff created this electronic version of the 1995 publication.

Death Investigation System Descriptions, Death Investigation Contacts, Vital Registrars, and Attorneys General

We receive updated information about system descriptions from individual offices of the medical examiner or coroner, medical examiner or coroner associations, and vital registrars, and attorneys general of individual states, territories, and provinces. We receive updated information about persons responsible for death investigation from individual offices of the medical examiner or coroner, medical examiner or coroner associations, and vital registrars, and attorneys general of individual states, territories, and provinces.

We obtain updated information about vital registrars and attorneys general from the National Center for Health Statistics and the National Association of Attorneys General, respectively.

Introduction

Medical examiners and coroners play a critical, although often unappreciated, role in the functioning of the judicial, public safety, and public health agencies of government. They are responsible for investigating sudden or violent deaths and providing accurate, legally defensible determinations of the manner and cause of these deaths.

Over the years, the CDC has collaborated with medical examiners and coroners to study deaths from homicide, suicide, poisoning and drug abuse, motor vehicle collisions, and occupational and unintentional injuries. CDC and other federal agencies continue to extend collaborative efforts to medical examiners and coroners in efforts to study various types of deaths that medical examiners and coroners investigate. Ultimately, it is CDC's goal to continue improving the collection and sharing of information generated by these investigations and to use this information to assist in planning public health policy.

Along with death investigation system descriptions, local jurisdiction lists are provided for states, counties within some states, U.S. territories, and Canadian provinces and territories. Although records are kept at centralized offices, the actual death investigation is often conducted locally by deputy medical examiners or coroners.

Use of Titles

In the jurisdiction listings, we have attempted to standardize titles to be consistent with general titles used in statutory language. Generally, we do not use the terms "Chief Medical Examiner" or "Chief Coroner" for local jurisdictions because each contact listed is the primary contact; therefore, "Chief" is implied.

Population

We have included the July 1994 population estimates for all death investigation jurisdictions except for the U.S. territories, for which 1990 population or 1992 estimates were included. For U.S. jurisdictions, state and county data were provided by the U.S. Bureau of the Census. For Canadian jurisdictions, data were provided by Statistics Canada.

Tables

See tables on following pages.

Table 4.1. State Death Investigation System by Type: United States

I. Medical Examiner Systems (22)

A. State Medical Examiner (19)

Connecticut	New Hampshire	Tennessee
Delaware	New Jersey	Utah
District of Columbia	New Mexico	Vermont
Iowa	North Carolina	Virginia
Maine	Oklahoma	West Virginia
Maryland	Oregon	
Massachusetts	Rhode Island	

B. District Medical Examiners (1)

Florida

C. County Medical Examiners (2)

Arizona	Michigan

II. Mixed Medical Examiner and Coroner Systems (18)

A. State Medical Examiner and County Coroners/Medical Examiners (7)

Alabama	Georgia	Mississippi
Alaska	Kentucky	Montana
Arkansas		

B. County Medical Examiners/Coroners (11)

California	Missouri	Texas
Hawaii	New York	Washington
Illinois	Pennsylvania	Wisconsin
Minnesota	South Carolina	

III. Coroner Systems (11)

A. District Coroners (2)

Kansas	Nevada

B. County Coroners (9)

Colorado	Louisiana	Ohio
Idaho	Nebraska	South Dakota
Indiana	North Dakota	Wyoming

Table 4.2. Territory Death Investigation System by Type: United States

I. Medical Examiner Systems (3)

  A. Territorial Medical Examiner (3)

   Guam   Puerto Rico   U.S. Virgin Islands

II. Mixed Medical Examiner and Coroner Systems (0)

III. Coroner Systems (2)

  A. Territorial Coroner (1)

   American Samoa

  B. Unknown (1)

   Northern Mariana Islands

Table 4.3. Province and Territory Death Investigation System by Type: Canada

I. Medical Examiner Systems (3)

  A. Provincial Medical Examiner (3)

   Alberta   Manitoba   Nova Scotia

II. Mixed Medical Examiner and Coroner Systems (0)

III. Coroner Systems (3)

  A. Provincial/Territorial Coroner (8)

   British Columbia   Ontario   Saskatchewan
   New Brunswick   Prince Edward Island   Yukon Territory
   Northwest Territories   Quebec

IV. Other (1)

   Newfoundland

Table 4.4a. (Continued in 4.4b.) Death Investigation Systems by State

State	# of Counties	# of Juris.	1994 Pop. (est.)	Type of Death Investigation System							
				Medical Examiner			Mixed		Coroner	
				State	Dist	Cty	State	Cty	Dist	Cty
AL	67	69	4,218,792				●			
AK	23	5	606,276				●			
AZ	15	15	4,075,052			●				
AR	75	76	2,452,671				●			
CA	58	58	31,430,697					●		
CO	63	63	3,655,647							●
CT	8	1	3,275,251	●						
DE	3	1	706,351	●						
DC	1	1	570,175	●						
FL	67	24	13,952,714		●					
GA	159	160	7,055,336					●		
HI	5	5	1,178,564						●	
ID	44	45	1,133,034							●
IL	102	102	11,751,774					●		
IN	92	92	5,752,073							●
IA	99	100	2,829,252	●						
KS	105	31	2,554,047						●	
KY	120	121	3,826,794				●			
LA	64	64	4,315,085							●
ME	16	1	1,240,209	●						
MD	23	1	5,006,265	●						
MA	14	65	6,041,123	●						
MI	83	84	9,496,147			●				
MN	87	87	4,567,267					●		
MS	82	83	2,669,111				●			
MO	115	115	5,277,640					●		

Table 4.4b. (Continued from 4.4a.) Death Investigation Systems by State

State	# of Counties	# of Juris.	1994 Pop. (Est.)	Medical Examiner			Mixed		Coroner	
				State	Dist	Cty	State	Cty	Dist	Cty
MT	56	57	856,047				●			
NE	93	93	1,622,858							●
NV	17	17	1,457,028						●	
NH	10	1	1,136,820	●						
NJ	21	22	7,903,925	●						
NM	33	1	1,653,521	●						
NY	62	58	18,169,051					●		
NC	100	1	7,069,836	●						
ND	53	53	637,988							●
OH	88	88	11,102,198							●
OK	77	1	3,258,069	●						
OR	36	37	3,086,188	●						
PA	67	67	12,052,367					●		
RI	5	1	996,757	●						
SC	46	46	3,663,984					●		
SD	66	66	721,164							●
TN	95	100	5,175,240	●						
TX	254	846	18,378,185					●		
UT	29	1	1,907,936	●						
VT	14	1	580,209	●						
VA	136	1	6,551,522	●						
WA	39	39	5,343,090					●		
WV	55	1	1,822,021	●						
WI	72	72	5,081,658					●		
WY	23	23	475,981							●
Total	**3,137**	**3,162**	**260,340,990**	19	1	2	7	11	2	9

33

Table 4.5. Death Investigation Systems by U. S. Territory

Territory	No. of Counties	No. of Jurisdictions	1990 Population	Type of Death Investigation System		
				Medical Examiner	Coroner	Other
American Samoa	5	1	46,743		●	
Guam	0	1	133,152	●		
Northern Mariana Islands	0	1	43,345			●
Puerto Rico	0	1	3,522,037	●		
U.S. Virgin Islands	2	2	101,809	●		
Total	7	6	3,847,086	3	1	1

Table 4.6. Death Investigation Systems by Canadian Province and Territory

Province or Territory	# of Counties	# of Juris.	1994 Pop. (est.)	Type of Death Investigation System		
				Medical Examiner	Coroner	Other
Alberta	68	1	2,716,200	AB		
British Columbia	0	1	3,668,400		BC	
Manitoba	0	1	1,131,100	MB		
New Brunswick	8	1	759,300		NB	
Newfoundland	56	1	582,400			NF
Northwest Territories	0	1	64,300		NT	
Nova Scotia	18	1	936,700	NS		
Ontario	27	1	10,927,800		ON	
Prince Edward Island	3	1	134,500		PI	
Quebec	16	1	7,281,100		QU	
Saskatchewan	0	1	1,016,200		SA	
Yukon Territory	0	1	30,100		YU	
Total	196	12	29,248,100	3	8	1

Chapter 5

Suspicious Death and Autopsy Statistics in the United States

Current Trends in Autopsy Frequency

In approximately 14% of the 2,089,378 deaths reported in the United States in 1985, an autopsy was performed. Recent reports indicate that the frequency of autopsy has been declining and that the decline may have adversely affected the accuracy of determining the underlying cause of death. To assess the recent variation in autopsy frequency, mortality data collected by the National Center for Health Statistics, CDC, for the period 1980-1985 were analyzed. During that time, the proportion of deaths involving an autopsy gradually declined from 17% to 14%. Within each year, however, autopsy frequency varied substantially by cause of death.

For this analysis, cause of death was grouped into six general categories: natural causes, unintentional injuries and poisonings, suicide, homicide, external causes with undetermined intent, and unknown or unspecified causes. These groups correspond to the codes in the International Classification of Diseases, Ninth Revision (ICD-9).

The proportion of autopsies performed ranged from 12% among natural deaths to 97% among homicide deaths. Deaths with unknown

From "Current Trends Autopsy Frequency—United States, 1980-1985," *Morbidity and Mortality Weekly Report* 37 (12): 191-4 (April 1, 1988) [Online]. Available: http://www.cdc.gov/epo/mmwr/preview/mmwrhtml/00000003.htm. And from "Fastats," National Center for Health Statistics [Online] May/June 1998. Available: http://www.cdc.gov/nchswww. Produced by the Centers for Disease Control and Prevention. For complete contact information, please refer to Chapter 56, "Resources."

autopsy status were enumerated separately and excluded from the calculations. Although 12% of all records lacked autopsy data, the proportion of records without autopsy data varied from 2% among homicide deaths to 13% among natural deaths. In general, larger autopsy percentages are associated with smaller percentages of missing data.

Autopsies for natural deaths declined at least 0.5% every year during the period 1980-1985, from 13% in 1980 to 10% in 1985. In contrast, the frequency of autopsies for deaths caused by unintentional injuries and poisoning increased from 46% to 51%, and the frequency among suicide deaths increased from 48% to 52%. Similarly, autopsies among deaths due to external causes of undetermined intent increased from 79% to 84%. The frequency of autopsy among homicide deaths was consistently high over this period (between 96% and 97%). The number of autopsies for deaths of unknown or unspecified cause fluctuated between 28% and 32%.

The distribution of cause of death for all autopsies has changed. In 1980, natural deaths accounted for 70% of all autopsies. By 1985, natural deaths accounted for 66% of all autopsies.

Autopsies for natural deaths or deaths occurring among patients under the care of a physician are usually performed at the hospital where the death occurred and with the permission of the decedent's next of kin. If the death is sudden, unexpected, or due to external causes, local statutes may require an autopsy. This autopsy is either requested by a coroner or performed by a medical examiner, depending upon the local medicolegal system. Since deaths due to other than natural causes require medicolegal investigation in most states, the number of autopsies performed was examined by type of medicolegal jurisdiction in the state. In 1980, 15 states had coroner systems; 18 states and the District of Columbia had medical examiner systems, and 17 states had both medical examiner systems and coroner systems. Approximately 44% of all deaths during the period 1980-1985 occurred in states with both medical examiners and coroners (a mixed medicolegal system); 29% of deaths occurred in states with a medical examiner system; the remaining 27% occurred in states with a coroner system. The percentage of deaths in which an autopsy was performed during this six-year period was greatest among states with a mixed medicolegal system, 16%. States with a medical examiner system had autopsies performed in 15% of deaths and states with coroners, 14%. States with a coroner system had the highest proportion of death records that did not indicate whether an autopsy was performed, 16%, and states with mixed systems had the smallest, 10%.

When autopsy frequency was examined by medicolegal system and cause of death, states with a medical examiner system had the highest autopsy frequency for deaths due to unintentional injuries and poisoning, homicide, suicide, undetermined intent, and unknown causes. States with mixed systems had higher autopsy frequencies for deaths due to unintentional injuries and poisoning, suicide, and undetermined intent than did states with coroners. The same pattern of annual trends was observed for each medicolegal system. Reported by: Surveillance and Programs Br, Div of Environmental Hazards and Health Effects, Center for Environmental Health and Injury Control. Editorial Note: Death certificates are the principal source of mortality statistics for the United States. Several studies, however, have raised questions concerning the accuracy of the recorded cause of death, and some investigators have advocated improving these statistics by performing more autopsies. Current data show a decline in the proportion of autopsy for natural causes of death and an increase in autopsy proportions for medicolegal deaths (homicides, suicides, and deaths caused by unintentional injuries and poisoning). As a result, 34% of autopsies performed in 1985 involved deaths due to other than natural causes, compared to 30% of autopsies performed in 1980.

State and local laws vary, but medical examiners and coroners typically have the legal authority to order autopsies for traumatic, sudden, or unexpected deaths. A more accurate picture of the frequency of autopsy among deaths outside of the medicolegal system would require separating the sudden or unexpected deaths from other natural deaths.

Death and Injury Statistics

Deaths/Mortality (All figures are for United States)

Number of Deaths Annually: 2,314,460 (1996)

Death Rate (age-adjusted): 491.6 deaths per 100,000 population (1996)

Ten Leading Causes of Death in the United States:

Heart Disease 733,361
Cancer 539,533
Stroke 160,431
Chronic Obstructive Pulmonary Disease 106,027
Accidents 94,948

Pneumonia/Influenza 83,727
Diabetes 61,767
HIV/AIDS 31,130
Suicide 30,903
Chronic Liver Disease and Cirrhosis 25,047

Source: *National Vital Statistics Reports,* Vol. 47, No. 9

Homicide (All figures are for United States)

Deaths Annually: 20,738 (1996)

Age-Adjusted Death Rate: 8.4 deaths per 100,000 population (1996)

Cause of Death Rank: 14 (1996)

Cause of Death Rank for 5-14-Year-Olds: 3 (1996)

Cause of Death Rank for 15-24-Year-Olds: 2 (1996)

Cause of Death Rank for 25-44-Year-Olds: 6 (1996)

Source: *Monthly Vital Statistics Report,* Vol. 46, No. 1 Supplement

Firearm Mortality (All figures are for United States)

Deaths Annually: 34,234 (1996)

Age-Adjusted Death Rate: 13.0 deaths per 100,000 population (1996)

Death Rate for Males, Ages 15-24: 47.6 deaths per 100,000 population (1995)

Source: *Monthly Vital Statistics Report,* Vol. 46, No. 1 Supplement 2

Death Rate for Black Males, Ages 15-24: 140 deaths per 100,000 population (1995)

Proportion of Firearm Deaths That Are Accidental: 3.4% (1995)

Proportion of Firearm Deaths That Are Suicides: 51% (1995)

Proportion of Firearm Deaths That Are Homicides: 44% (1995)

Source: *Monthly Vital Statistics Report,* Vol. 45, No. 11 Supplement 2

Annual Estimated Number of Persons Treated for Non-Fatal Firearm Injuries in Hospital Emergency Departments: 100,000 (1994)

Source: *Health, United States: 1996-97*

Suicide (All figures are for United States.)

Deaths Annually: 30,862 (1996)

Age-Adjusted Death Rate: 11 deaths per 100,000 population (1996)

Cause of Death Rank: 9 (1996)

Cause of Death Rank for 5-14-Year-Olds: 5 (1996)

Cause of Death Rank for 15-24-Year-Olds: 3 (1996)

Cause of Death Rank for 25-44-Year-Olds: 5 (1996)

Source: *Monthly Vital Statistics Report,* Vol. 46, No. 1 Supplement

Injuries (All figures are for United States)

Deaths Annually: 147,891 (1995)

Hospital Discharges: 2,591,000 (1995)

Emergency Department Visits: 36,961,000 (1995)

Episodes of Injuries Reported: 59,127,000 (1995)

Source: *Health, United States: 1996-97 Injury Chartbook*

Accidents/Unintentional Injuries (All figures are for United States)

Deaths Annually: 93,874 (1996)

Death Rate: 30 deaths per 100,000 population (1996)

Cause of Death Rank: 5 (1996)

Motor Vehicle Deaths: 43,449 (1996)

Motor Vehicle Fatality Rates: 16 deaths per 100,000 population (1996)

Source: *Monthly Vital Statistics Report,* Vol. 46, No. 1 Supplement

Motor Vehicle Accident-Related Emergency Department Visits: 4,200,000 (1995)

Source: *Advance Data 285*

Occupational Injuries (All figures are for United States)

Deaths from Work-Related Injuries: 5,687 (1996)

Age-Adjusted Death Rate: 2 deaths per 100,000 population (1996)

Source: *Monthly Vital Statistics Report,* Vol. 46, No. 1 Supplement

Number of Work-Loss Days Related to Acute Conditions: 384 million (1994)

Source: *Vital and Health Statistics Series 10, No. 193*

Number of Emergency Department Visits for Work-Related Injuries: 4.8 million (1995)

Source: *Advance Data 285*

Alcohol Use (All figures are for United States)

Number of Alcohol-Induced Deaths in the United States Each Year, Not Including Motor Vehicle Fatalities (1995): >20,000

Source: *Monthly Vital Statistics Report,* Vol. 45, No. 11 Supplement 2

Number of Deaths in the United States Each Year from Chronic Liver Disease and Cirrhosis: >25,000

10th Leading Cause of Death in the United States (1996): Chronic Liver Disease and Cirrhosis

Source: *Monthly Vital Statistics Report,* Vol. 46, No. 1 Supplement

Percentage of Americans, Ages 12 and over, Who Have Drunk Alcohol in the Past Month (1995): 52%

Percentage of These Who Are "Binge Drinkers" (five or more drinks on the same occasion at least once in the past month): 16%

Percentage of Men between Ages 18 and 25 Who Drink: 68%

Percentage of Women between Ages 18 and 25 Who Drink: 55%

Source: *Health, United States: 1996-97*

Illegal Drug Use (All figures are for United States)

Number of Deaths from Drug-Induced Causes in 1995 (legal and illegal drugs): 14,218

Source: *Monthly Vital Statistics Report,* Vol. 45, No. 11 Supplement 2

Percentage of Youth, Ages 12-17, Who Have Smoked Marijuana in the Past Month (1995): 8%

Percentage of High School Seniors Who Have Smoked Marijuana in the Past Month (1995): 22%

Percentage of Persons, Ages 18-25, Who Have Used Cocaine in the Past Month (1995): >1%

Percentage of High School Seniors Who Have Used Cocaine in the Past Month (1995): 2%

Percentage of High School Seniors Who Have Used Inhalants in the Past Month (1995): >2%

Number of Cocaine-Related Emergency Room Episodes in 1995: 142,164

Source: *Health, United States: 1996-97*

Part Two

Crime Scene and Laboratory Investigation

Chapter 6

Collection and Preservation of Evidence

Protecting the Crime Scene

The most important aspect of evidence collection and preservation is protecting the crime scene. This is to keep the pertinent evidence uncontaminated until it can be recorded and collected. The successful prosecution of a case can hinge on the state of the physical evidence at the time it is collected. The protection of the scene begins with the arrival of the first police officer at the scene and ends when the scene is released from police custody.

All police departments and sheriffs' offices should include intensive training for their personnel on how to properly protect crime scenes. Potentially, any police officer can be put into the position of first responding officer to a crime scene. The first officer on the scene of a crime should approach the scene slowly and methodically. In some cases this is not altogether practical. The first officer may also be involved in arresting an uncooperative suspect or performing lifesaving measures on an injured victim. In either ease the officer should make mental or written notes (as is practical in each situation) about the condition of the scene as it was upon the officer's arrival and after the scene has been stabilized. The officer should keep notes on the

From, "Collection and Preservation of Evidence," [Online] undated. Available: http://police2ucr.edu. Produced by George Schiro, Forensic Scientist, Louisiana State Police Crime Laboratory, P.O. Box 66614, Baton Rouge, LA 70896. For complete contact information, please refer to Chapter 56, "Resources." Reprinted with permission.

significant times involved in responding to the crime scene (time dispatched to scene, time left for scene, time arrived at scene, time left scene, etc.). An effort must be made to disturb things as little as possible in assessing the situation. Particular attention should be paid to the floor since this is the most common repository for evidence and it poses the greatest potential for contamination. Notes should also be taken if the officer has to alter something in the investigation. Some things the officer should note include: the condition of the doors, windows, and lighting (both natural and manmade); if there are any odors present; if there are any signs of activity; how EMS [(Emergency Medical Services)] or fire personnel have altered the scene; anything essential about the suspect (description, statements, physical condition, mental condition, intoxication, etc.); and anything essential about the victim. Once the scene has been stabilized, the scene and any other areas which may yield valuable evidence (driveways, surrounding yards, pathways, etc.) should be roped off to prevent unauthorized people from entering the area and potentially contaminating it. Investigators and other necessary personnel should be contacted and dispatched to the scene, however, under no circumstances should the telephone at the scene be used. Once the officer has secured the scene, he or she could do the following: record witness names and others who may have entered or been at the scene; separate witnesses and suspect(s); do not discuss the events or the crime with witnesses or bystanders or let the witnesses discuss these events; listen attentively but discreetly; and protect evidence which may be in danger of being destroyed. Any actions taken should be reported to the investigators.

Many times the arrival of additional personnel can cause problems in protecting the scene. Only those people responsible for the immediate investigation of the crime, the securing of the crime scene, and the processing of the crime scene should be present. Nonessential police officers, district attorney investigators, federal agents, politicians, etc. should never be allowed into a secured crime scene unless they can add something (other than contamination) to the crime scene investigation. One way to dissuade unnecessary people from entering the crime scene is to have only one entrance/exit into the crime scene. An officer can be placed here with a notebook to take the names of all of the people entering the crime scene. The officer can then inform them that by entering the crime scene they may pose a problem by adding potential contamination, and the reason that the officer is taking their names is in case the crime scene investigators need to collect fingerprints, shoes, fibers, blood, saliva, pulled head hair, and/

or pulled pubic hair from all those entering the crime scene. This will sometimes discourage nonessential personnel from entering the crime scene. The officer can also stop unwanted visitors from entering the restricted areas. If extraneous people do have to enter the scene, then make sure that they are escorted by someone who is working the scene. This is to make sure that they will not inadvertently destroy any valuable evidence or leave any worthless evidence.

Eating, drinking, or smoking should never be allowed at a crime scene. Not only can this wreck a crime scene, but it can also be a health hazard. A command post should be set up for such purposes. The post is to be set up somewhere outside the restricted areas. It could be a vehicle, picnic table, hotel room, tent, etc. It can be used as a gathering place for noninvolved personnel, a place for investigators to take breaks, eat, drink, or smoke, a communication center, a place for press conferences, a central intelligence area, etc. The best thing about it is that it is away from the crime scene.

Protection of the crime scene also includes protection of the crime scene investigators. One person, whether a civilian or a police crime scene investigator, should never be left alone while processing the scene. This is especially true if the suspect has not been apprehended. There are many stories of suspects still hiding at or near their area of misdeed. That is why there should always be at least two people working the scene. At least one of these people should have a radio and a firearm.

Examination and Documentation of the Crime Scene

Before the investigators begin examining the scene of the crime, they should gather as much information as possible about the scene. Once again, a slow and methodical approach is recommended. Information is gathered to prevent destruction of valuable and/or fragile evidence such as shoeprints, trace evidence, etc. Once all of the information is gathered, a mental plan is formulated as to how the crime scene will be analyzed. Copious notes and relevant times should be kept on every aspect of the crime scene investigation. The examination of the scene will usually begin with a walk-through of the area along the "trail" of the crime. The trail is that area which all apparent actions associated with the crime took place. The trail is usually marked by the presence of physical evidence. This may include the point of entry, the location of the crime, areas where a suspect may have cleaned up, and the point of exit. In some cases, a walk-through may become secondary if potential evidence is in danger of being destroyed.

In that case, this evidence should be preserved, or documented and collected as quickly as possible.

The purpose of the walk-through is to note the location of potential evidence and to mentally outline how the scene will be examined. The walk-through begins as close to the point of entry as possible. The first place the investigators should examine is the ground on which they are about to tread. If any evidence is observed, then a marker should be placed at the location as a warning to others not to step on the item of interest.

A good technique to use indoors on hard floors is the oblique lighting technique (also known as side lighting). A good flashlight with a strong concentrated beam is the only tool needed. The room should be darkened as much as possible. If a light switch which a suspect may have touched needs to be turned off, then make sure the switch has been dusted for fingerprints first. Do not close any blinds or shades until after all general photographs have been taken. In the side lighting technique, a flashlight is held about one inch from the floor. The beam is then angled so that it just sweeps over the floor surface and is almost parallel to the surface. The light is then fanned back and forth. Any evidence, such as trace evidence and shoeprints, will show up dramatically. Under normal lighting conditions, this evidence may be barely visible or completely invisible.

As the walk-through progresses, the investigators should make sure their hands are occupied by either carrying notebooks, flashlights, pens, etc., or by keeping them in their pockets. This is to prevent depositing of unwanted fingerprints at the scene. As a final note on the walk-through, the investigators should examine whatever is over their heads (ceiling, tree branches, etc.). These areas may yield such valuable evidence as blood spatters and bullet holes. Once the walk-through is completed, the scene should be documented with videotape, photographs, and/or sketches.

If available, a video camera is the first step to documenting a crime scene. Videotape can provide a perspective on the crime scene layout which cannot be as easily perceived in photographs and sketches. It is a more natural viewing medium to which people can readily relate, especially in demonstrating the structure of the crime scene and how the evidence relates to the crime. The video camera should have a fully charged battery as well as date and time videotape display functions. A title generator and "shake free" operations are also nice options. If a title generator is not available, then about 15 seconds at the beginning of the tape should be left blank. This will allow the addition of a title card with any pertinent information to the beginning of the crime scene tape. The condition of the scene should remain unaltered with the exception of markers placed by the investigators and any lights turned on during the walk-through. These alterations can be noted on the audio portion of the tape. Before taping, the camera range should be cleared of all personnel. Any people in the area should be forewarned that taping is about to commence and they should remain silent for the duration of the tape. This prevents recording any potentially embarrassing statements.

Once the video camera begins recording, it should not be stopped until the taping is complete. The key to good videotaping is slow camera movement. A person can never move too slowly when videotaping, yet it is all too easy to move the camera fast without realizing it. This is why videotaping is not ideal for viewing detail. People have a tendency to pan past objects in a manner that does not allow the camera to properly capture the object. This is why slow panning of an area is necessary and it should be panned twice in order to prevent unnecessary rewinding of the tape when viewing.

The taping should begin with a general overview of the scene and surrounding area. The taping should continue throughout the crime scene using wide angle, close up, and even macro (extreme close-up) shots to demonstrate the layout of the evidence and its relevance to the crime scene. If videotaping in a residence, the camera can show how the pertinent rooms are laid out in relation to each other and how they can be accessed. This is sometimes lost in photographs and sketches. After the taping is complete, it is wise to leave about 15 seconds of blank tape to prevent the crime scene tape from running into anything else previously recorded on the tape. The tape should then be transferred to a high quality master tape. The recording tabs should be removed from the master tape after transferring the crime scene tape and the master should be stored in a safe place. This is to prevent accidental erasure of the crime scene tape. Copies can then be made from the master tape.

Whether a video camera is available or not, it is absolutely essential that still photographs be taken to document the crime scene. If a video camera is available, then photographs will be the second step in recording the crime scene. If video is not available, then still photography will be the first step. Photographs can demonstrate the same type of things that the videotape does, but photographs from the crime scene can also be used in direct comparison situations. For example, actual size photographs (also known as one-to-one photos) can be used to compare fingerprints and shoeprints photographed at the crime scene to known fingerprints or shoes from a suspect. This is the advantage of photographs over videotape.

Almost any type of camera with interchangeable lenses and a format of 35mm or larger will do in crime scene photography. The lenses should include a 28mm wide angle lens, a normal 55mm lens, and a lens with macro capabilities (1:4 or better). The flash unit used with the camera should be one that is not fixed to the camera. It should be able to function at various angles and distances from the camera. This is to allow lighting of certain areas to provide maximum contrast, place the flash in hard-to-reach areas, and reduce flash wash out which can render the item photographed invisible. Print and/or slide color film (25-400 ISO) should be used. A tripod, a level, and a small ruler should also be available for one-to-one photography. It may be of help to the investigation to have a Polaroid camera handy for instant photographs. For example, an instant photograph of a shoeprint found at a crime scene can be provided to investigators who are running a search warrant on a suspect's residence. The photo will tell them the type of shoe for which they are searching.

The photography of the crime scene should begin with wide-angle photos of the crime scene and surrounding areas. When shooting the general overall scene, the photos should show the layout of the crime scene and the overall spatial relationships of the various pieces of evidence to each other. A good technique to use indoors is to shoot from all four corners of a room to show its overall arrangement. The next set of photos should be medium range to show the relationships of individual pieces of evidence to other pieces of evidence or structures in the crime scene. Finally, close-up photos should be taken of key pieces of evidence. A ruler should be photographed with items where relative size is important or on items which need to have one-to-one comparison photographs. The object should first be photographed as is, then photographed with the ruler. It is important that when doing one-to-one photography that the ruler is on the same plane as the object being photographed and the film plane is parallel to the ruler. This is why a level and a tripod are necessary. Notes should also be taken as to what the investigator is photographing or wishes to demonstrate in each photograph. This is to prevent the investigator from getting the picture back at a later date and trying to figure out what he or she was trying to accomplish with the photo. The same areas should be photographed in the same sequence as mentioned above in the paragraphs on videotaping.

The final phase in documenting the scene is making a crime scene sketch. The drawback of photographs is that they are two-dimensional representations of three-dimensional objects. As a result, most photographs can distort the spatial relationships of the photographed objects causing items to appear closer together or farther apart than they actually are. If spatial relationships of the evidence are important or if something needs to have proportional measurements included in it for calculations (such as bullet trajectory angles, accident reconstructions, etc.) then a sketch must be made of the crime scene.

A sketch is usually made of the scene as if one is looking straight down (overhead sketch) or straight ahead (elevation sketch) at a crime scene. A rough sketch at the scene is usually made first on graph paper in pencil with so many squares representing so many square feet or inches. Directionality of the overhead view is determined by using a compass. Using a tape measure or other measuring devices, measurements are taken at crime scene of the distances between objects and/or structures at the crime scene. These measurements are proportionally reduced on the rough sketch and the objects are drawn in. Two measurements taken at right angles to each other or from two reference points will usually suffice in placing the objects where they belong in a sketch. Double measurements should also be taken to make sure they are correct. This is especially true where calculations will later be used. A final sketch can be made later using inks, paper, and ruler, or a computer. The original rough sketch should be retained and preserved in case it is needed at a later date. Once the scene has been thoroughly documented then the evidence collection can commence.

Collection and Preservation of Evidence

Once the crime scene has been thoroughly documented and the locations of the evidence noted, then the collection process can begin. The collection process will usually start with the collection of the most fragile or most easily lost evidence. Special consideration can also be given to any evidence or objects which need to be moved. Collection can then continue along the crime scene trail or in some other logical manner. Photographs should also continue to be taken if the investigator is revealing layers of evidence which were not previously documented because they were hidden from sight.

Most items of evidence will be collected in paper containers such as packets, envelopes, and bags. Liquid items can be transported in non-breakable, leakproof containers. Arson evidence is usually collected in air-tight, clean metal cans. Only large quantities of dry powder should be collected and stored in plastic bags. Moist or wet evidence (blood, plants, etc.) from a crime scene can be collected in plastic containers at the scene and transported back to an evidence receiving area if the storage time in plastic is two hours or less and this is done to prevent contamination of other evidence. Once in a secure location, wet evidence, whether packaged in plastic or paper, must be removed and allowed to completely air-dry. That evidence can then be repackaged in a new, dry paper container. UNDER NO CIRCUMSTANCES SHOULD EVIDENCE CONTAINING MOISTURE BE PACKAGED IN PLASTIC OR PAPER CONTAINERS FOR MORE THAN TWO HOURS. Moisture allows the growth of microorganisms which can destroy or alter evidence.

Any items which may cross contaminate each other must be packaged separately. The containers should be closed and secured to prevent the mixture of evidence during transportation. Each container should have: the collecting person's initials; the date and time it was collected; a complete description of the evidence and where it was found; and the investigating agency's name and their file number.

Each type of evidence has a specific value in an investigation. The value of evidence should be kept in mind by the investigator when doing a crime scene investigation. For example, when investigating a crime, he or she should spend more time on collecting good fingerprints than trying to find fibers left by a suspect's clothing. The reason is that fingerprints can positively identify a person as having been at the scene of a crime, whereas fibers could have come from anyone wearing clothes made out of the same material. Of course, if obvious or numerous fibers are found at the point of entry, on a victim's body, etc., then they should be collected in case no fingerprints of value are found. It is also wise to collect more evidence at a crime scene than not to collect enough evidence. An investigator usually only has one shot at a crime scene, so the most should be made of it.

The following is a breakdown of the types of evidence encountered and how the evidence should be handled:

Fingerprints. (also includes palm prints and bare footprints)—the best evidence to place an individual at the scene of a crime. Collecting fingerprints at a crime scene requires very few materials, making it ideal from a cost standpoint. All nonmovable items at a crime scene should be processed at the scene using gray powder, black powder, or black magnetic powder. Polaroid 665 black and white film loaded in a Polaroid CU-5 camera with detachable flash should be used to make one-to-one photographs of prints which do not readily lift. All small transportable items should be packaged in paper bags or envelopes and sent to the crime lab for processing. Because of the "package it up and send it to the lab" mentality, some investigators skim over collecting prints at a crime scene. Collecting prints at the crime scene should be every investigator's top priority. Fingerprints from the suspect as well as elimination fingerprints from the victim will also be needed for comparison (the same holds true for palm [prints] and bare footprints).

Bite marks.—found many times in sexual assaults and can be matched back to the individual who did the biting. They should be photographed using an ABFO No. 2 Scale with normal lighting conditions, side lighting, UV light, and alternate light sources. Color slide and print film as well as black and white film should be used. The more photographs under a variety of conditions, the better. Older bite marks which are no longer visible on the skin may sometimes be visualized and photographed using UV light and alternate light sources. If the bite mark has left an impression then maybe a cast can be made of it. Casts and photographs of the suspect's teeth and maybe the victim's teeth will be needed for comparison. For more information, consult a forensic odontologist. [Also see Chapter 20, "Forensic Odontology," and Chapter 30, "Bite Mark Evidence."]

Broken fingernails.—much like a bullet that has individualizing striations on it, natural fingernails have individualizing striations on them. A broken fingernail found at a crime scene can be matched to the individual it came from many months after the crime has been committed. Broken fingernails should be placed in a paper packet which is then placed in a paper envelope. It can then be transported to the crime lab for analysis. Known samples from the suspect and maybe from the victim will be needed for comparison.

Questioned documents.—handwriting samples can also be matched back to the individual that produced them. Known exemplars of the suspected person's handwriting must be submitted for comparison to the unknown samples. Questioned documents can also be processed for fingerprints. All items should be collected in paper containers. For more information consult a questioned documents examiner. [Also see Chapter 26, "Questioned Document Examination."]

Blood and body fluids.—if using the RFLP [(Restriction Fragment Length Polymorphism)] method of DNA analysis, then blood and seminal fluid can be matched back to an individual with a high degree of probability. Currently, if using the PCR [(Polymerase Chain Reaction)] method of DNA analysis or conventional serological techniques, then blood and some body fluids can be said to come from a certain population group to which the individual belongs. As PCR technology advances, these population groups will become smaller, eventually giving it the same discriminating power as RFLP analysis has today. Dried blood and body fluid stains should be collected in the following manner: If the stained object can be transported back to the crime lab, then package it in a paper bag or envelope and send it to the lab; if the object cannot be transported, then either use fingerprint tape and lift it like a fingerprint and place the tape on a lift back; scrape the stain into a paper packet and package it in a paper envelope; or absorb the stain onto ½" long threads moistened with distilled water. The threads must be air-dried before permanently packaging. For transportation purposes and to prevent cross contamination, the threads may be placed into a plastic container for no more than two hours. Once in a secure location, the threads must be removed from the plastic and allowed to air-dry. They may then be repackaged into a paper packet and placed in a paper envelope. Wet blood and body fluid stains should be collected in the following manner: all items should be packaged separately to prevent cross contamination, if the item can be transported to the crime lab, then package it in a paper bag (or plastic bag if the transportation time is under two hours), bring it to a secure place and allow it to thoroughly air-dry, then repackage it in a paper bag. If the item cannot be transported back to the lab, then absorb the stain onto a small (1" x 1") square of precleaned, 100% cotton sheeting. Package it in paper (or plastic if the transportation time is less than two hours), bring it to a secure place and allow it to thoroughly air-dry; then repackage it in a paper envelope. UNDER NO CIRCUMSTANCES SHOULD WET OR MOIST ITEMS REMAIN IN PLASTIC OR PAPER CONTAINERS FOR MORE THAN TWO HOURS. Victim and suspect's known whole blood samples will have to be collected in yellow, red, or purple top "Vacutainers." Contact the lab to which the samples will be submitted for specific information.

Firearms and toolmarks.—bullets and casings found at the crime scene can be positively matched back to a gun in the possession of a suspect. Bullets and casings can also be examined at the crime lab and sometimes tell an investigator what make and model of weapons may have expended the casing or bullet. A bullet found at the crime scene can sometimes be matched back to the same lot of ammunition found in a suspect's possession. Toolmarks can be positively matched to a tool in the suspect's possession. Firearm safety is a must at any crime scene. If a firearm must be moved at a crime scene, never move it by placing a pencil in the barrel or inside the trigger guard. Not only is this unsafe, but it could damage potential evidence. The gun can be picked up by the textured surface on the grips without fear of placing unnecessary fingerprints on the weapon. Before picking up the gun, make sure that the gun barrel is not pointed at anyone. Keep notes on the condition of the weapon as found and stops taken to render it as safe as possible without damaging potential evidence. The firearm can then be processed for prints and finally rendered completely safe. FIREARMS MUST BE RENDERED SAFE BEFORE SUBMISSION TO THE CRIME LAB. The firearm should be packaged in an envelope or paper bag separately from the ammunition and/or magazine. The ammunition and/or magazine should be placed in a paper envelope or bag. It is important that the ammunition found in the gun be submitted to the crime lab. Any boxes of similar ammunition found in a suspect's possession should also be placed in a paper container and sent to the crime lab. Casings and/or bullets found at the crime scene should be packaged separately and placed in paper envelopes or small cardboard pillboxes. If knives (or other sharp objects) are being submitted to the lab (for toolmarks, fingerprints, serology, etc.), then the blade and point should be wrapped in stiff unmovable cardboard and placed in a paper bag or envelope. The container should be labeled to warn that the contents are sharp and precautions should be taken. This is to prevent anyone from being injured.

Shoeprints and tire tracks. — can be matched positively to a pair of shoes or to tires in a suspect's possession. Shoeprints and tire tracks can sometimes tell investigators what type of shoes or tires to look for when searching a suspect's residence or vehicles. Before any attempt is made at collecting shoeprints or tire tracks, one-to-one photographs should be made using a tripod, ruler, and level. The flash should be held at about 45 degree angles from the surface containing an impression. Casts can be made of impressions using dental stone. Once hardened, the cast can be packaged in paper and submitted to the lab. When photographing prints on hard flat surfaces, the flash should be used as side lighting. Shoeprints on hard flat surfaces can also sometimes be lifted like a fingerprint. Dust prints on certain surfaces can be lifted with an electrostatic dustprint lifter.

Fracture matches.—can positively link broken pieces at the scene with pieces found in the possession of a suspect. For example, headlight fragments found at the scene of a hit-and-run could be positively matched to a broken headlight (just like putting together a jigsaw puzzle) on a suspect's vehicle. Larger fragments should be placed in paper bags or envelopes. Smaller fragments should be placed in a paper packet and then placed in an envelope.

Hair.—if a root sheath is attached, then DNA analysis using PCR technology can say that this hair came from a certain percentage of the population to which the suspect belongs. If there is no root sheath, then a microscopic analysis can say that the hair has the same characteristics as the suspect's hair and is similar to his or her hair. At this point, no one can say that a hair came from a particular individual. Hair found at the scene should be placed in a paper packet and then placed in an envelope. If a microscopic examination is required, then 15-20 representative hairs from the suspect must be submitted to the lab for comparison. If DNA analysis if going to be used, then a whole blood sample from the suspect must be submitted to the lab in a "Vacutainer." Contact a DNA lab for more information.

Fibers.—can be said to be the same type and color as those found in a suspect's clothes, residence, vehicle, etc. Fibers should be collected in a paper packet and placed in an envelope. Representative fibers should be collected from a suspect and submitted to the lab for comparison.

Paint.—can be said to be the same type and color as paint found in the possession of a suspect. Paint fragments should be collected in a paper packet and placed in an envelope. Representative paint chips or samples should be collected from the suspect and submitted to the lab for comparison.

Glass.—can be said to have the same characteristics as glass found in the possession of a suspect. Smaller glass fragments should be placed in a paper packet and then in an envelope. Larger pieces should be wrapped securely in paper or cardboard and then placed in a padded cardboard box to prevent further breakage. Representative samples from the suspect should be submitted to the lab for comparison.

Other trace evidence.—sometimes during the commission of a crime, there are other items which may be transferred to a perpetrator from the scene or from the perpetrator to the scene (sheetrock, safe insulation. etc.). The guidelines for collecting the evidence and obtaining known samples is about the same as for paint and fibers. For specific information, contact your crime lab.

Special Considerations for Sexual Assault Evidence

When dealing with sexual assaults, the investigator usually has a living victim who can provide the investigator with information which will help in collecting and preserving the pertinent evidence. The investigator should glean as much information as possible, so he or she will know which evidence to collect. For example, if the victim tells the investigator (which in this case may be the examining physician) that no oral penetration occurred, then the investigator knows that no oral swabs will need to be taken. Any information should be passed on to the crime lab, so the forensic scientists will know how to process the evidence submitted. Evidence should never be submitted without communicating relevant information.

When dealing with sex crimes, the victim should be taken to the hospital immediately and the examination started as soon as possible. Photographs should be taken to document any injuries which the victim received. If necessary, oral, vaginal, and/or anal swabs should be taken from the victim and air-dried for one hour in a moving air source as soon as possible. They should be collected as soon as possible because the body begins breaking down the various components in seminal fluid through drainage, enzyme activity, pH, etc. The swabs should be air-dried under a fan for at least one hour. This can either be accomplished by the doctor at the hospital, or, upon collecting the kit from the doctor, the investigator should bring it immediately to a secure place and air-dry it. The reason for this is that the moisture in the swabs allows microorganisms to grow which can destroy the evidentiary value of the swabs. Known saliva samples from the victim must also be air-dried along with any other wet or moist samples (not including whole blood samples, vaginal washing, or any other liquid samples collected).

Usually, the best sample of seminal fluid comes from the swabs, as long as they are preserved properly. The next best place is usually the victim's panties because the seminal fluid will drain into the panties (if the assault was vaginal or anal in nature). The stain will sometimes be better preserved because the seminal fluid tends to dry faster in the panties. If the panties have wet stains, then they should be air-dried as soon as possible before packaging. Clothes can be a good source of seminal fluid if the assailant ejaculated on the victim's clothes. The clothes can also be a source for the suspect's blood, hairs, fibers, or other evidence transferred to the victim from the suspect. Clothing should be air-dried before permanent packaging, and each article of clothing should be packaged separately.

Bed sheets, comforters, spreads, etc., can also be a source of evidence from the suspect. The value of this type of evidence should be carefully considered by the investigator before collecting it. If the bed is a "high traffic" area, meaning that numerous people have had access to the bed and the bed sheets haven't been cleaned in a long time, then it won't have as much evidentiary value as a bed where only one person had access to it and the sheets have been cleaned recently. The investigator should use the side lighting technique to look for any loose trace evidence on the sheets which may be lost during handling and packaging. This evidence should be placed in a paper packet and then placed in an envelope. If the sheets have wet stains and these can be attributed to the rape, then the investigator should circle these stains and inform the crime lab that those are the relevant stains to be examined. The investigator should note that he or she circled the stains and as always, air-dry the evidence before permanently packaging it. The investigator should neatly fold the sheets inward to prevent the loss of any other loose evidence. The sheets can then be packaged separately in paper bags, air-dried if necessary, and submitted to the crime lab.

If a suspect is established in a rape case, then reference samples should be collected from the suspect for comparison. These samples should include: a whole blood sample in a red, yellow, or purple top "Vacutainer"; a saliva sample (air-dried); 15-20 pulled head hairs; and 15-20 pulled pubic hairs. If the suspect is captured within 24 hours and it can be established which clothes and/or shoes he wore during the attack, then the items should be packaged separately and submitted to the crime lab. Sometimes trace evidence from the victim such as hairs, fibers, blood, etc., can be found on the suspect's clothing.

The key to proper collection, preservation, analysis, and overall usefulness of evidence is open and plentiful communication between investigators, forensic scientists, and prosecutors. This will make the most of the evidence which can make or break a case. This [chapter] has presented general guidelines on the collection and preservation of evidence. The investigator should remember that each crime scene is different and each crime scene is a learning process. The investigator should also keep in mind that different crime labs may like their evidence collected in different manners. This is why the investigator should not hesitate to call his or her crime lab if he or has a question or a problem on the collection or preservation of evidence.

Recommended Reading

Evidence Handling Guide. Louisiana Dept. of Public Safety and Corrections, Office of State Police, Crime Laboratory.

Fisher, Barry A.J., Arne Svensson, and Otto Wendell. *Techniques of Crime Scene Investigation*. New York: Elsevier, 1981.

Moreau, Dale M. *Fundamental Principles and Theory of Crime Scene Photography*. Quantico: Forensic Science Training Unit, FBI Academy.

Redsicker, David R. *The Practical Methodology of Forensic Photography*. Elsevier: New York, 1991.

Sketching Crime Scenes. U.S. Dept. of Justice, FBI.

— by George Schiro, Forensic Scientist,
Louisiana State Police Crime Laboratory

Chapter 7

Bloodstain Photography

Once the walk-through is completed, the notes must be supplemented with other forms of documentation, such as videotape, photographs, and/or sketches.

Videotape can be an excellent medium for documenting bloodstains at a crime scene. If a video camera is available, it is best used after the initial walk-through. This is to record the evidence before any major alterations have occurred at the scene. Videotape provides a perspective on the crime scene layout that cannot be as easily perceived in photographs and sketches. It is a more natural viewing medium to which people can readily relate, especially in demonstrating the structure of the crime scene and how the evidence relates to those structures.

The value of videotaping blood evidence is that the overall relationship of various blood spatters and patterns can be demonstrated. One example of this could be a beating homicide. In this case, videotape can show the overall blood spatter patterns and how these spatters are interrelated. The videotape can also show the relationship of the spatters to the various structures at the crime scene. In cases where the suspect may have been injured (such as stabbing homicides), the video camera can be used to document any blood trails that

From "Bloodstain Photography," [Online] undated. Available: http://police2ucr.edu/phoblood.html. Produced by George Schiro, Forensic Scientist, Louisiana State Police Crime Laboratory, P.O. Box 66614, Baton Rouge, LA 70896. For complete contact information, please refer to Chapter 56, "Resources." Reprinted with permission.

may lead away from the scene. If videotaping indoors, the camera can show how the various areas are laid out in relation to each other and how they can be accessed. This is particularly valuable when recording peripheral bloodstains that may be found in other rooms. The high intensity light source can also be used for illuminating the bloodstains to make them more visible on the videotape.

Whether a video camera is available or not, it is absolutely essential that still photographs are taken to document the crime scene and any associated blood evidence. If a video camera is available, then still photography will be the second step in recording the crime scene. If video is not available, then still photography will be the first step. Photographs can demonstrate the same type of things that the videotape does, but crime scene photographs can also be used to record close-up details, record objects at any scaled size, and record objects at actual size. These measurements and recordings are more difficult to achieve with videotape.

Blood evidence can be photographed using color print film and/or color slide film. Infrared film can also be used for documenting bloodstains on dark surfaces. Overall, medium range, and close-up photographs should be taken of pertinent bloodstains. Scaled photographs (photographs with a ruler next to the evidence) must also be taken of items in cases where size relevance is significant or when direct (one-to-one) comparisons will be made, such as with bloody shoeprints, fingerprints, high-velocity blood spatter patterns, etc. A good technique for recording a large area of blood spatter on a light colored wall is to measure and record the heights of some of the individual blood spatters. The overall pattern on the wall including a yard stick as a scale is then photographed with slide film. After the slide is developed, it can be projected onto a blank wall or onto the actual wall many years after the original incident. By using a yardstick, the original blood spatters can be viewed at their actual size and placed in their original positions. Measurements and projections can then be made to determine the spatters' points of origin.

—by George Schiro, Forensic Scientist,
Louisiana State Police Crime Laboratory

Chapter 8

Domestic Violence Cases

The scenario plays out innumerable times in jurisdictions across America. In response to a 911 call, officers rush to the site of a domestic disturbance, where they encounter the suspect and his girlfriend. The sobbing victim holds an ice pack to her swollen face and claims that her boyfriend struck her during an argument. When an officer asks for the offender's account, he replies that a disagreement had "gotten out of hand" but that everything is fine now.

The officers arrest the offender and call for a unit to transport him to a holding center. An officer then photographs the victim's injuries and obtains a written statement from her, requesting that she report to the police station the following day for additional photographs. Other department personnel arrive and provide the victim with the telephone number of a local shelter and with information on securing a protective order against her boyfriend. They also suggest that the victim have a doctor examine her injuries.

Three days after the assault, the victim calls the station to inform one of the arresting officers that she wishes to drop the assault charge. She tells the officer that the dispute had been her fault and that her boyfriend was merely defending himself when he struck her. Although the victim did not admit to it, the officer had an idea of what actually had led to her change of heart: The defendant had returned with the

From "Focus on Domestic Violence: Prosecuting Cases without Victim Cooperation," in the FBI *Law Enforcement Bulletin,* April 1996. Produced by George Wattendorf, J.D.

63

rent money, a bouquet of flowers, and a promise that "nothing like this will ever happen again."

But to the victim's surprise, the officer calmly advises her that the evidence collected in the case will enable prosecution efforts to proceed despite her lack of cooperation. Like a growing number of domestic abuse victims who decide to disavow statements and drop charges against their abusers, this victim has discovered that the criminal justice system may not be as willing to forgive and forget. In fact, with the right evidence, prosecutors can gain a conviction, even if the victim testifies on the abuser's behalf.

Aside from protecting victims from further abuse, law enforcement agencies have a vested interest in pursuing such cases. Departments often respond to repeated domestic disturbance calls from the same address. A manipulative offender who can convince a frightened and vulnerable victim to drop her charges may be deterred from violence if he knows that the police and prosecutors can pursue the case without the victim's testimony.

Law enforcement agencies can obtain sufficient evidence to secure convictions without the assistance of victims by carefully prioritizing evidence collection in domestic assault cases. In a case like the one described above, evidence collected by police officers enabled prosecutors in New Hampshire to win a conviction without calling the victim as a witness.

Evidence Collection

The Dover, New Hampshire, Police Department began prioritizing evidence collection for domestic assault cases in June 1993. Since implementation of the policy based on a similar approach used in San Diego, the conviction rate for domestic violence assault cases has increased significantly.

As part of the policy, officers use a checklist to ensure that all evidence is preserved for later use by the prosecution. Together, the different types of evidence can more than compensate for the lack of a victim's testimony. However, the fact that conviction may depend solely on this evidence underscores the need for officers to collect and save all relevant documentation regarding the case.

Secure Emergency 911 Tape

Investigating officers should secure a recording of any 911 call made by the victim. Calls to the 911 dispatcher reporting the assault can be presented at trial under the hearsay exception or as impeachment.

64

Often, these tapes will include the defendant in the background, yelling or threatening the victim.

Record Excited Statements by the Victim

Any statement made while the victim is still under stress from the assault can be admitted into court through responding officers as a hearsay exception. It is important that officers document the victim's condition and note her exact statements concerning the assault. Officers can testify to such remarks as, "He punched me!" under the excited utterance exception.

Take Photographs

Photographs are critical pieces of evidence. In court, pictures truly do say a thousand words, and two or three photographs can have more impact than hours of testimony from officers describing a victim's condition after an assault.

Recent advances in instant camera technology allow for highly detailed close-up shots. Instant photographs also reveal immediately any problems in focusing or lighting, so that corrections can be made before the opportunity is lost. Because full bruising coloration may take at least 24 hours, responding officers should encourage the victim to report to the police station the day after the assault for followup photographs.

Officers also should photograph the crime scene to provide a record of damaged property or to show evidence of a struggle. If the defendant pleads self-defense in court, prosecutors may choose to introduce booking photographs in court to rebut such claims.

Request a Statement from the Victim

While a victim is cooperating, responding officers should request that she provide a detailed, written account of the assault. If the victim appears too traumatized to write, an officer should transcribe her exact words as she dictates the statement. Officers should make sure that the victim's statement references any prior abuse. The victim also should be encouraged to file a petition for a protective order.

If the victim later becomes uncooperative, the written statement can be used to refresh her memory or to impeach her testimony. If the victim has indicated past instances of abuse, prosecutors can request that the court admit the prior acts as character evidence. Prosecutors can even file additional charges if corroborating evidence supports the claims. The victim's sworn petition for a protective order can be used to impeach her testimony if she becomes a hostile witness.

Interview the Offender

Officers should record all spontaneous remarks the offender makes at the scene. While the officers are conducting their probable cause investigation, they should request that the offender provide his version of the incident. Such noncustodial interviews do not require a Miranda warning. However, even when officers issue a Miranda warning upon arrest, offenders usually respond to questions. Admissions by the offender are the best type of evidence.

Interview Other Witnesses

Unlike some other crimes, domestic violence is difficult to hide. Unfortunately, children often are the primary witnesses. Officers should not overlook taking statements from children who were present during the assault. Neighbors also can provide statements that could be introduced later by prosecutors to rebut claims of accidental injury or self-defense.

Secure Medical Records

Responding officers should request that the victim sign a medical records release. If she later proves uncooperative, the prosecution can still obtain medical records relevant to the case.

Similarly, officers should not overlook reports made by the emergency medical team. These reports generally contain very detailed information regarding the victim's injuries and can provide necessary documentation that confirms the assault.

Seize Plain-View Evidence

Responding officers should seize any evidence in plain view, such as blood-stained or torn clothing, and look for indications of a struggle, such as hair clumps, bloodstains, torn buttons, etc. Officers also should seize as evidence any weapon used in the assault.

Conclusion

Domestic violence represents one of the most vexing problems facing law enforcement agencies. Domestic disturbance calls are especially stress-inducing for responding officers, not only because of the potential for violence but also because officers know their efforts on behalf of the victim will probably prove futile. After a cooling down period, battered victims often reconcile with their abusive partner and refuse to support prosecution efforts. The cumulative effect of responding to repeated calls involving the same parties also takes a considerable toll on officers' morale.

But, law enforcement agencies do not need to be passive players in a cycle of violence. By collecting sufficient evidence, law enforcement officers can help prosecutors prove assault, even if the victim testifies on the assailant's behalf. Such proactive efforts on the part of the criminal justice system send a clear message to potential abusers. At the very least, the real threat of prosecution may deter some offenders. At best, courts can use the threat of jail time to divert abusers into treatment programs.

The more evidence that officers collect, the better the chance that prosecutors can prove assault. Not every case can be won. But by collecting the right evidence and using it wisely, law enforcement officers and prosecutors can take a more active role in curbing domestic violence.

— by George Wattendorf, J.D.

Lieutenant Wattendorf serves as a legal advisor to the Dover, New Hampshire, Police Department on liability and labor issues.

Chapter 9

Domestic Violence Photography

Documentation by photography is an important and powerful tool in the investigation of domestic violence crimes. When injuries resulting from domestic violence are promptly and adequately documented, it is possible for prosecution to occur without the victim's testimony.

Often, victims of domestic violence are dependent upon the abuser for food and shelter. If the abuser is only jailed temporarily after the initial arrest, it is possible for an abuser to coerce the victim into not testifying. Therefore, the importance of documentation becomes relevant in preventing the recurring abuse of victims. The pictures can be used in the event that the victim later becomes unwilling to testify.

The objective of this article is to provide some basic knowledge of photography and illustrate four photographic techniques that have proven to be successful in domestic violence cases: color photography, alternative light source (narrow band light source) photography, reflective ultraviolet (UV) photography, and infrared (IR) photography. In addition, affordability of the necessary equipment is a concern, and the illustrated techniques were developed with this in mind.

From "Domestic Violence Photography," [Online] undated. Available: http://police2.ucr.edu/dv-photo.html. Produced by Lt. James O. Pex, Oregon State Police Forensic Laboratory, 3334 S. 4th, Coos Bay, OR 97420. For complete contact information, please refer to Chapter 56, "Resources." Reprinted with permission.

Understanding Photography

The Light Spectrum

The colors that are visible to the eye represent only a small portion of the light spectrum, also known as the electromagnetic spectrum. Visible light, or white light, is a combination of all the visible colors. A beam of white light can be separated into the visible spectrum using a prism. The band of colors range from violet to blue, blue-green, green, yellow, orange, red and deep red. Each color represents a different wavelength of light. These wavelengths increase in the direction from blue to red along the length of the spectrum. The visible region of the light spectrum ranges from 400 to 700 nanometers (nm) in wavelength.

The areas extending in either direction beyond the visible spectrum are the invisible regions of light. Below violet from 200 to 400 nm is the ultraviolet region. Although we cannot see this light, it is reactive with photographic materials. Therefore, it is possible to produce images that may only be observed using photography. Extending just beyond the visible region in the other direction from 700 nm and higher is the infrared region of light radiation. The range of infrared light close to the visible spectrum is also photographically reactive.

Film

There are basically three common types of film: black and white, color negative, and transparency. Film has varying degrees of sensitivity to the amount and intensity of light. These degrees of sensitivity are referred to as ASA. The higher the ASA number the "faster" the film. Faster film reacts quicker to light, therefore it requires less light for proper exposure. The drawback of using higher ASA film is that enlarged photos may appear grainy and less detailed.

Although slide film has accurate color rendition, it lacks "latitude." Latitude in photography is the ability to produce a good picture from a negative that is slightly underexposed or slightly overexposed. These corrections can be made to print film through adjustments in the print processing. Slide film is not designed for print processing and thus lacks latitude. This means that the exposure must be exact for the photo to turn out correctly. In addition, for use in trial situations, slides are more expensive to convert to enlargements than print film.

70

Since print film offers considerable latitude in exposure, it provides a definite advantage for those who are not expert photographers. Because documentation of evidence requires the reproduction to be as accurate as possible, color film is the best medium.

Yet in domestic violence photography, UV and IR techniques are often used to see images that our eyes cannot see. These techniques are useful because of the way our skin interacts differently with UV and IR light compared to visible light. For these techniques black and white film offers the best results.

There are two reasons for this. First, the top emulsion layer of all color film which is blue, contains UV blockers preventing the exposure of the bottom layers. Second, the blue layer that does react does not provide as much contrast as black and white film. In addition, there is no "color" in the UV and IR region so nothing is gained using color films.

It should also be noted that special IR film is needed for IR photography. Normal black and white film is not sensitive to the near IR region. IR film is sensitive from the IR region to the UV region and may be used for both techniques.

Polaroid Corporation has an active market in domestic abuse photography by utilizing their pack films and instant cameras. These systems work well when instant results are necessary. However, the color balance is not comparable to print film, and either duplicates or enlargements must be made by re-photographing the Polaroid picture with print film. Despite its shortcomings, the simplicity of the instant camera may be critical if the alternative equipment and necessary skills are not available.

Cameras and Lenses

For the photographic techniques illustrated in this article a 35mm single lens reflex (SLR) camera is needed. SLR cameras are versatile because of interchangeable lens and filter adapters which are necessary for abuse photography.

To obtain adequate detail, close-up photography is essential for the techniques that will be outlined. The SLR camera incorporates a mirror and a prism that enables the subject to be viewed through the camera lens. This allows the photographer to document exactly what is framed by the viewfinder without "chopping off" the subject or getting out of focus.

35mm point-and-shoot cameras will not work. The minimum focusing distance (approximately 3 feet) is not adequate to fill a frame.

A built-in wide angle lens and the viewfinder optics used for framing and focusing are separate from the lens. With a point-and-shoot camera, the photographer may be able to focus the subject in the viewfinder, but the picture will be either out of focus or "chopped off" because the lens is not able to focus.

For domestic violence photography a shorter focal length (fl) is better. A fl.4 to fl.8 normal or macro lens is good enough to get close to the subject for detailed pictures. Most of the photographs taken in domestic violence photography will be taken at the minimum focusing distance to "fill the frame."

For UV photography, the lens must transmit light into the UV region. However, most lenses have been treated with a coating that blocks UV light. If money is not an issue, then an expensive quartz lens may be purchased. On the other hand, if money is a concern, the alternative is to check the ability of a lens to transmit UV light. This is accomplished by performing an analysis to determine the percent transmittance of light less than 400 nm with a spectrophotometer. If the lens does not transmit light in this region of the spectrum, it will not work for UV photography.

In photography, controlling light is essential to obtain the proper exposure of film. This is achieved by manipulating the reciprocity law of photochemistry. The law states that exposure (E) is equal to the product of intensity (I) multiplied by the time (T). $E = I \times T$

The shutter speed on a camera determines the amount of time the film is exposed. The settings on a given camera may range from 1 second to 1/1000 of a second. Proceeding from 1 second each step down reduces the time by one half. An example of shutter-scale markings would be as follows: 1, 2, 4, 8, 15, 30, 60, 125, 250, 500, 1000.

Intensity is dependent on the maximum amount of light available and may be reduced by adjusting the aperture on the camera. The aperture is a diaphragm of metal leaves forming a nearly circular opening that the light has to pass through in order to reach the film. The range of aperture sizes are adjusted by turning a ring on the outside of the lens. The aperture settings (f-stops or f/numbers) usually consist of the following sequence: 1.4, 2, 2.8, 4, 5.6, 8, 11, 16, . . . The smallest f/number is the largest opening, while the largest number is the smallest opening. For every consecutive increase in the f/number, the amount of light is decreased by half.

Because domestic violence photography is done indoors, the light sources used have relatively low intensities compared to sunlight. Therefore the choice of film and the settings for the aperture and shutter speed need to be adjusted to allow enough light to reach the film while still being able to hold the camera. It is possible to "blur" a picture when holding a camera if the film and the shutter speed are too slow. This problem may be avoided by choosing a fast film such as 1600 ASA, in addition to setting the aperture shutter speed pairing based on the camera's built-in light meter. It is important that the camera has a built in light-meter, as photographing without one will be nearly impossible.

The light source is another variable that may need to be manipulated in order to obtain enough light for proper exposure. Because light waves spread out as they travel away from the source, the farther away the light source is from the subject the less light there is being focused on the subject.

The relationship between light intensity and distance is as follows: the light that falls on the subject is inversely proportional to the square of the distance. This relationship is known as the inverse square law. What this means to the photographer is that the intensity of light falling on the subject can be doubled by decreasing the distance from the source to the subject by half.

Photographing Injuries to the Skin

UV Photography

Penetration and reflection of light on the skin is a function of wavelength. Shorter wavelengths such as UV do not penetrate the skin very far before it is reflected back to the camera. Therefore a high resolution picture of the skin surface is possible. This works well for bite marks, cuts, scratches, and scars. This is not a good technique to apply to bruises unless the blood accumulation is very close to the skin surface.

UV Photography can be accomplished with an ordinary 35mm SLR if the lens is capable of transmitting light somewhere between 300 nm and 400 nm. The easiest way to make that determination is to place the lens in a spectrophotometer and test it. Most clinical, university, or forensic laboratories have one available. Manufacturers coat most lenses to prevent excess UV penetration. Excess UV will unbalance a color photograph with excess blue. There isn't a common lens manufacturer that can be recommended. Some lenses will allow UV light transmission down to the 350 nm range and some will not. A simple test in the absence of a spectrophotometer is to photograph someone with freckles. The appearance of freckles in UV light is considerably enhanced compared to standard visible range light photography. No focus correction is necessary. Success in UV photography is also a function of light intensity (I) in the absence of the other wavelengths. To handhold photograph a living object requires a high intensity source such as an Omnichrome 1000 or Omnichrome FLS 5000 and a dark room. Photography with small handheld UV sources is possible, but standardization of source-to-target and lens-to-target distance is critical. The following features are a good starting point for UV photography:

1. 35mm SLR with f1.4 or 1.8 normal lens

2. 3200 ASA Black and White film

3. UV source

4. Room without windows to turn out the room lights

5. Measuring scale-to-place near injuries

If there is a need for macro photography, avoid complex lenses and use extension tubes. Proper light metering with a through-the-lens light meter is close enough that bracketing your shots will lead to a quality photograph.

Visible Light Region

After an assault, the victim's injuries may be photographed any time within the next two to five days. Visible light penetrates deeper into the skin than UV light and is sufficient to document most bruises. The addition of special wavelength sources and special filters can improve the visualization of the injuries by enhancing the blue color and improving the contrast against the normal skin tones.

The equipment of choice again is a 35mm SLR with a fast lens. No special wavelength considerations are necessary. Most of the shots are at the minimum focusing position on the lens and available light as opposed to flash. If the room has fluorescent lights, be sure to use a correction filter such as the Cokin A.036. Standard documentation with available light is usually followed with special wavelength photography that is sometimes called "Alternate light photography" (ALP). The Omnichrome 1000 or the Omnichrome FLS 5000 have positions for 450 and 485 nm that emit a blue light that improves the visibility of bruises. High ASA films such as Kodak Gold 1600, Ektapress 1600, or Fujicolor Super HG 1600 are the films of choice. ALP in combination with an orange filter (Cokin A.002) requires a fast film for handheld photography.

Through-the-lens light metering is accurate with visible and ALP photography. Beware of using a white ruler or measuring tape in close-up pictures. The meter may take the light reading of the scale and the skin tones and injury will be too dark. This can be avoided by keeping the scales at the edge of the photo since most light meters are center weighted.

The crime victim should be accompanied by a Victim's Assistant from the District Attorney's office when being transported to the laboratory. A short interview is conducted to determine the location of the injuries and how the injuries occurred. Bruises are transfer patterns. The victim's statements may be supported by placing fingers on the finger marks or blunt instruments over blunt injury bruises. If a weapon was used, be sure to bring it to the photo session whenever possible. Rough anatomical drawings and a standardized form are used to determine the time interval for each injury. Any scars or birthmarks are also noted.

After the interview, the photographic procedure is as follows:

1. Place an 18% gray scale against the arm of the victim to aid the developer in assigning the proper skin tones. Also identify the victim and include a case number for reference.

2. Starting with visible light photo techniques, photograph the upper half of the victim for identification purposes.

3. Photograph the general area or appendage where the injury occurs.

4. Adjust the lens to the minimum focusing distance and photograph the injury. (Small injuries may require the use of extension tubes). Place a scale in the photos.

5. Look for patterns in the bruising. Re-photograph with suspect's weapon adjacent to the bruise, then directly over the bruise. If the finger marks are on one side, look for the thumb mark on the other side.

6. Repeat the sequence with the ALP source and appropriate filters with the room lights out.

7. If UV photography is a consideration, change to 3200 ASA black and white film and repeat the sequence with a UV source. Bracket these shots extensively.

The methods discussed above have been employed for the last year in casework and are the result of extensive literature review and research on how to best represent the victims of domestic violence. All cases are by appointment to contain the labor costs. The methods have found application not only to spousal abuse or child abuse, but also to rape victims and homicide victims prior to autopsy and homicide suspects to document their injuries or lack of injuries. These techniques could be applied to elder abuse and fatal traffic accidents to identify the driver.

Most of the domestic abuse cases that have been photographed in the laboratory have been prosecuted or resolved in a positive manner. This is a direct reversal to the national statistics associated with domestic violence. One surprise that has occurred is the upgrade of charges when ligature marks can be documented. In one recent case, the photography resulted in the grand jury upgrading the charges from Assault IV to Attempted Murder. The case went to trial and the suspect was found guilty of Attempted Murder. Of course this is the exception as most cases end with the abuser pleading guilty and getting a diversion to counseling. If the photography is done properly, the abuser has lost his leverage over the victim and the case may proceed without the victim's testimony. After all, let's look at the reality of the circumstance, "Mrs. Smith, is this you in the photograph?" or, "Mr. Smith, is this your wife?"

References

Hyzer, W. G., and Krauss, T. C. "The Bite Mark Standard Reference Scale—ABFO No. 2." *Journal of Forensic Sciences* 33 (2): 498-506 (March 1988).

Krauss, T. C. "Forensic Evidence Documentation Using Reflective Ultraviolet Photography." *Photo Electronic Imaging* 18-23 (February 1993).

Krauss, T. C., and Warlen, S. C. "The Forensic Science Use of Reflective Ultra-Violet Photography." *Journal of Forensic Sciences* 30 (1): 262-8 (January 1985).

McEvoy, R T. *Reflective UV Photography*. IX Log 911, Rochester, NY: Eastman Kodak, 1987.

Redsicker, David R. *The Practical Methodology of Forensic Photography*. New York: Elsevier, 1991.

Ultra-Violet and Fluorescence Photography. Eastman Kodak Publication M-27.

West, M. H., Barsley, R. E., Hall, J. E., Hayne, S., and Cimrmancic, M. "The Detection and Documentation of Trace Wound Patterns by the Use of Alternative Light Source." *Journal of Forensic Sciences* 37 (6): 1480-8 (November 1992).

—by Lt. James O. Pex,
Oregon State Police Forensic Laboratory

Chapter 10

Arson Investigation

Introduction

Damage from fire is Australia's most costly public safety problem. Losses due to fire, in life and injury, are exceeded only by those due to traffic accidents. The cost of fire damage to the Australian community has been estimated to be $600 million per year. Our own experience over recent years suggests that this may be a conservative estimate. Arson, the willful and malicious burning of property, accounts for approximately 30% of this figure.

The most effective way to try to reduce this appalling cost, and to reduce the damage caused by fire, is effective fire investigation. It should then be possible to reduce the number of accidental fires by improving building codes, and by identifying and eliminating dangerous products. Arson is said to be the easiest crime to commit (even young children can do it), but the most difficult to detect and prove. It needs to be combated by finding and prosecuting those responsible.

Fire Investigation

A fire investigation is an unenviable task. The devastation, charred debris, collapsed structures, water soaked ashes, together with the

Excerpted from "Is It an Accidental Fire or Arson?" by Tony Cafe and Prof. Wal Stern; and "Aids Used for Detecting Accelerants at Fire Scenes," by Tony Cafe [Online]. Available: http://www.ozemail.com.au/~tcforen. © 1995-1996 by T. C. Forensic Pty Ltd., P.O. Box 8, NSW Australia 2168. For complete contact information, please refer to Chapter 56, "Resources." Reprinted with permission.

smoke and stench, makes the task uninviting and seemingly impossible. In the past, many investigators appear to have come to the task with inherent biases; fire brigade members have decided that all unexplained fires were due to electrical faults, whilst police and insurance investigators leaned towards "arson, by person or persons unknown."

There are different types of fires; in homes or factories, in the bush or a forest. The best investigation would use a team of trained personnel; fire brigade staff, with their experience of fires at first hand, police and insurance investigators, with their skills for determining motive and opportunities. An electrical engineer or electrician is required to investigate electrical systems. The scientist also has a most valuable role to play. The scientist should he able to arrive at a fire scene without any predetermined ideas. An analytical approach, using patient, thorough, and systematic techniques should reveal critical and vital information. The knowledge of a chemist is invaluable. A chemist should understand the properties of fuels and building materials, and have an understanding of the combustion process. In addition, an analytical chemist should also be able to identify in the laboratory materials found at the fire scene, even if they are only present as trace amounts.

Methodology

The basic role of an investigator at a fire scene is twofold; firstly, to determine the origin of the fire (the site where the fire began), and secondly, to examine closely the site of origin to try and determine what it was that caused a fire to start at or around that location. An examination would typically begin by trying to gain an overall impression of the site and the fire damage; this could be done at ground level or from an elevated position. From this, one might proceed to an examination of the materials present, the fuel load, and the state of the debris at various places. The search for the fire's origin should be based on elementary rules such as:

- Fire tends to burn upwards and outwards (look for V-patterns along walls).

- The presence of combustible materials will increase the intensity and extent of the fire; the fire will rise faster as it gets hotter (look for different temperature conditions).

- The fire needs fuel and oxygen to continue.

- A fire's spread will be influenced by factors such as air currents, walls, and stairways. Falling, burning debris and the effect of fire fighters will also have an influence.

A knowledge of the colour and state of various materials at elevated temperatures is required to help determine the temperature of the fire in different locations. An examination is also carried out of structural deformations, char depths, smoke patterns. It is important to try to discover if the fire started at floor level, as from a cigarette butt, or at elevated level, as for a gas explosion. This summary attempts only to indicate some of the steps typically undertaken. A more detailed list can be obtained from a number of texts.[1, 2]

These procedures are designed to locate the site of origin of the fire. Multiple sites of origin suggest a deliberately lit fire. Assuming that the site of origin has been found, a thorough examination of the debris in this area is then necessary. All electrical appliances in the vicinity should be examined. The presence of any flammable liquids, trails, or spalling of concrete or intense burn-marks in the floor should be checked. No fire can commence without an ignition source. One should therefore be on the lookout for matches, lighters, sources of sparks, hot objects, chemicals, gas and electrical lines, cigarettes, fireplaces, and chimneys.

A knowledge of spontaneous combustion, and its likely sources, is needed. It may be necessary to collect samples and carry out experiments in the laboratory (it is not difficult to show that loose rags with linseed oil on them cause spontaneous combustion). The collection of samples requires a chemist's knowledge of sampling procedures and the need to obtain uncontaminated materials.

Provided the investigation has been patiently and scientifically carried out, when combined with the evidence of eyewitnesses or fire officers, it may be possible at this stage to draw a conclusion about the fire. Typical causes of accidental fires are cooking accidents, overheated or short circuited electrical connections, spontaneous combustion of oils, welding sparks, burst gas lines, sparks from fireplaces, lightning, cigarette butts, left-on appliances, reacting chemicals. The list of all the possible causes is very long.

Arson

If a fire is not the result of an accident, it must have been deliberately lit; arson. The motives to commit arson include vandalism, fraud, revenge, sabotage, and pyromania. A major objective in any suspected case of arson would be to search for, locate, sample, and analyse residual accelerants. Most, though certainly not all incendiary fires involve the use of an accelerant to speed the ignition and rate of spread of fire. A rapid and intense fire, inconsistent with the natural fuel loading is indicative of an accelerated fire. Such a fire is likely to be initiated at ground level, possibly in a number of sites and may produce trail marks, burn-throughs, or spalling of concrete.

The accelerants most commonly used, on account of their flammability and ready availability are petrol, kerosene, mineral turpentine and diesel. Other accelerants such as alcohols, acetone, and industrial solvents are less commonly used. It might be thought (certainly many arsonists assume) that after an intense fire there will be negligible amounts of such accelerants remaining. Given our current sophistication of analytical techniques, this is not true. The amount of accelerant remaining after a fire will depend on factors such as the quantity and type of compound used, but also on the nature of material it is poured on, the elapsed time since the fire, and the severity of the fire. Chemists have been able to locate and detect trace amounts of liquid hydrocarbons in soil beneath a gutted house several months after a fire.

Detection of trace quantities of materials requires careful attention to sampling techniques and analysis. The most frequently sampled material is flooring material such as wood, carpet, soil, and linoleum. Porous material is best. There is a need to take control samples in some cases, away from the area where the accelerant is suspected, but preferably of the same material as the sample.

Some investigators use "sniffers" at fire scenes. These portable detectors usually note changes in oxygen level on a semiconductor. They are not specific for liquid hydrocarbons, responding to a variety of vapours, and need to be used with caution. They can be used as a guide as to the best place from which to collect samples, for removal to, and analysis in, the chemical laboratory.

Sampling

The materials found to give the most positive analyses for accelerants are porous samples; carpet and underlay, cardboard, paper, felt, cloth, and soil. At all stages, because of the sensitivity of the analysis, care must be taken to avoid contamination. In our experience unlined metal cans have been found to be the best containers.

Lined cans may have a coating which contains volatile components and should not be used. Plastic bags may allow diffusion of volatile components either into or out of the sample and are not recommended. Glass containers may be used, but the cleanliness of lids needs to be assured. Cans need to be clean and well sealed, and clearly labelled, for transport to the laboratory. At the laboratory, they need to be documented and kept secure prior to analysis.

Extraction

The methods of extraction most commonly used for fire debris samples, are distillation, solvent extraction, and headspace analysis. The distillation techniques used have included steam distillation, ethylene glycol distillation, ethanol distillation, and vacuum distillation. Of these, steam distillation has been the most widely used, and is still used, particularly where reasonably large quantities of accelerant are suspected to be present. Solvent extraction is not used except in special cases. Both static and dynamic headspace analysis are now in common use, in both cases at and above room temperatures. In the former case, a needle of a gas syringe is placed into a container containing fire debris, and a volume of vapour is withdrawn for analysis.

Our own preferred method, on the basis of experience and experimentation, is for dynamic headspace extraction equipment. The fire debris, in its original container is placed into an oven and heated at 150° C for approximately one hour, whilst at the same time a continuous flow of filtered nitrogen gas flushes the headspace and sweeps any volatile components through a water trap onto an absorbent. This method in effect samples 3000 times more gas than does a static headspace sample. It has the advantage that the can is always vented, so that pressure does not build up in the can. Water present will volatilise, and essentially steam-distill the sample.

Absorption and Desorption

The absorbents in most common use are activated charcoal, Tenax G.C., and Porapak Q. All three absorb accelerant components, but do not absorb water or nitrogen. Tenax is stable up to 350° C and is ideal for rapid thermal desorption. It is used for most fire samples by the London Metropolitan Police Laboratories (Scotland Yard). An advantage of thermal desorption is that the material to be analysed can proceed directly from the absorbent into a gas chromatogram. One disadvantage is that when this happens the sample is used up, and the evidence is no longer present.

In the case of solvent desorption, one obtains a liquid sample which can be reanalysed many times and retained as evidence. A variety of solvents have been used for desorption, but we have found carbon disulfide to be the best, because of its high desorption efficiency for the components commonly found, its low detector response, and its high volatility. We use 1 mL A.R. grade carbon disulfide for extraction, and store liquid samples in a glass vial to which we add 1 mL water to prevent loss by evaporation.

Detection and Identification

Ultraviolet, infrared, and nuclear magnetic resonance spectroscopy have all been used for identifying accelerant components, but by far the most widely used technique is gas liquid chromatography. It is able to separate and detect trace amounts of volatile hydrocarbons in complex mixtures. The flame ionisation detector has been widely used because of its great sensitivity for these components. The introduction of capillary columns allows for smaller samples and produces sharper peaks and greater resolution. The number of different columns now available is quite large, but we have found that a 25m. BP-1 capillary column, 0.33mm. i.d. to be widely applicable. In our laboratory, we run unknown samples on a dual plotter against standard samples, so that a comparison can be made of samples run under similar conditions.

The four most commonly found accelerants (petrol, kerosene, mineral turpentine, and diesel) are all highly complex mixtures of many components, in very different ratios. Most forensic laboratories feel confident in identifying these compounds on the basis of their gas chromatograms alone, even if the samples are evaporated and contaminated.

In order to make a positive identification, it is necessary to identify a large number of the components present, and to note that their ratios are very similar to that of a standard. The use of evaporated and burnt standards may aid this comparison. To make absolutely sure of the identity of any component we have relied on gas chromatography/mass spectrometry (GC/MS). We have been fortunate to have available an AEI MS902, fitted with a Pye Unicam GC, and more recently a Hewlett Packard GC/MS, the 5970 MSD. This latter instrument contains a data library of some 42,000 compounds. It is possible to conduct searches for particular fragments, groups of fragments, or molecular ions, and is particularly well suited to identify aliphatic and aromatic hydrocarbon peaks and mixtures.

We have had a number of honours students working on finding the best experimental conditions, and on identifying as many as possible of the straight and branched chain aliphatic hydrocarbons, the xylenes, tri and tetramethylbenzenes, naphthalenes and methylnaphthalenes, styrene, and indanes. In the case of petrol, it is also possible to detect and identify, under different conditions, the organo-lead additives. At the same time consideration has also been given to the effects of evaporating and burning accelerants. A study has also been made of likely contaminants, particularly the pyrolysis products from various plastics, carpet, wood, tiles, glues and other adhesives, lacquers, thinners, vegetable oils. We have built up a library of possible contaminants. The techniques described are capable of detecting $1\ \mu L$ of accelerant. In fact, it is possible to detect $0.1\ \mu L$, but we have set a minimum level of $1\ \mu L$, because of the possibility of background material which may be present. At this level one must be very careful about contamination and pyrolysis compounds, so that they are not confused with accelerant. It is necessary to clean all equipment before use and to run blanks at regular intervals to ensure that there is no contamination present.

Conclusion

Fires present a major social and economic problem. A thorough investigation of any large-scale fire, be it accidental or deliberate, is warranted. Chemists have expertise which can be used in an on-the-spot investigation, and in the analytical laboratory. This is not an area for which many scientists in Australia have been specifically trained, but is an area where the chemist's skills and expertise can be of great benefit.

Aids Used for Detecting Accelerants at Fire Scenes

Introduction

Recently some members of the NSW Chapter of the IAAI witnessed demonstrations of aids which could be used to assist an investigator at the fire scene in selecting samples for later laboratory analysis. A sniffer dog trained to detect accelerants was demonstrated, as well as a portable gas chromatograph.

The use of various aids and techniques to detect accelerants at fire scenes has attracted controversy during the previous ten years. The much maligned sniffer has suffered continual criticism, yet the author has found it to be invaluable on some occasions. The use of physical indicators such as floor burn through to indicate the presence of accelerants continues to be debated in court. Experts using this sort of evidence without the support of positive laboratory evidence are often heard resorting to hyperbole and analogy to support their case, which usually ends in indignation. The fact is, these techniques are solely used as aids to detect the presence of accelerants, and samples should be submitted to the laboratory for confirmation of the presence and identification of the accelerant.

The aim of this section is to discuss the properties of accelerants and to give an overview and evaluation of the various techniques which can be used to assist the investigator in sampling debris at the fire scene. As the topic is regularly debated at seminars, views opposite to those in this section will inevitably surface.

The Common Accelerants

The most commonly used accelerants are petrol, kerosene, mineral turps, and diesel. These accelerants are generally complex mixtures of hydrocarbon molecules. These hydrocarbons have similar chemical properties, however their boiling points vary and cover a wide range of values. This variation causes the accelerants to alter their composition during the evaporation process. The more volatile hydrocarbons evaporate at a faster rate leaving the heavier hydrocarbons in the debris and after a period of time the accelerant becomes less volatile and less abundant.

During the evaporation process, the headspace above the accelerant becomes concentrated with the more volatile hydrocarbons and so has a different composition than the accelerant left in the debris. It is this headspace which is tested by the various techniques to detect the presence of an accelerant amongst the debris.

Heavy accelerants such as diesel, or accelerant residues which are heavily evaporated will be difficult to detect as they provide little vapour in the headspace. Accelerants trapped under compacted soil and debris will also be difficult to detect so the debris must be disturbed or a very sensitive technique used. If the detection technique is too sensitive, then hydrocarbons from a material such as rubber backed carpet could be detected and wrongly interpreted as indicating the presence of an accelerant.

Most of the volatile hydrocarbons found in the headspace of the common accelerants are also found in the headspace above most burnt plastics and synthetics, but accelerant hydrocarbons are found in different ratios. A chromatographic fingerprint prepared in the laboratory must be used to determine if the hydrocarbons came from an accelerant.

The extraction technique used in the laboratory to prepare the sample for chromatographic analysis also relies on sampling and concentrating the headspace above the debris. During the extraction process it is important to recover as much of the heavier components of the accelerant as possible to avoid analytical discrimination. Extraction techniques such as purge and trap, which rely on a modified version of steam distillation give the least amount of discrimination.

Methylated spirits and acetone are also used as accelerants however they differ from the common accelerants as they are water soluble and composed of essentially a single compound. Being water soluble, they are frequently washed from the fire scene by the fire fighting operations. They are also common pyrolysis products so their presence in debris must be quantitatively assessed.

The techniques used for detecting accelerants are outlined below and discussed. The techniques are listed according to the author's opinion of their degree of usage and relative merit.

Physical Indicators

Physical indicators are listed first as they prove the accelerant was present at the time of the fire and was not placed there after the fire was extinguished. Investigators armed with even the most sophisticated hydrocarbon detector should not overlook the physical evidence.

Physical indicators used to detect the presence of accelerants are localised burn patterns to floors and surfaces and overhead damage inconsistent with the naturally available fuel. Reports from fire fighters or eyewitnesses of a rapid fire or of suspicious odours can also indicate the presence of an accelerant.

These physical indicators, if initially present, can often be destroyed during the course of the fire. If the roof or ceiling has collapsed, then evidence such as localised burn patterns on the floor can be concealed. The investigator should excavate the debris around doorways or in the centre of open spaces as these are areas where accelerants are normally used. If a wooden floor is involved, the investigator can hit the floor with a shovel and excavate the areas where the floor appears weakened.

Physical evidence which indicates a hot and intense fire such as a colour change or spalling in concrete, melted aluminium, and deformation of steel are unreliable indicators of the presence of an accelerant, as the temperature reached during the course of a fire is governed by the amount of both fuel and oxygen available. Many combustible materials tend to burn with the same intensity as accelerants, given an appropriate supply of oxygen.

Use of One's Sense of Smell

The human sense of smell can quite correctly identify the presence of accelerants, even in trace amounts. This ability varies amongst investigators as the sense of smell is like most other senses and can become highly developed through experience, or it can become impaired both temporarily or permanently.

When one smells fire debris, they are actually sampling the headspace above the debris and noting the chemical fingerprint of the headspace. Then using one's discriminatory powers by comparing the fingerprint with those stored in one's memory, a decision can be made as to the possible presence of an accelerant.

Wine tasters use a similar technique, and their highly developed sense of smell can detect extremely minute variations in the chemical fingerprint of a wine amongst a background of water and ethanol. The same test performed by scientific analysis and scientific interpretation requires a considerable amount of time and expertise.

The human sense of smell suffers from fatigue which causes a loss of sensitivity and also the ability to discriminate accelerant vapours. The vapours found at fire scenes may be harmful so debris should only be smelt when necessary. Continually smelling these toxic vapours will cause the smelling senses to become less effective. On cold still mornings when the sense of smell is quite sharp, accelerant odours can sometimes be smelt while the investigator is making his initial inspection of the fire scene. As the debris becomes disturbed during the course of the investigation, the sense of smell becomes less effective due to the contamination of the atmosphere.

If dangerous chemicals are known to be at the fire scene, it is imperative to avoid smelling debris. Residues from copper chrome arsenic treated logs, if inhaled, could cause serious health problems. All fire scenes have noxious gases and soot particles present which can lodge in the respiratory system and cause problems. Asbestos fibres and mineral fibres from insulation are also a problem. Because of these dangers, fire investigators should not examine a fire scene soon after the fire is extinguished. At this time the concentration of toxic vapours will be at a maximum and these vapours, if trapped in pockets under debris, could be released during the excavation. The investigation should ideally be made a day after the fire as by that time the scene will have cooled and the toxic vapours held in pockets will have dispersed.

Cartridge respirators should be worn whenever possible during fire scene excavations. These have been considered by some to be expensive and uncomfortable, but designs have improved in recent years and a good respirator can now be purchased for approximately $25 from most hardware stores.

Sniffers

Sniffers (or portable gas detectors) are best employed when toxic dust or vapours are present or if the investigator's sense of smell is impaired. They do not have the same discriminatory powers as the sense of smell as they respond to a wide variety of compounds in the headspace including nonaccelerant vapours.

A range of portable gas detectors is available on the market as industry has a need for these types of instruments to detect gas leaks, or flammable or toxic atmospheres. Various types of detection techniques are employed in sniffers and the price reflects the type of detector used in the instrument.

The cheapest type of sniffer uses a detector which measures changes in the oxygen concentration. These instruments lack specificity as they respond to all types of hydrocarbons and also gases such as ammonia, alcohols, carbon monoxide, carbon dioxide, and even water vapour. The advantages of using these instruments are they are small, cheap, and robust. The best instruments are those which have a control to vary the sensitivity of the instrument. They can be used very effectively if the operator is familiar with the instrument and aware of their shortcomings.

A more expensive sniffer employs a detector such as a flame ionisation (FID) or photo ionisation (PID) which will respond to hydrocarbons but not inorganic vapours. The instrument is extremely sensitive but cannot discriminate between hydrocarbons originating from accelerants or those from burnt plastics. Because of their high sensitivity, the investigator could easily misinterpret the results and could, for example, believe he is following an accelerant trail when in fact the investigator is simply following a trail where a synthetic carpet has become more severely burnt.

Sniffers do not respond to the quantity of accelerant present in the debris but to the quantity of accelerant present in the headspace above the debris. Therefore the debris needs to be disturbed before the sniffer probe is inserted amongst the debris. A large area of the fire scene can be scanned in a relatively short time by using techniques such as continuously lifting the debris with a shovel and inserting the sniffer probe under the shovel blade and noting the detector's response. Sniffers are invaluable when tracing the source of a gas leak.

Sniffer Dogs

Sniffer dogs are used for the detection of drugs, explosives, corpse location, termites, contraband food, and for tracking purposes. Dogs have a sense of smell which is much more sensitive than the human sense of smell. They also have much greater discriminatory powers and can therefore respond much more quickly to target scents. Their physical abilities and their desire to please their handlers enable dogs to thoroughly scan a large area at a fire scene in a relatively short time.

Dogs sample the headspace above the fire debris with their smelling senses and use their discriminatory powers to determine if the detected hydrocarbons originated from an accelerant. Their discriminatory powers are learnt through training. Training generally involves a series of exercises where the dog routinely retrieves a hidden toy or object which carries the target scent. Upon successfully retrieving the object, the dog is rewarded with affection or a favourite food. When the dog locates the target, the handler notes a change in the dog's behaviour and then calls the dog so the area is not disturbed.

Dogs need to be able to discriminate between accelerant vapours and vapours such as those originating from burnt plastics and paints. They must reliably perform this task amongst a background composed of thousands of different chemicals originating from burnt furniture and building materials. Dogs should therefore be trained and rated at fire scenes.

The effectiveness of sniffer dogs is entirely dependent on the level of training the dog has been given. Drug detection dogs, for instance, are trained to detect drugs when a masking agent such as curry powder or pepper has been used. Criminals in an attempt to avoid pursuit by tracking dogs have been known to place urine obtained from a bitch in heat across their escape route.

Sniffer dogs have only recently been used at fire scenes but I'm sure that given the correct training they will be the greatest advancement made in recent years in accelerant detection. The use of sniffer dogs at fire scenes where the damage is widespread, such as a furniture factory fire, would be extremely cost-effective as compared to using a forensic expert to dig out and inspect the entire scene.

Portable Gas Chromatographs

At a recent demonstration a portable gas chromatograph was used for accelerant analysis. The instrument was equipped with an FID detector and a small packed separation column. The instrument was versatile as it could be used as a sniffer where the air sample is introduced directly into the detector or as a chromatograph where the sample is introduced into the column for separation before reaching the detector and a chromatogram produced of the analysis.

The instrument was quite sensitive, however, the analytical column available at the time of testing was lacking in resolving power. Further developments in this area are being undertaken by the manufacturer. These developments could lead to the instrument being quite valuable to investigators as the instrument is capable of not only detecting hydrocarbons at trace levels, but can also discriminate whether these hydrocarbons originated from an accelerant or from a burnt plastic. The result obtained from the machine should be verified by laboratory analysis as the machine samples the headspace above the debris which can lead to discrimination.

Chemical Tests

Two types of hydrocarbon chemical tests have been used for accelerant detection. Draegar tubes are routinely used for detecting hydrocarbons in the atmosphere and hydrocarbon field test kits are used for soil and water analysis and both have been used at fire scenes.

Both tests rely on a colour change as a result of the hydrocarbon reacting with a developing agent. They are generally used for the quantitative analysis of hydrocarbons and cannot discriminate between hydrocarbons originating from accelerants or those originating from burnt plastics. Both techniques are expensive to use and can only be used for a single analysis.

Conclusion

Of the techniques discussed above, the sniffer and the chemical tests cannot discriminate between hydrocarbons emanating from accelerants or those emanating from materials such as burnt plastics. The human sense of smell, the sniffer dog, and the portable gas chromatograph have this discriminating ability.

Regardless of the technique used to detect the presence of an accelerant, the findings must be verified by the available physical evidence and by laboratory tests.

Notes

1. John D. Dehaan, *Kirk's Fire Investigation,* 2nd ed. (John Wiley, 1983).

2. Roy A. Cooke and Rodger Fl. Ide, *Principles of Fire Investigation* (The Institution of Fire Engineers, 1985).

Chapter 11

The Corpse

(Note: Authorization for all the principles stated below can be found in the Medical Examiner/Coroner Official Office Policy Manual; State or Federal Statutory Authority.)

Documenting and Evaluating the Body

Photograph the Body

The photographic documentation of the body at the scene [of death] creates a permanent record that preserves essential details of the body position, appearance, identity, and final movements. Photographs allow sharing of information with other agencies investigating the death.

Upon arrival at the scene, and prior to moving the body or evidence, the investigator should:

- Photograph the body and immediate scene (including the decedent as initially found).

- Photograph the decedent's face.

Excerpted from the NIJ Research Report (NCJ No. 167568), "National Guidelines for Death Investigation," December 1997. Produced by the National Medicolegal Review Panel; Executive Director, Steven C. Clark, Ph.D. This project was cosponsored by the CDC (Centers for Disease Control and Prevention) and the Bureau of Justice Assistance. For complete contact information, please refer to Chapter 56, "Resources."

- Take additional photographs after removal of objects/items that interfere with photographic documentation of the decedent (e.g., body removed from car).

- Photograph the decedent with and without measurements (as appropriate).

- Photograph the surface beneath the body (after the body has been removed, as appropriate).

Note: Never clean face, do not change condition. Take multiple shots if possible.

Summary. The photographic documentation of the body at the scene provides for documentation of the body position, identity, and appearance. The details of the body at the scene provide investigators with pertinent information of the terminal events.

Conduct External Body Examination (Superficial)

Conducting the external body examination provides the investigator with objective data regarding the single most important piece of evidence at the scene, the body. This documentation provides detailed information regarding the decedent's physical attributes, his/her relationship to the scene, and possible cause, manner, and circumstances of death.

After arrival at the scene and prior to moving the decedent, the investigator should, without removing decedent's clothing:

- Document the decedent's physical characteristics.

- Document the presence or absence of clothing and personal effects.

- Document the presence or absence of any items/objects that may be relevant.

- Document the presence or absence of marks, scars, and tattoos.

- Document the presence or absence of injury/trauma, petechiae, etc.

- Document the presence of treatment or resuscitative efforts.

- Based on the findings, determine the need for further evaluation/assistance of forensic specialists (e.g., pathologists, odontologists).

Summary. Thorough evaluation and documentation (photographic and written) of the deceased at the scene is essential to determine the depth and direction the investigation will take.

Preserve Evidence (on Body)

The photographic and written documentation of evidence on the body allows the investigator to obtain a permanent historical record of that evidence. To maintain chain of custody, evidence must be collected, preserved, and transported properly. In addition to all of the physical evidence visible on the body, blood and other body fluids present must be photographed and documented prior to collection and transport. Fragile evidence (that which can be easily contaminated, lost, or altered) must also be collected and/or preserved to maintain chain of custody and to assist in determination of cause, manner, and circumstances of death.

Once evidence on the body is recognized, the investigator should:

- Photograph the evidence.
- Document blood/body fluid on the body (froth/purge, substances from orifices), location, and pattern before transporting.
- Place decedent's hands and/or feet in unused paper bags (as determined by the scene).
- Collect trace evidence before transporting the body (e.g., blood, hair, fibers, etc.).
- Arrange for the collection and transport of evidence at the scene (when necessary).
- Ensure the proper collection of blood and body fluids for subsequent analysis (if body will be released from scene to an outside agency without an autopsy).

Summary. It is essential that evidence be collected, preserved, transported, and documented in an orderly and proper fashion to ensure the chain of custody and admissibility in a legal action. The preservation and documentation of the evidence on the body must be initiated by the investigator at the scene to prevent alterations or contamination.

Establish Decedent Identification

The establishment or confirmation of the decedent's identity is paramount to the death investigation. Proper identification allows notification of next of kin, settlement of estates, resolution of criminal and civil litigation, and the proper completion of the death certificate.

To establish identity, the investigator should document use of the following methods:

- Direct visual or photographic identification of the decedent if visually recognizable.

- Scientific methods such as fingerprints, dental, radiographic, and DNA comparisons.

- Circumstantial methods such as (but not restricted to) personal effects, circumstances, physical characteristics, tattoos, and anthropologic data.

Summary. There are several methods available that can be used to properly identify deceased persons. This is essential for investigative, judicial, family, and vital records issues.

Document Postmortem Changes

The documenting of postmortem changes to the body assists the investigator in explaining body appearance in the interval following death. Inconsistencies between postmortem changes and body location may indicate movement of body and validate or invalidate witness statements. In addition, postmortem changes to the body, when correlated with circumstantial information, can assist the investigators in estimating the approximate time of death.

Upon arrival at the scene and prior to moving the body, the investigator should note the presence of each of the following in his/her report:

- Livor (color, location, blanchability, Tardieu spots) consistent/inconsistent with position of the body.

- Rigor (stage/intensity, location on the body, broken, inconsistent with the scene).

- Degree of decomposition (putrefaction, adipocere, mummification, skeletonization, as appropriate).

- Insect and animal activity.

- Scene temperature (document method used and time estimated).

- Description of body temperature (e.g., warm, cold, frozen) or measurement of body temperature (document method used and time of measurement).

Summary. Documentation of post mortem changes in every report is essential to determine an accurate cause and manner of death, provide information as to the time of death, corroborate witness statements, and indicate that the body may have been moved after death.

Participate in Scene Debriefing

The scene debriefing helps investigators from all participating agencies to establish post-scene responsibilities by sharing data regarding particular scene findings. The scene debriefing provides each agency the opportunity for input regarding special requests for assistance, additional information, special examinations, and other requests requiring interagency communication, cooperation, and education.

When participating in scene debriefing, the investigator should:

- Determine post-scene responsibilities (identification, notification, press relations, and evidence transportation).
- Determine/identify the need for a specialist (e.g., crime laboratory technicians, social services, entomologists, OSHA).
- Communicate with the pathologist about responding to the scene or to the autopsy schedule (as needed).
- Share investigative data (as required in furtherance of the investigation).
- Communicate special requests to appropriate agencies, being mindful of the necessity for confidentiality.

Summary. The scene debriefing is the best opportunity for investigative participants to communicate special requests and confirm all current and additional scene responsibilities. The debriefing allows participants the opportunity to establish clear lines of responsibility for a successful investigation.

Determine Notification Procedures (Next of Kin)

Every reasonable effort should be made to notify the next of kin as soon as possible. Notification of next of kin initiates closure for the family, disposition of remains, and facilitates the collection of additional information relative to the case.

When determining notification procedures, the investigator should:

- Identify next of kin (determine who will perform task).

- Locate next of kin (determine who will perform task).

- Notify next of kin (assign person(s) to perform task) and record time of notification, or, if delegated to another agency, gain confirmation when notification is made.

- Notify concerned agencies of status of the notification.

Summary. The investigator is responsible for ensuring that the next of kin is identified, located, and notified in a timely manner. The time and method of notification should be documented. Failure to locate next of kin and efforts to do so should be a matter of record. This ensures that every reasonable effort has been made to contact the family.

Ensure Security of Remains

Ensuring security of the body requires the investigator to supervise the labeling, packaging, and removal of the remains. An appropriate identification tag is placed on the body to preclude misidentification upon receipt at the examining agency. This function also includes safeguarding all potential physical evidence and/or property and clothing that remain on the body.

Prior to leaving the scene, the investigator should:

- Ensure that the body is protected from further trauma or contamination (if not, document) and unauthorized removal of therapeutic and resuscitative equipment.

- Inventory and secure property, clothing, and personal effects that are on the body (remove in a controlled environment with witness present).

- Identify property and clothing to be retained as evidence (in a controlled environment).

- Recover blood and/or vitreous samples prior to release of remains.

- Place identification on the body and body bag.

- Ensure/supervise the placement of the body into the bag.

- Ensure/supervise the removal of the body from the scene.

- Secure transportation.

Summary. Ensuring the security of the remains facilitates proper identification of the remains, maintains a proper chain of custody, and safeguards property and evidence.

Establishing and Recording Decedent Profile Information

Document the Discovery History

Establishing a decedent profile includes documenting a discovery history and circumstances surrounding the discovery. The basic profile will dictate subsequent levels of investigation, jurisdiction, and authority. The focus (breadth/depth) of further investigation is dependent on this information.

For an investigator to correctly document the discovery history, he/she should:

- Establish and record person(s) who discovered the body and when.

- Document the circumstances surrounding the discovery (who, what, where, when, how).

Summary. The investigator must produce clear, concise, documented information concerning who discovered the body, what are the circumstances of discovery, where the discovery occurred, when the discovery was made, and how the discovery was made.

Determine Terminal Episode History

Pre-terminal circumstances play a significant role in determining cause and manner of death. Documentation of medical intervention and/or procurement of antemortem specimens help to establish the decedent's condition prior to death.

In order for the investigator to determine terminal episode history, he/she should:

- Document when, where, how, and by whom decedent was last known to be alive.

- Document the incidents prior to the death.

- Document complaints/symptoms prior to the death.

- Document and review complete EMS [Emergency Medical Services] records (including the initial electrocardiogram).

- Obtain relevant medical records (copies).

- Obtain relevant antemortem specimens.

Summary. Obtaining records of pre-terminal circumstances and medical history distinguishes medical treatment from trauma. This history and relevant antemortem specimens assist the medical examiner/coroner in determining cause and manner of death.

Document Decedent Medical History

The majority of deaths referred to the medical examiner/coroner are natural deaths. Establishing the decedent's medical history helps to focus the investigation. Documenting the decedent's medical signs or symptoms prior to death determines the need for subsequent examinations. The relationship between disease and injury may play a role in the cause, manner, and circumstances of death.

Through interviews and review of the written records, the investigator should:

- Document medical history, including medications taken, alcohol and drug use, and family medical history from family members and witnesses.

- Document information from treating physicians and/or hospitals to confirm history and treatment.

- Document physical characteristics and traits (e.g., left-/right-handedness, missing appendages, tattoos, etc.).

Summary. Obtaining a thorough medical history focuses the investigation, aids in disposition of the case, and helps determine the need for a postmortem examination or other laboratory tests or studies.

Document Decedent Mental Health History

The decedent's mental health history can provide insight into the behavior/state of mind of the individual. That insight may produce clues that will aid in establishing the cause, manner, and circumstances of the death.

The investigator should:

- Document the decedent's mental health history, including hospitalizations and medications.

- Document the history of suicidal ideations, gestures, and/or attempts.

- Document mental health professionals (e.g., psychiatrists, psychologists, counselors, etc.) who treated the decedent.

- Document family mental health history.

Summary. Knowledge of the mental health history allows the investigator to evaluate properly the decedent's state of mind and contributes to the determination of cause, manner, and circumstances of death.

Document Social History

Social history includes marital, family, sexual, educational, employment, and financial information. Daily routines, habits and activities, and friends and associates of the decedent help in developing the decedent's profile. This information will aid in establishing the cause, manner, and circumstances of death.

When collecting relevant social history information, the investigator should:

- Document marital/domestic history.

- Document family history (similar deaths, significant dates).

- Document sexual history.

- Document employment history.

- Document financial history.

- Document daily routines, habits, and activities.

- Document relationships, friends, and associates.

- Document religious, ethnic, or other pertinent information (e.g., religious objection to autopsy).

- Document educational background.

- Document criminal history.

Summary. Information from sources familiar with the decedent pertaining to the decedent's social history assists in determining cause, manner, and circumstances of death.

Completing the Scene Investigation

Maintain Jurisdiction over the Body

Maintaining jurisdiction over the body allows the investigator to protect the chain of custody as the body is transported from the scene for autopsy, specimen collection, or storage.

When maintaining jurisdiction over the body, the investigator should:

- Arrange for, and document, secure transportation of the body to a medical or autopsy facility for further examination or storage.

- Coordinate and document procedures to be performed when the body is received at the facility.

Summary. By providing documented secure transportation of the body from the scene to an authorized receiving facility, the investigator maintains jurisdiction and protects chain of custody of the body.

Release Jurisdiction of the Body

Prior to releasing jurisdiction of the body to an authorized receiving agent or funeral director, it is necessary to determine the person responsible for certification of the death. Information to complete the death certificate includes demographic information and the date, time, and location of death.

When releasing jurisdiction over the body, the investigator should:

- Determine who will sign the death certificate (name, agency, etc.).

- Confirm the date, time, and location of death.

- Collect, when appropriate, blood, vitreous fluid, and other evidence prior to release of the body from the scene.

- Document and arrange with the authorized receiving agent to reconcile all death certificate information.

- Release the body to a funeral director or other authorized receiving agent.

Summary. The investigator releases jurisdiction only after determining who will sign the death certificate; documenting the date, time, and location of death; collecting appropriate specimens; and releasing the body to the funeral director or other authorized receiving agent.

Perform Exit Procedures

Bringing closure to the scene investigation ensures that important evidence has been collected and the scene has been processed. In addition, a systematic review of the scene ensures that artifacts or equipment are not inadvertently left behind (e.g., used disposable gloves, paramedical debris, film wrappers, etc.), and any dangerous materials or conditions have been reported.

When performing exit procedures, the investigator should:

- Identify, inventory, and remove all evidence collected at the scene.

- Remove all personal equipment and materials from the scene.

- Report and document any dangerous materials or conditions.

Summary. Conducting a scene "walk-through" upon exit ensures that all evidence has been collected, that materials are not inadvertently left behind, and that any dangerous materials or conditions have been reported to the proper entities.

Assist the Family

The investigator provides the family with a timetable so they can arrange for final disposition and provides information on available community and professional resources that may assist the family.

When the investigator is assisting the family, it is important to:

- Inform the family if an autopsy is required.
- Inform the family of available support services (e.g., victim assistance, police, social services, etc.).
- Inform the family of appropriate agencies to contact with questions (medical examiner/coroner offices, law enforcement, SIDS support group, etc.).
- Ensure family is not left alone with body (if circumstances warrant).
- Inform the family of approximate body release timetable.
- Inform the family of information release timetable (toxicology, autopsy results, etc., as required).
- Inform the family of available reports, including cost, if any.

Summary. The interaction with the family allows the investigator to assist and direct them to appropriate resources. It is essential that families be given a timetable of events so that they can make necessary arrangements. In addition, the investigator needs to make them aware of what and when information will be available.

Chapter 12

Rapid Anoxial Deaths ('Asphyxia')

Introduction

The expression 'rapid anoxial death' is probably new to you although the term 'asphyxia' is readily understood. The reason for the preference of rapid anoxia to that of asphyxia is that not all cases of rapid anoxial death show the pathological features of asphyxia.

Anoxia means lack of oxygen. This lack of oxygen can develop rapidly or over a period of time. The slow and progressive development of anoxia is seen in a variety of diseases—diseases mainly of the heart and lungs. Heart failure of various types, progressive lung disease (e.g., emphysema, chronic bronchitis, cancer, and some industrial diseases) and chronic or long-standing anemia all have the same effect. These cases are rarely of medicolegal importance. However, the lack of oxygen coming on rapidly has great medicolegal significance and these are properly referred to as 'rapid anoxial deaths.'

A clear understanding of rapid anoxial death can only be achieved by understanding the mechanism of breathing. If the flow of oxygen from the atmosphere to the tissues is interrupted suddenly at any stage of its pathway, then we have the makings of a rapid anoxial death. It is possible to classify rapid anoxial deaths on the basis of

From "Rapid Anoxial Deaths ('Asphyxia')," [Online] undated. Available: http://www.erin.utoronto.ca/academic/FSC/FSC239Y_STRANGULATION.htm. Produced by Michael S. Pollanen, Ph.D., Forensic Pathology Unit, Office of the Chief Coroner, 26 Grenville St., Toronto, ON M7A 2G9 Canada. For complete contact information, please refer to Chapter 56, "Resources." Reprinted with permission.

the mechanism causing the lack of oxygen. In addition, it is essential that we all use the correct terms in order that we all know what the other is talking about. These terms are based upon the definitions and mechanics of the various causes of rapid anoxial death.

Classification of Rapid Anoxial Deaths

1. Atmosphere suddenly becomes deficient in oxygen.

2. Obstruction of nose and mouth, (e.g., suffocation).

3. Obstruction of the larger air passages, (e.g., choking).

4. Obstruction to air passages by pressure on neck, (e.g., strangulation, hanging).

5. Compression of chest, (e.g., traumatic asphyxia).

6. Positional restriction of breathing (e.g., positional asphyxia).

7. Inability of blood to carry oxygen to tissues, (e.g., carbon monoxide poisoning).

8. Inability of tissues to use oxygen, (e.g., cyanide poisoning).

9. Inhalation of fluids into air passages, (e.g., drowning).

Although all these cases come into the category of rapid anoxial death, some are more rapid than others. Death or unconsciousness may occur in as few as seven seconds or take as long as a few minutes. However, the findings at the scene and at autopsy are to some extent related to the speed of onset of unconsciousness or death.

In very rapid deaths, the oxygen supply to the body (brain) is cut off and the 'victim' immediately becomes quiet and possibly pale and passes into unconsciousness followed by death. Thus at the scene, the body, unless otherwise disturbed, is found where the incident occurred and there is not likely to be any evidence of a disturbance. However, in the more slowly progressing rapid anoxial deaths, the situation is different. Once anoxia has been started, the victim struggles for breath, his face turns blue and becomes congested. He then passes into a stage of convulsions during which

1. He may cause great disturbance at the scene.

2. The features looked upon as being typical of 'asphyxia' develop on and in the body, e.g., bluish-black congestion of the face, pin-point hemorrhages (petechial) over the whites of the

eyes and about the forehead and cheeks, and internally as petechiae over the surfaces of the heart and lungs and dark fluid blood. Because these so-called classical features of asphyxia are not present in all cases of rapid anoxial deaths, the latter term is preferable to that of asphyxia.

Classes of Rapid Anoxial Deaths of Medicolegal Importance

Suffocation

Definition: Obstruction of the nose and mouth and as such can be divided into accidental, suicidal and homicidal origin.

1. Accidental

   - Infants: overlaying; deaths (not SIDS)—mattress, pillow, or plastic bags over face.

   - Adults: variants of autoerotic deaths.

2. Suicidal

   - Impervious material/wet material wrapped around face occluding nose and mouth.

   - Plastic bag: over face in drug overdose.

3. Homicidal

   - Victims: the old, enfeebled, or intoxicated; infants.

   - Methods: handkerchief—gagging; wet material over head; hands over mouth and nose; (if with chest compression—'burking'); pillow, palm of hand.

Suffocation is relatively slow anoxia—therefore, will usually show the classical signs of asphyxia.

In the case of homicide—fingernail marks and scratches may be found around nose and mouth together with other injuries consistent with a struggle. In the same cases, the lips may be dry and parchment-like due to postmortem drying of abrasions.

Choking

Definition: Airway obstruction by a foreign object.

1. Accidental: witnessed choking on food ('cafe coronary').

2. Homicidal: usually gagging or forceful insertion of foreign object in mouth which is usually a cloth pushed into back of throat.

Strangulation

There are two classical types of strangulation:

1. manual—use of hands;

2. ligature—use of ligature.

Manual Strangulation (throttling): always homicidal. The forceful application of one or both hands to the neck causing compression of the neck structures.

External Examination of Throttling

Neck. Marks on the neck from the fingernails or tips of the fingers may be present or absent—much more frequently they are present to varying degrees. These marks may take the form of classical curved or crescent shaped abrasions or superficial splits of the skin. In most cases these fingernail marks are not so clearly defined and present as a few or many scratches over the front of the neck. The number and distribution of such marks is often related to the use of one or both hands, from the front or the back of the neck. The thumb usually exerts more pressure than the fingers and so marks due to the thumb are more pronounced. If, as happens often, there is a struggle, the grip on the neck is likely to be relaxed and reapplied—sometimes many times. This increases the number of the marks on the neck and often involves a large surface area of the neck skin.

In addition to these scratch marks, there may be small, roughly circular bruises of the skin of the neck due to pressure of the tips of the fingers.

Head. As a part of the asphyxial process there is usually

1. petechial hemorrhages in the whites of the eyes, over the cheeks and forehead;

2. cyanosis or deep blue congestion of the face and neck above the compressed area of the neck;

3. the tongue may protrude, and the eyeballs may bulge;

4. bloody mucus may be present between the lips.

Remainder of Body. Examination may show

1. other injuries suggestive of a struggle;
2. bite marks on neck or breasts in throttling associated with sexual assaults;
3. evidence of rape.

Internal Examination of Throttling

1. Fracture of the hyoid bone—at the tip or base of the cornu with local hemorrhage at the fracture site. Occasionally the larynx is fractured.
2. Bruises in the 'strap' muscles of the neck, hemorrhages at the base of the tongue, in the epiglottis, and in the mucosa of the larynx.
3. The internal features of asphyxia (such as petechiae, fluidity of blood, empty blood).

Strangulation by Ligature

This is compression of the neck by a ligature, the pressure being exerted directly by the hands usually of another person.

As opposed to manual strangulation, strangulation by ligature can be very occasionally accidental or rarely suicidal, but of course, is almost universally homicidal.

The Features of Homicidal Ligature Strangulation

Ligature mark: A pressure mark on the neck is usually present—depending upon ligature material used. This mark is usually horizontally placed around the neck, at a level of the thyroid prominence or below and is complete (i.e., it extends around the entire circumference of the neck). If a knot has been tied, this often leaves an area of abrasion and depression beneath it. The ligature mark varies in width according to the material used, may reveal a pattern corresponding to the weave of the ligature material and is usually depressed, yellowish in colour and 'dry' like parchment with reddish edges.

Other features: petechial hemorrhages—face and eyes; cyanosis of face and neck above ligature; protrusion of tongue and bulging of eyes;

hemorrhage in mastoid air cells; other injuries associated with assault, rape, or other sexual assaults.

The internal findings are similar to those of manual strangulation except that

1. the hyoid bone is not usually fractured;

2. the distribution of bruising of the neck tissues (if present) follows the line of the ligature.

Hanging

Definition: Compression of the neck by a ligature, the compressive force being exerted by the weight of the body in a gravitational field. The features of hanging are

1. A ligature mark around the neck which is

    *   usually incomplete—where the weight of the body pulls the knot away from the neck nearest to the point of suspension;

    *   situated between the larynx and the hyoid bone, i.e., well above that seen in strangulation by ligature;

    *   the mark can vary from almost complete totally around the neck to a mere few inches at the front depending upon position and degree of suspension;

    *   the mark is depressed, pale, parchment-like, and may reproduce the weave or pattern of the ligature used;

    *   at least one component of the ligature (or its furrow) rises on the side of the neck.

2. Postmortem lividity is found in the forearms, hands, legs below the knees, and the feet unless [the corpse is]cut down soon after death. If [the corpse is] suspended for more than 3-4 hours—lividity is well marked and may show large hemorrhages into its substance due to bursting of blood vessels after death by the effects of gravity (Tardieu's spots).

Manner of Death in Hanging

1. Accidental (children; autoerotic hanging)

2. Suicidal (common)

3. Homicidal (very rare)

Traumatic Asphyxia

Definition: The acute compression and immobilization of the chest resulting in rapid anoxia, due to the instability of breath (e.g., crown disasters, industrial accidents with cave-in of earth).

A recently recognized variant is positional asphyxia in which the body's position restricts respiration.

Carbon Monoxide Poisoning

Mechanism: Oxygen is carried by hemoglobin in red blood cells from lungs to tissues where oxygen is given up to the cells—the whole reason for breathing.

Hemoglobin: HB has 300 times the liking or affinity for carbon monoxide than it has for oxygen. Therefore it takes it up in preference to oxygen depriving tissues of oxygen. [The result is] rapid anoxial death.

Manner of Death

1. Accidental: incomplete combustion of carbon fires or smoke; car exhausts; or mine accidents.

2. Suicide: exhaust fumes.

3. Homicide: rare, usually murder-suicide pact.

Postmortem Findings in CO Toxicity

Lividity is cherry pink in colour.

Cyanide Poisoning (Rare)

Mechanism: CN binds to cytochromes inhibiting oxidative phosphorylation in mitochondria.

Drowning

A separate topic of study.

> —*by Michael S. Pollanen, Ph.D., Forensic Pathology Unit,*
> *Office of the Chief Coroner of Ontario, Canada.*

Chapter 13

Age Determination from Skeletal Remains

The determination of age relies on the assessment of the physiological age of the skeleton, as opposed to the chronological age of the individual. The physiological age is based upon relative growth patterns, and is hoped to give an accurate estimate of chronological age, but environmental, nutritional, and disease stresses often cause changes in the skeleton which will mask the true age of the individual. In addition, the accuracy with which age can be estimated varies inversely with the age of the individual at death. In younger years, with age being estimated primarily upon observed developmental changes, more precise estimates are possible, whereas in older individuals, age estimates are more often accomplished via the observation of degenerative changes, which offer less accuracy.

Age determination can be accomplished through many means, and a holistic analysis of all possible age-related attributes is best for an overall estimate. Some of the more typically utilized attributes include:

1. Dental Eruption and Occlusion
2. Cortical Bone Histology
3. Cranial Suture Closures

From "The Determination of the Age of the Individual from Skeletal Remains," [Online] 1994. Available: http://www.doitnow.com/~cerci/agelect.htm. Produced by John A. Giacobbe, Stantec Consulting, Inc., 1440 W. Lobster Trap Dr., Gilbert, AZ 85233. For complete contact information, please refer to Chapter 56, "Resources." Reprinted with permission.

4. Postcranial Epiphysial Unions

5. Pubic Symphysial Face Morphology

6. Age-Related Degenerative Conditions

7. Phase Changes in the Sternal Rib

8. Potpourri

Dental Eruption and Occlusion

Age estimates are based on the age of eruption of the deciduous and permanent dentition. This method is useful in age estimates of up to about 15 years. The third molar (wisdom tooth) erupts after this time, but is so variable in age of eruption, if it erupts at all, that it is not a very reliable age indicator. (See Bass, pp. 289-90 for an illustration of Ubelaker's eruptive phases, noting the standard deviations.) Occlusal wear has also been offered as an indicator of age, but this has been shown to be highly inaccurate, especially in archaeological context, where high-grit content diets (such as from the use of natural stone mano and metate) can wear down the occlusal surface of the tooth by the end of puberty (Bass, pp. 286-7).

Cortical Bone Histology

Kerley (1984) developed a system of aging based on osteon counts taken from midshaft long bone sections. This process involves counting the number of whole osteons and osteon fragments (which increase in number with age), and nonhaversian canals and the percentage of circumferential lamellar bone in the cortex (which decreases with age, completely disappearing around age fifty). These estimates are taken from the outer one third on the cortex, with a normal light microscope in four fields at 100X. A percentage estimate is calculated, and what is sought after is the rate of osteon turnover or replacement. These percentages are plugged into either a regression formula or a precalculated age/profile chart. Kerley has obtained a reliability of almost 90% with a standard deviation of +/- 5 years, with the best correlation coming from the fibula, then the femur and the tibia.

Cranial Suture Closures

This method bases age upon the degree of closure, union, or ossification of the cranial sutures. These methods have until recently been considered inaccurate, but Meindl and Lovejoy (1985) have introduced new evidence to indicate parietal ectocranial sutures are reliable indicators of age over 40 years. In addition, Mann, et al., (1987) have offered the four maxillary sutures and their rates of closure as reliable age estimators (Bass, pp. 47-8).

Postcranial Epiphysial Unions

Endochondral bones of the postcranium form via the union and ossification of cartilaginous bridges between growing bones. This process can be seen to occur along a growth algorithm, and can be used to estimate age at death. Bass (1987) lists some of these locations of epiphysial union, as well as the approximate age ranges for which these unions occur. This data can be used on a union/non-union basis, and McKern and Stewart have defined five grades of epiphysial union: unobservable (0), beginning (1), active (2), recent (3), and complete (4), and these offer a possibly more accurate estimate of age.

Pubic Symphysial Face Morphology

The pubic symphysial face in the young is characterized by an undulating surface, such as the crenulated surface of a typical nonfused epiphysial plate. This surface undergoes a regular progressive metamorphosis from age 18 onwards.

Age-Related Degenerative Changes in Skeletal Features

Many nonpathogenic conditions such as certain expressions of arthritis and osteoporosis become more prevalent and pronounced in old age, and can be used to give corroborative evidence in the determination of age. These occurrences are not entirely reliable in themselves, however, as injury and pathological expressions of these conditions can mimic the degenerative condition. An illustrative case can be seen in the osteophytic growths of the vertebral body (via osteoarthritis). These growths form on the outer margins of the centra, and Stewart (1958) has computed an age progression histogram for humans over 21 years based on the percentage of extra-central lipping as a function of age for the lumbar and thoracic vertebra (Bass, pp. 20-1).

Phase Changes in the Sternal Ribs

M. Y. Iscan and Susan Loth have developed a system of age estimation based on sequential changes at the sternal end of the fourth rib. These changes are similar to those that occur on the pubic symphysial face. They are of a specific morphological nature and occur on the costochondral joint between the rib and sternum. They consider that these phases are not as subject to variation due to sex, pregnancy and activity patterns as is the pubic symphysial face. See Bass, pp. 135-142 for photos of Iscan and Loth's phases, with the general progression illustrated as an increase in the depth of the articular depression and the degenerative fragmentation, thinning and increased porosity at the edges of the articular surface over time.

Potpourri

- Note that generally females are more advanced than males with regard to physiological age, being about two years advanced at puberty, five years at maturity, and seven to ten years in old age.

- The sacroiliac joint undergoes changes in morphology similar to those at the pubic symphysis, Lovejoy et al. (1985) offers a phase system based on these morphological changes.

- W. M. Krogman (1949) offers a system of aging based on transillumination through the scapular body to chart the occurrence and amount of atrophic (thinning) centers, basically, the more that are present, the older the individual.

- Various radiographic analysis techniques focus on age related changes to interior bone structures, such as at the costochondral juncture, the metaphysial plates of the long bones, and Walker and Lovejoy's (1985) radiographic analysis of trabecular bone involution in the clavicle.

- Bass (1987) and Ubelaker (1989) offer age estimates based on long bone lengths, but these have a wide range of variation even within a single relatively homogenous population.

References

Bass, William M. *Human Osteology: A Laboratory and Field Manual*, 3rd ed., Special Publication No. 2. Columbia, MO.: Missouri Archaeological Society, 1987.

Kerley, Ellis R. "Microscopic Aging of Human Bone." Chap. 21 in *Human Identification: Case Studies in Forensic Anthropology*, edited by T. A. Rathbun and J. E. Buikstra. Springfield, IL.: Charles C. Thomas Company, 1984.

Mann, R. W., S. A. Symes, and W. M. Bass. "Maxillary Suture Obliteration: Aging the Human Skeleton Based on Intact or Fragmentary Maxilla." *Journal of Fosensic Sciences* 32: 148-57, 1987.

McKern, T. W., and T. D. Stewart. *Skeletal Age Changes in Young American Males, Technical Report EP-45.* Natick, MA: U.S. Army Quartermaster Research and Development Center, 1957.

Meindl, Richard S., and C. Owen Lovejoy. "Ectocranial Suture Closure: A Revised Method for the Determination of Skeletal Age at Death Based on the Lateral-Anterior Sutures." *American Journal of Physical Anthropology* 86: 57-66, 1985.

Ubelaker, Douglas H. *Human Skeletal Remains: Excavation, Analysis, Interpretation.* Washington, D.C.: Taraxacum, 1989.

Walker, Robert A., and C. Owen Lovejoy. "Radiographic Changes in the Clavicle and Proximal Femur and Their Use in the Determination of Skeletal Age at Death." *American Journal of Physical Anthropology* 68: 67-78, 1985.

—*by John A. Giacobbe*

Chapter 14

Analytical Tools

Forensic chemistry deals with trace evidence; when two objects come into contact, be it a person and a car or bicycle, or a broken window, there is a transfer of materials between the two objects. Examples of trace evidence include paint, glass, fire accelerants, and soil.

Thus the broad range of trace evidence that a forensic chemist may be asked to examine requires familiarity with various analytical techniques. The instrumentation available ranges from the very simple tools to modern computer-controlled analytical instruments.

Microscope

The microscope is the basic tool for examining and finding trace evidence. The first comparison between a questioned sample and known sample is visual (microscopic), followed thereafter by chemical analyses. In some instances, a microscopic examination is all that is necessary.

The stereomicroscope is the most common microscope used in a forensic laboratory. Specialized microscopes such as the polarizing microscope is used to identify the polarizing properties of materials.

From "Overview of Instrumental Analysis (Chemistry)," [Online] November 6, 1997. Available: http://www.erin.utoronto.ca/library/reserve/notes/FSC/ FSC239Y/nov6.html. Produced by Karen L. Kwek, Forensic Chemist, Centre of Forensic Sciences, University of Toronto at Mississauga, 3359 Mississauga Rd., Mississauga, ON, Canada L5L 1C6. Reprinted with permission.

Scanning Electron Microscope/Energy Dispersive X-Ray (SEM/EDX)

Trace metal analysis for barium, lead, and antimony (in any combination) is an established procedure for gunshot residue (GSR) analysis. SEM/EDX is the technique employed for the detection and identification of GSR particles formed by the condensation of vapourized bullet and primer materials. The particles possess a characteristic spheroidal shape and a unique composition.

SEM utilizes a focused beam of electrons in an evacuated sample chamber to image samples of material (magnification range from 5X to 100,000X). The SEM has the advantage of producing images with great depth of field which allows one to examine surface morphology. The EDX is an X-ray detector system which analyses X-rays generated by the electron imaging beam in the SEM. The X-rays produced are characteristic of the elements present in the analysed sample.

X-Ray Diffraction (XRD)

Unlike most other techniques that allow only the analysis of elemental composition, XRD gives the identification of the sample based on its crystal structure which allows conclusive identification of compounds. The technique is used for both inorganic and organic analysis, the requirement being that the sample contains crystalline compounds.

This application is based upon the fact that an X-ray diffraction pattern is unique for each crystalline substance. The technique relies on the establishment of a database or the availability of an authentic comparison sample. There are commercial databases available, and computerized search routines are used.

Fourier Transform Infrared (FTIR)

The theory of infrared spectroscopy is based upon differential absorption of infrared radiation by different molecules. A graph of energy absorbed versus frequency is the absorption spectrum of the sample. The spectrum is characteristic of the particular molecule and its molecular motions.

The main drawback to forensic applications was the sample size requirements, however, with an FTIR and the adaptation of various accessories (for example a microscope), this technique is used by the forensic chemist. It finds application in the analysis of

- polymers, including paint and fibres in trace analysis
- explosive substances such as nitrocellulose and nitroglycerine
- lacrimators
- unknown organic compounds encountered in sexual assault and homicide cases.

Glass Refractive Index Measurement (GRIM)

Measurement of the refractive index of glass is the only routine physical measurement (other than size measurements) done in our forensic chemistry laboratory. It is a measure of how light bends as it passes through the glass, and is dependent upon the chemical composition and thermal history of the glass.

Preliminary examination of glass samples includes a surface examination, measurement of thickness, and colour description.

Gas Chromatography

This technique is widely used in many diverse applications of forensic science in both Chemistry and Toxicology. Gas chromatography is essentially a separation technique which allows the separation of the components of a mixture of organic chemicals. The instrumentation consists of

- an injector to allow the introduction of the sample
- a column which has properties to enable the separation of the components of the mixture
- an oven over which a microprocessor allows precise temperature control
- a detector to allow a visual display of the separated chemicals.

Since the separation process can be very well controlled, a relationship can be established between the time that a component is retained in an instrument and its identity by comparison to standards; this is called the retention time. While this relationship is not sufficient for the unequivocal identification of a single component, as you might require in the analysis of drugs or their metabolites, the fortuitous match of retention times for multiple components of a mixture is unlikely; therefore, the technique can produce a fingerprint identification of things such as petroleum products and paint pyrograms.

121

A number of detectors have been developed to sense the components as they emerge from the chromatograph in order to display the results in a graphical manner. If the detector adds specificity, this may contribute to the likelihood of an identification.

In chemistry, the main detector remains the flame ionization detector which tends to be universal and particularly good for petroleum products.

GC/Mass Spectrometry (GC/MS) has become the instrument of choice for the detection of drugs since it has very high sensitivity and gives the identification of the compound from its mass spectral fragmentation pattern. In addition, it can be used to scan a chromatogram for specific ions to eliminate the effects of contamination— this is a technique that is the subject of recent research in improving the sensitivity of arson investigations in which there is a high level of background contamination from other organic substrates such as rubber-backed carpets. GC/MS also finds applications in explosive cases and lachrymator cases (including pepper spray, tear gas, and mace). For the latter, GC/MS is used to analyze the active ingredient(s), solvents, and propellants used in the aerosol dispensers. The active ingredients encountered are CN, CS, capsaicin, or capsaicinoids from the natural oleoresin of capsicum. In addition, GC/MS is used to a lesser extent in the analysis of paints and plastics.

GC is readily adapted to take advantage of automation and extraction techniques that enhance detection sensitivity by pre-concentration. An example of both of these together is the Perkin Elmer ATD-400 instrument which we use for the headspace analysis of fire debris samples.

— by Karen L. Kwek, Forensic Chemist

Part Three

Forensic Medicine/Science Subspecialties

Chapter 15

Forensic Pathology

What is a pathologist?

A pathologist is a physician trained in the medical specialty of pathology. Pathology is the branch of medicine that deals with the diagnosis of disease and causes of death by means of laboratory examination of body fluids (clinical pathology), cell samples (cytology), and tissues (pathologic anatomy). The autopsy is the procedure utilized to study the dead. It is primarily a systematic external and internal examination for the purposes of diagnosing disease and determining the presence or absence of injury. In modern times chemical analysis of body fluids for medical information as well as analysis for drugs and poisons should be part of any autopsy on a dead body coming under the jurisdiction of the medical examiner or coroner.

What is a forensic pathologist?

The forensic pathologist is a subspecialist in pathology whose area of special competence is the examination of persons who die sudden, unexpected or violent death. The forensic pathologist is an expert in determining cause and manner of death. The forensic pathologist is specially trained: to perform autopsies to determine the presence or absence of disease, injury or poisoning; to evaluate historical and law enforcement investigative information relating to the manner of death; to collect medical evidence, such as trace evidence and secretions, to document sexual assault; and to reconstruct how a person received injuries. Forensic pathologists are trained in multiple nonmedical sciences as well as traditional medicine. Other areas of science that the forensic pathologist must have a working knowledge of the applicability of are toxicology, firearms examination (wound ballistics), trace evidence, forensic serology, and DNA technology. The forensic pathologist acts as the case coordinator for the medical and forensic scientific assessment of a given death, making sure that the appropriate procedures and evidence collection techniques are applied to the body. When forensic pathologists are employed as death investigators, they bring their expertise to bear upon the interpretation of the scene of death, in the assessment of the consistency of witnesses' statements with injuries, and the interpretation of injury patterns or patterned injuries. In jurisdictions where there are medical examiner systems, forensic pathologists are usually employed to perform autopsies to determine cause of death.

Specifically what does a forensic pathologist do?

As a physician who specializes in the investigation of sudden, unexpected, and violent deaths, the forensic pathologist attempts to determine the identification of the deceased, the time of death, the manner of death (natural, accident, suicide, or homicide), the cause of death, and if the death was by injury, the nature of the instrument used to cause the death.

First, the forensic pathologist gathers a history as to how the death occurred and often obtains the past medical history of the deceased as well. Next, the forensic pathologist examines the body externally and then internally taking biopsies of tissues to further examine under the microscope for disease not visible to the naked eye. This postmortem examination is known as an autopsy.

During the course of the autopsy, various laboratory tests may be undertaken, including x-rays, retention of body fluids such as blood and urine for toxicologic analysis, and cultures of body fluids and organs for evidence of infection.

When all of the information including the history, the results of the autopsy, and the laboratory tests are completed, the forensic pathologist correlates all the information and draws conclusions as to the cause and manner of death. A report is then prepared summarizing these findings. The forensic pathologist can expect to be subpoenaed to testify before courts and other tribunals about the pathologic findings and conclusions. Coroners, medical examiners, and pathologists provide copies of their official reports to parties, such as insurers or public agencies, having a legitimate interest in the cause and manner of death of citizens.

How does the forensic pathologist use the history, external physical examination, autopsy, and laboratory studies to determine the cause and manner of death?

The history is the beginning of the investigation and is of utmost importance in making the determination of cause of death. The scene investigation may disclose drugs or toxins which may be related to the cause of death. Some poisonous agents are not detected in routine drug screens; therefore, the pathologist must have knowledge of medications and toxins in order to request the specific analytical tests needed to detect them. An example would include the "sniffing" of aerosol propellants, a risky activity which has been frequently reported in teenagers. Sniffing of propellent substances can cause sudden death by precipitating lethal cardiac arrhythmias. A special analysis (gas chromatography by headspace analysis) is required to detect the chemicals in the blood. In other cases, there may be sufficient natural disease to account for death, but the individual may, in fact, have died of a drug overdose or other subtle cause. In the case of drowning and suffocation, the autopsy findings may not be specific, and police investigation may be critical to the understanding of the death. Data developed by coroners, medical examiners, and pathologists is studied by medical epidemiologists and health and safety agencies to develop strategies to prevent disease and injury, thereby saving lives. The data developed about motor vehicle injuries and fire deaths lead to legislation requiring seat belts in vehicles and smoke detectors in building construction.

In the examination of skeletonized or severely decomposed remains, the forensic pathologist needs a working knowledge of multiple methods of identification including forensic anthropology in order to establish identity. If sufficient skeletal parts remain, the pathologist may be able to determine the age, race, and sex of the individual, and sometimes estimate the length of time since death. Occasionally, specific markings on the bones may enable the pathologist to come to a conclusion as to the cause of death.

What is the importance of performing an autopsy in some-one in whom the cause of death is "obvious"?

The importance of examining people in whom the cause of death appears obvious is several fold. In the case of shootings or other fatal assaults, the forensic pathologist, during the course of the examination, may recover bullets or other important trace evidence. In the case of motor vehicle occupants, it is important to determine who was driving and to assess driver factors, vehicle factors, or environmental factors that might have caused or contributed to the crash. Forensic autopsies may identify inherited diseases that constitute a risk for next of kin. Examples include certain types of heart disease (premature atherosclerosis, hypertrophic cardiomyopathy) and certain kinds of kidney disease (adult polycystic kidney disease). Notifying the family would be an important service to the living. In individuals who have undergone medical treatment after collapse or injury, it is important to share the findings with the treating physicians for educational purposes.

How does an autopsy authorized by the next of kin on a patient dying in the hospital of a natural disease differ from an autopsy authorized by law as part of a medicolegal investigation?

The hospital autopsy is often performed on individuals in whom the disease causing death is known. The purpose of the autopsy is to determine the extent of the disease and/or the effects of therapy and the presence of any undiagnosed disease of interest or that might have contributed to death.

The next of kin must give permission for the autopsy and may limit the extent of the dissection (for example the chest and abdomen only, excluding the head).

A medicolegal (forensic) autopsy is ordered by the coroner or medical examiner as authorized by law with the statutory purpose of establishing the cause of death and answering other medicolegal questions. The next of kin do not authorize and may not limit the extent of the autopsy. Common questions include the identity of the deceased person, the time of injury and death, and the presence of medical evidence (for example, bullets, hair, fibers, semen). Observations made at autopsy elucidate how and by what weapon lethal injury was inflicted. During the course of the forensic autopsy, blood and other body fluids are routinely obtained in order to check for alcohol and other drugs. The forensic autopsy should be complete (including the head, chest, abdomen, and other parts of the body as indicated.

What is clinical forensic pathology?

Because of their expertise in interpreting methods of injury, many forensic pathologists also examine, upon request, living patients including individuals who have been sexually assaulted (rape) and children who have been injured to assist in determining if child abuse or neglect has occurred. The forensic pathologist also examines patients to determine whether the pattern of injuries is consistent with accidental or intentionally inflicted injuries. During these examinations, a forensic pathologist may collect evidence for analysis. Examination of living patients is customarily performed on behalf of law enforcement agencies needing the same information on the living as required on dead victims of injury.

Where do forensic pathologists work?

Forensic pathologists are employed by states, counties, groups of counties, or cities, as well as by medical schools, the military services, and the federal government. In some setting such as medium-sized and smaller counties, the forensic pathologist may work for a private group or hospital which contracts with the county to perform forensic autopsies.

How does one become a forensic pathologist?

1. After high school, the future forensic pathologist attends college for four years and receives a bachelor's degree.

2. After undergraduate school, the aspiring forensic pathologist spends four years in medical school, earning an M.D. or D.O. degree.

3. After medical school, there are several routes by which one may become a forensic pathologist. One may spend five years training in anatomic and clinical pathology followed by one year of residency or fellowship in forensic pathology. A second option is to train for four years in anatomic pathology and train for one year in forensic pathology. The residency training in forensic pathology involves practical (on-the-job) experience supervised by a trained forensic pathologist. The forensic

pathology resident actually performs autopsies and partici-
pates in death investigation. To become certified, one then
must pass an examination given by the American Board of Pathology certifying special competence in forensic pathology.

Forensic pathologists practice medicine in the finest tradition of
preventive medicine and public health by making the study of the
dead benefit the living.

Chapter 16

Forensic Psychiatry

A physician trained as a forensic psychiatrist integrates clinical experience and scientific knowledge of medicine and mental health to formulate an objective evaluation of questions posed to clinical and scientific experts by the law. The applications of forensic psychiatry are not widely known to the general public, or even to many attorneys. A few of the more common areas of expertise are briefly described below.

A forensic psychiatrist is helpful to individuals who need evaluation of medical and mental health issues related to claims such as medical malpractice, employment issues (e.g., disability, sexual harassment), and many other areas. Relevant data are gathered, reviewed, and analyzed, then communicated by written report, deposition, courtroom testimony, or all of these. Without a forensic psychiatrist as an expert witness, the court may not be able to determine the validity of a claim. Insurance companies can benefit from a forensic psychiatric/medical expert consultation to determine the legitimacy of employment-related claims, supervisory responsibility, or the level of maintenance of health care standards.

For example, when there is a question of psychiatric or medical malpractice, a forensic psychiatrist with a special interest in medical

Excerpted from "Forensic Psychiatry and Medicine," [Online] October 27, 1997. Available: http://www.forensic-psych.com/newhome.html. Produced by Harold J. Bursztajn, M.D., Associate Clinical Professor, Harvard Medical School, Cambridge, MA 02138. For complete contact information, please refer to Chapter 56, "Resources." Reprinted with permission.

decision analysis can evaluate whether the standard of care for medical decision making and informed consent has been met. Where appropriate, a forensic psychiatrist can team up with other medical specialists to formulate a comprehensive set of expert opinions applicable to the specific questions. This objective analysis can address the professional pressures and public suspicions that have become commonplace with the advent of managed care. Moreover, such analysis can also be helpful toward preventing the recurrence of critical incidents.

This [chapter] has been developed to answer some of the basic questions about forensic psychiatry and medicine, as well as to provide a deeper overview of its objectives and applications. Additionally, it offers news of recent case decisions and publications that are relevant to forensic psychiatry and medicine. By providing such information to the public as well as to health and law professionals, the author hopes to contribute to the understanding of everyday issues in medicine, mental health, and the law.

Employment Issues

Employment issues, including worker's compensation and disability law, supervisory negligence, workplace discrimination, and wrongful termination can benefit from a forensic pre-neuropsychiatric evaluation. Such an evaluation begins with a review and analysis of medical records, depositions, and supporting documents. Initial working hypotheses may be supplemented by a forensic psychiatric examination of the plaintiff or the insured. This process can result in the formulation of an expert opinion as to the validity, nature, and extent of the claims at issue. Areas of interest include risk factors for misdiagnosis, misattribution, malingering, or motivation for secondary gain.

Disability and Workers' Compensation

Questionable claims of pain or impairment are sometimes presented in workers' compensation or disability laws. An expert in medical decision analysis and forensic neuropsychiatry can evaluate the following factors: that a treating physician maintained established reliability standards in the diagnostic process; emotional factors that could complicate physical illness have been addressed; and the ruling out of common psychiatric mimics of physical illness (e.g., somatization, conversion disorders, substance abuse, and personality traits such as malingering, exaggeration, misattribution of pain and impairment).

132

Case. *Mayotte M. Jones* v. *MetroWest Medical, Inc.* In this case, on behalf of the defense, Dr. Bursztajn performed a forensic psychiatric evaluation of the plaintiff's claim of multiple chemical sensitivity-induced impairment. In its favorable ruling, the court cited Dr. Bursztajn's expert report critiquing the diagnostic reasoning relied upon by the plaintiff's treating physician.

Sexual Harassment

Both true and false allegations of sexual harassment are made in the workplace. The presence or absence of psychological trauma is not enough to prove sexual harassment. False memories, desire for attention or revenge, and later reconsideration of consent can all lead to false allegations. At the same time, true allegations may not initially be considered credible. While a treating psychiatrist's goal is to help alleviate the presenting emotional and psychological pain and trauma without necessarily determining the facts of the incident, a forensic psychiatrist is trained to objectively evaluate claims such as that of sexual harassment. Such an evaluation yields more accurate testimony regarding the grounds on which the claim of sexual harassment is made, and potential emotional and physical damages.

In 1991, the Equal Employment Opportunity Commission (EEOC), the federal agency that deals with such complaints, handled 6,127 of them (sexual harassment cases) and settled cases worth $7.7m in damages to victims. In 1997, it handled 15,889 complaints and won $49.4m for victims (*The Economist,* February 14, 1998, p. 25).

Case. *Oncale* v. *Sundowner Offshore Services, Inc., et al.:*

1. This ruling of the U.S. Supreme Court (March 4, 1998) clarifies the sexual harassment law as it applies to same-sex relationships.

2. "Reasonableness Key: The social context in which particular behavior occurs [Justice Scalia] is the key to distinguishing between simple teasing and genuinely abusive behavior." This distinction can be explored in the course of forensic psychiatric examination, evaluation, and opinion formation.

Case. *Azzaro* v. *County of Allegheny.* In this sexual harassment case, the plaintiff alleged that she lost her job because she reported the incident to her supervisor; the court ruled that her reporting the incident, even privately, made it a public concern.

133

Americans with Disabilities Act (ADA)

The Americans with Disabilities Act shields disabled persons from discrimination in the workplace. Claims of having a protected disability status and allegations of disability-related discrimination in hiring, firing, or workplace practices must be supportable. A forensic neuropsychiatric evaluation and investigation into the discrimination claim can help to determine whether the alleged discrimination actually arose from the employee's claimed disability.

The ADA and Mental Impairment. [The following table] summarizes the relationship between mental impairments and the ADA based on the EEOC (Equal Employment Opportunity Commission) Notice No. 915.002 [on state workers' compensation laws], *Texas Trial Lawyer,* June 30, 1997 (source: EEOC Notice No. 915.002).

On March 27, 1997, the EEOC issued guidelines concerning mental and psychiatric disabilities under the ADA. The guidelines list what is and is not considered an impairment.

The Guidelines also list major life activities and require employers to determine if a mental impairment substantially limits one of these activities. The guidelines discuss the effects of medication as well as the effects of not taking medication that would help the impairment if taken correctly.

Finally, the guidelines consider appropriate ways in which an employer may take disciplinary action against a person with a psychiatric disability without violating the ADA.

Age Discrimination

EEOC Clarifies Job Termination Rules. The Equal Employment Opportunity Commission issued a regulation clarifying what companies have to tell older workers who are terminated and asked to sign waivers giving up their right to sue for age discrimination.

Among the areas addressed is how companies should provide statistical data regarding the job classifications and ages of those being terminated and those who aren't (*Wall Street Journal,* June 8, 1998, p. B12).

Managed Health Care and Malpractice

Managed health care organizations are more numerous and pervasive today. As they have grown in influence, many patients and professionals have claimed that medical care, while increasing in sophistication, has declined in quality. At the same time, the large-business

Table 16.1a. Mental Impairments and Life Activities

What are mental impairments?	What are not mental impairments?
Any mental, emotional, or psychological disorder	Various sexual behaviors
Major depression	Compulsive gambling
Bipolar disorders	Kleptomania
Anxiety disorders (e.g., obsessive compulsive disorders, panic disorders, and post traumatic stress disorder	Pyromania
Schizophrenia	Psychoactive substance abuse disorders resulting from the current illegal use of drugs
Personality disorders	Certain behavioral traits (e.g., irritability, chronic lateness, and poor judgement)

Table 16.1b. Mental Impairments and Life Activities

What major life activities are affected by mental impairment?	Employee discipline
Learning	An employer may take disciplinary action against an employee with a psychiatric disability "provided that the workplace conduct standard is job-related for the position in question and is consistent with business necessity."
Thinking	
Concentrating	
Interacting with others	
Caring for oneself	
Speaking	
Performing manual tasks	
Sleeping	
Working	

and third-party aspects of managed care organizations can make medical decision-making an impersonal process, and increase the need for organizations and clinics to exercise joint responsibility with the treating physician for informed patient care.

Malpractice

Health services often involve an element of risk and consequently decision-making on the part of the provider/practitioner. Whether a treating physician could and should reasonably have made a more informed decision can be addressed by consultation with a physician with a special interest in medical decision-making and the informed consent process.

Forensic psychiatric experts include physicians with training and expertise who consult regularly to physicians in other specialties regarding standards for informed clinical decision making. The following cases illustrate how forensic psychiatric and medical expertise can be useful in objectively evaluating malpractice claims.

Case. *Elaine Kennedy* v. *Dr. Ferroll Sams, III;* U.S. District Court, District of Georgia. A forty-eight-year-old physician was awarded $3.4 million by a federal jury. The physician alleged that she was wrongly committed to a psychiatric hospital by the defendant internist.

She was hospitalized for five days, which ultimately led to her loss of her medical license. Her license was restored after further evaluation found no evidence of a mental disorder.

The plantiff had come to the defendant to see the medical records of an elderly aunt. While in the office, the defendant told her she was mentally impaired and had an ambulance take her to a psychiatric facility.

The defendant maintained that the plaintiff was hostile and demanding in regard to the aunt's care. His commitment form identified the plaintiff as 'delusional,' 'hyperactive,' and suggested that she was manic-depressive.

The plaintiff claimed that the physician did not examine her before deciding that she was mentally ill and that she did not meet the criteria for involuntary commitment.

The verdict included $1.6 million for pain and suffering, $1.3 million for loss of income and $500,000 in punitive damages. Post-trial motions were expected (*Mental Health Law News,* Vol. 13, No. 6, June 1998, p. 4).

Case. Notable Malpractice Verdict. The state of Florida has agreed to indemnify 13 of its state mental hospital employees who have been ordered to pay 17.99 million dollars for medical malpractice and civil rights violations. Aaron Wynn developed schizophrenia-like symptoms after a 1985 head injury, and he spent from 1988 to 1991 committed to the Florida Department of Health and Rehabilitation Services. While hospitalized, he reportedly was kept in seclusion and restraint for over 19,000 hours and 'medicated on drugs contraindicated for brain injuries.' His mother filed suit on his behalf alleging that his treatment aggravated his injury to the point that he will need institutional care for the rest of his life (*Journal of the American Academy of Psychiatry Law,* Vol. 26, No. 3, 1998, pp. 519-20).

Benefit Denial

Disabilities, including psychiatric disabilities, are controversial reasons for denial of health benefits or health insurance altogether.

Case. Mental Health Benefits/Parity. A federal court in New York last month denied a motion to dismiss a lawsuit challenging an insurer's mental illness coverage limit for disability insurance (*Leonard F.* v. *Israel Discount Bank of New York,* 95 Civ. 6964). The suit is among the first to challenge discrimination in the long-term disability insurance against people with psychiatric disabilities under the Americans with Disabilities Act (ADA).

In refusing to dismiss the suit, U.S. District Judge Charles Brieant cites the opinion expressed by the EEOC in its friend-of-the-court brief. The EEOC suggested that the plaintiff meets the definition of a "Qualified Individual with a Disability" in Title I of ADA.

Organizational Responsibility

Under some circumstances, managed health care organizations can be liable for employee conduct at their facilities or by plan physicians, as in the cases below.

Case. *Group Home Resident Sexually Assaulted by Employee Niece* v. *Elmview Group Home* (929 P. 2d 42-Wash. 1/16/97). The Court concluded that Elmview had a duty to take reasonable precautions to protect Niece from the foreseeable consequences of her impairments, including possible sexual assaults by staff. The Court noted that a special relationship existed between Elmview and its vulnerable residents, from which the duty to protect arose. The fact that Quevedo was acting outside the scope of his employment when he sexually assaulted the plaintiff did not limit Elmview's liability for a breach of its own duty of care. The court held further that sexual assault by a staff member was not a legally unforeseeable harm. Indeed, prior sexual assaults at Elmview, Elmview's earlier policy prohibiting male staff members from being left alone with female residents, the opinion of Niece's expert that unsupervised contact between male staff members and female residents violated the standard of care for group homes with disabled residents, and the Legislature's recognition of the problem of sexual abuse in residential care facilities, all demonstrated that sexual abuse by staff at Elmview was foreseeable (*Crime Liability Monthly,* Vol. 2, No. 7, July 1997, pp 9-10).

Case. HMO Liability. A California Jury recently awarded $3 million to the family of Joyce Ching, who died of colon cancer that went undiagnosed for months while her primary care physicians, under contract to MetLife HMO, ignored her requests to be referred to a specialist. Ching's lawyer, Mark Hiepler, argued that by the time Ching was referred to a specialist, who diagnosed the cancer immediately, the tumor had perforated her colon, reducing her odds of survival from 60-80% to 11-35% (*Ching* v. *Gaines,* Calif Super Ct—Ventura County—No. 137878, 15 November 1995). In 1993, Hielper won a ground-breaking jury award against HMO Net, for refusing to pay for bone marrow treatment for his now-deceased sister's breast cancer.

ERISA

According to the *Pocket Guide to Managed Care,* the Employee Retirement Income Security Act (ERISA) is a federal law that governs the rights of employees to employer-sponsored pension and health benefits. It is supposed to protect patients by preempting state laws that regulate or tax employee benefits provided by employers. . . . In theory, ERISA can protect managed care organizations that are sued for (a) Malpractice, (b) Refusal to preauthorize care, and (c) Denying payment through their utilization management process. In practice, ERISA's actual protection of MCOs is variable (La Puma, J., and D. Schiedermayer. New York: McGraw Hill, 1996, pp. 24-5).

Political activity has recently increased to address the need for patient protection.

Case. *Shea* v. *Esensten.* HMO Can Be Sued under ERISA for Failure to Inform. In a case of first impression, a federal appeals court has reversed the dismissal of a case against an HMO, holding that the HMO can be sued under the Employee Retirement Income Security Act for failure to inform a patient that it penalized physicians if they made too many referrals. *Shea* v. *Esensten,* No. 95-4029MN (8th Cir. Feb. 26). The plaintiff claimed that the HMO had a 'fiduciary duty' under ERISA to disclose its policy. The court agreed, stating that 'an ERISA fiduciary has a duty to speak out if it knows that silence might be harmful.' It is yet unclear what damages the plaintiff can recover, as ERISA provides only for 'equitable relief' (*Medical Malpractice Law & Strategy,* April 1997).

Informed Consent

It is important for the individual patient to be involved in the decision-making process of choosing appropriate treatment. Informed consent can not only help the patient maintain control over his or her health care; it can help to prevent medical malpractice litigation. Lack of adequate information or influence over one's treatment can result in a lawsuit.

Care for the Dying

Terminally ill patients are often denied certain kinds of medical treatment. While the process of dying is often depressing, such depression is rarely treated. Often, this depression leads to giving up on life rather than the desire to make one's last months feel worthwhile. There are serious ethical and medical considerations in regard to best practice treatment for the terminally ill.

Emotional and Physical Damages

Forensic psychiatrists evaluate the validity of psychological and emotional suffering attributed to alleged physical damages.

Conscious Pain and Suffering

Claims of conscious pain and suffering may be difficult to support. The task of the forensic psychiatrist in such cases is to reconstruct the state of mind along scientifically acceptable principles. The following case demonstrates the forensic psychiatric evaluation of conscious pain and suffering.

Case. *Nonaka* v. *D'Urso,* Mass., Middlesex County Superior Court, No., 90-5227-B, May 31, 1991. Nonaka, 30, went to D'Urso's house to complain about his barking dogs. While Nonaka was standing on the steps talking with D'Urso's wife and son, D'Urso went into the house and returned with a shotgun. As Nonaka fled D'Urso's property, D'Urso shot him in the back.

Nonaka underwent surgery to remove the shotgun pellets and a portion of his small intestine. About 150 pellets remain lodged in his body, presenting a danger of lead poisoning, intestinal obstruction, and pancreatis. He suffers post-traumatic stress disorder that requires therapy. He incurred about $32,700 in medical expenses. A computer science graduate student who had earned about $40,000 annually, Nonaka cannot return to work.

Nonaka sued D'Urso, alleging assault, battery, and negligence in handling a loaded shotgun.

D'Urso tendered defense of the action to his homeowner insurance carrier, which initially agreed to defend without reserving its rights. However, during the pendency of the underlying action, the insurer filed a declaratory judgment action against D'Urso and Nonaka, alleging that it was not liable for coverage because D'Urso had acted intentionally.

The jury in the underlying action awarded $900,000. The trial court, hearing the declaratory judgment action, then found that the insurer had waived its right to disclaim coverage by undertaking defense of the action without reserving its rights. *Merrimack Mut. Fire Ins. Co.* v. *Nonaka,* Mass., Middlesex County Superior Court, No. 91-1588-B, June 10, 1991.

Post-Traumatic Stress Disorder (PTSD)

The courts recognize Post-Traumatic Stress Disorder as a type of damages. The cause and effects of PTSD must be distinguished from causes and effects of other symptoms and/or conditions. Therefore, the presence of PTSD can be verified or disclaimed only by a trained evaluator. The following [case] used forensic psychiatric testimony to support or refute claims of PTSD related injury.

Case. *Paul P. Sullivan and Mary J. McDonald* v. *Boston Gas Company* (605 N.E.2d 805 (Mass. 1993). Homeowners brought action against a natural gas utility, seeking damages for lost property, lost wages, and financial expenses related to gas explosion which caused destruction of their home, and also seeking compensation for negligent infliction of emotional distress. The court ruled that Post-Traumatic Stress Disorder meets the "physical harm rule."

Family and Custody Issues

Allegations such as lack of parental fitness or intentional infliction of emotional harm disputes sometimes arise in divorce and custody issues. Resolution of such charges may be helped by a forensic psychiatric examination.

Product Liability and Toxic Tort

Product liability and toxic tort issues often raise the question of the patient/injured party's ability to give informed consent or assume risk.

Also, in suits involving product liability and toxic tort, the plaintiff sometimes claims new psychiatric damages. The testimony of a forensic psychiatrist can support or refute such claims. Further, a forensic psychiatrist can shed light on the reasonableness of risk perception and pre-existing condition's influence on the capacity to give informed consent or assume risk.

Viagra, the first oval pill to treat male sexual impotence, has generated not only excitement, but also concern. The importance of informed consent and choice for physicians and patients alike is crucial to avoid both tragic outcomes and litigations:

FDA Asked to Increase Cautions on Viagra Warning Label. After two cardiology groups urged physicians to exercise caution when prescribing Viagra to their patients, the consumer advocacy group Public Citizen has asked the Food and Drug Administration to review the drug's side effects and strengthen its warning label.

As of Aug. 25, the FDA had confirmed the deaths of 69 men who took Viagra. Forty-six of these men died of cardiovascular events and two from strokes; the cause of death of the others had not been determined. All but five of the deaths occurred among patients who had known risk factors, including obesity, hypertension, and a history of heart problems (*Medical Malpractice*, Vol. 15, No. 11, September 1998, p.12).

Criminal Justice

Forensic psychiatrists are trained to evaluate defendants for evidence or absence of psychiatric disorders that impair competence or diminish capacity. Following the Daubert decision, guidelines for reliability and relevance of expert evidence have evolved. Thus, experts today need additional preparation (e.g. literature review) prior to offering courtroom testimony. The following [sections] provide a deeper analysis of forensic psychiatry.

Diminished Capacity

Case. *United States* v. *Johnson* (Maine Federal District Court, November 27, 1996). Apparently agreeing that government agents entrapped a naïve, hard-working marina owner from Hancock, a federal jury of four woman and eight men Tuesday found Philip Johnson not guilty of felony drug charges.

The jury took about 2.50 hours to acquit the 45-year-old of the charges stemming from an alleged conspiracy to smuggle $10 million worth of marijuana into Maine through the secluded port.

Allowing expert mental health testimony as part of the entrapment defense has never before been allowed in the federal court region that encompasses Maine, New Hampshire, Rhode Island, Massachusetts, and Puerto Rico.

Sentencing Guidelines

Forensic psychiatric testimony can affect sentencing. Since a defendant found to be suffering from a psychiatric symptom often receives a less severe sentence, accurately determining a defendant's psychiatric health is important in judging the severity of the offense and the potential for rehabilitation and future offense prevention.

Jury Instruction

Brunner v. *Florida,* 683 So. 2d 1129 (Fla. Dist. Ct. App. 1996), held that jurors needed instruction on the fact that insanity can result from intoxication by prescribed medication.

Public Safety

Safety First. After a wave of job-site violence, including the murder of a housing inspector on the job and shootings in hospitals, the American Federation of State, County and Municipal Employees published a handbook for union reps, "Preventing Workplace Violence" (*Wall Street Journal,* February 17, 1998).

Violence Prevention

Violence is sometimes a problem in legal proceedings:

Suspect's Killing of Cats Was an Ominous Sign. What initially piqued psychiatrists' interest in Russell Eugene Weston Jr., charged with gunning down two policemen at the U.S. Capitol on Friday, was another shooting that Weston committed the previous day in America's heartland, 1,000 miles away.

His father said Weston picked up a shotgun and killed a dozen or more cats in his hometown of Valmeyer, Ill., although he maintained yesterday the younger man had been asked to "to do something" about the felines on the family property (*Boston Herald,* July 27, 1998).

Testamentary and Contractual Capacity

Wills and contracts are sometimes contested on the claim that the testator was not mentally competent to draw up the will or contract in question. Another question raised regarding each is the presence of undue influence or duress limiting voluntariness. The resulting lawsuits focus on reconstructing the state of mind of the testator at the time the will was created.

Case. *Goddard* v. *Dupree*, Mass. Sup. Jud. Ct., (1948). Testamentary capacity requires ability on the part of the testator to understand and carry in mind, in a general way, the nature and situation of his property and his relations to those persons who would naturally have some claim to his remembrance. It requires freedom from delusion which is the effect of disease or weakness and which might influence the disposition of his property. And it requires ability at the time of execution of the alleged will to comprehend the nature of the act of making a will (*ElderLaw Services,* Vol. 2, No. 6, February 5, 1996).

With respect to testamentary capacity, as with other forms of competence, the treating clinician should refer the patient to someone in a position to make an objective evaluation. The treating clinician's proper concern with relieving the patient's suffering precludes objectivity in conducting a competency evaluation for deathbed will revisions. The clinician may confuse competence to consent to treatment with competence to dispose of property, each of which must be assessed independently.

Professional Ethics

Professional ethics, perched on the border between science and humanity, has undergone public scrutiny in modern times. One of the most notable examinations of professional ethics occurred during the Nuremberg trial of Nazi medical atrocities in 1946. In recent years, increasing use of medical technology and the formation of health maintenance organizations have created a new environment in which medical ethics are questioned. "Right to Die" debates and health professionals' sexual misconduct with patients are often in the news.

Administrative bodies struggle with maintaining a balance between protecting the public and liberty interests.

Case. *Tank* v. *Chronister,* 941 F.Supp. 969 (1996). The husband of a deceased patient failed to allege that a hospital and physician failed to apply its emergency patient screening procedures, as required to maintain a cause of action against them pursuant to the Emergency Medical Treatment and Active Labor Act (EMTALA), ruled the U.S. District Court in Kansas. The husband sought to present the case to the jury through evidence of malpractice, based upon what the physician should have inferred from the patient's respiratory symptoms, and failure of the attending nurse to recheck the patient's vital signs was not an EMTALA violation absent allegations that the initial readings were false, the court explained. In addition, the court said the patient did not have a constitutional right to medical treatment, as required to maintain a federal civil rights action for the patient's failure to receive treatment. However, the court also held that, under Kansas law, the husband substantially complied with the notice statute, as required to maintain state claims.

In this case, the husband of a deceased patient brought action against a hospital under EMTALA alleging violation of state and federal laws. The hospital moved for dismissal. The district court granted the motion in regard to the federal claims but denied as to the claim for medical malpractice.

Trial Consulting and Forensic Psychiatry

Medical, particularly psychological, evidence is challenging to present to judges and juries. Forensic psychiatrists are trained to evaluate individuals for evidence or absence of psychiatric disorders and to present this information to the court. They also inform and work with counsel toward presenting clear and convincing testimony. In light of the Daubert decision, in which the relevance and reliability of medical testimony is determined at the discretion of the court, the role of forensic psychiatry has achieved an important standing in the field of expert testimony.

When O. J. Didn't Have His Game Face. Did O. J. Simpson murder Nicole Simpson and Ron Goldman as a result of a chronic steroid addiction? The evidence for this theory—strangely overlooked by both the prosecution and defense—is compelling. According to a confidante of A. C. Cowlings, Simpson began abusing anabolic steroids during his football career and has been taking cortisone for pain ever since. If Simpson were indeed addicted to these drugs, it would help explain how a genial and popular man could have violently murdered two people. According to Harvard Medical School forensic psychiatrist Dr. Harold Bursztajn, abuse of these drugs is known to cause sudden bouts of violence and amnesia. Even stopping the medicine abruptly, Bursztajn points out, may result in 'depression, paranoia, and fluctuating psychotic outbreaks.' Though the LAPD lab tested Simpson's blood for eight substances including cocaine and heroin, it concedes it never tested for steroids. Says Dr. Bursztajn: 'Longtime steroid use or abuse can't be found unless you test for it specifically.' But evidence of Simpson's possible drug problem shows up in much of the trial testimony. Limo driver Allan Park testified that Simpson was "hot" and demanded both air-conditioning and open windows on the way to the airport the night of the murders even though it was a mild evening. Cortisone abuse, according to experts, often causes excessive sweating. On the flight to Chicago, Simpson went to the bathroom every fifteen minutes, a flight attendant later reported to the police. 'Even if he had stopped using steroids abruptly, he would pee and pee and drink and drink [water],' says Dr. Bursztajn. And finally, on the evening of the Bronco 'chase,' defense lawyer Robert Shapiro called in steroid specialist Dr. Robert Huizenga when Simpson was feared suicidal. Since then, the former L.A. Raiders team doctor has been Simpson's personal physician (*New York Magazine*, July 24, 1995).

— by Harold J. Bursztajn, M.D.

Harold J. Bursztajn, M.D., a senior clinical faculty member at Harvard Medical School and codirector of the Program in Psychiatry and the Law at the Massachusetts Mental Health Center, consults, teaches, and testifies nationwide as an expert in medical decision analysis, professional ethics, and general and forensic psychiatry. As well as maintaining an active clinical practice, Dr. Bursztajn publishes numerous articles and authors chapters in standard texts in these areas.

Chapter 17

Forensic Nursing

Violence and its associated trauma are widely recognized as a critical health problem in North America and throughout the world. Forensic nursing represents a new era of nursing practice that is evolving in direct response to the sequelae of criminal and interpersonal violence. The application of the principles and standards of the forensic specialist in nursing has been recognized as a vital new role in trauma care in the 1990s.[1] Daily, nurses encounter the results of human behavior extremes: abused children, individuals suffering from blatant neglect and maltreatment or self-inflicted injury, and victims of firearm injuries, knife wounds, and other assaults. These cases must, by law, be reported to a legal agency for investigation and follow-up. As trends in crime and violence change, new antiviolence legislation is being implemented; consequently, new personnel resources are required to ensure that these legislative mandates are effectively meeting the needs of society.

Nurses have been challenged to share responsibility with the legal system to augment the resources available to patients with liability-related injuries, crime victims, and perpetrators or suspects in police custody. The mutual responsibility concept represents a new

From "Clinical Forensic Nursing: A New Perspective in the Management of Crime Victims from Trauma to Trial," [Online] September 1995. Available: http://members.aol.com/COCFCI/Vart.html. Produced by Virginia A. Lynch, M.S.N., R.N., F.A.A.F.S., University of Colorado, 644 Brewer Dr., Fort Collins, CO 80524. For complete contact information, please refer to Chapter 56, "Resources." Reprinted with permission.

perspective in the holistic approach to legal issues surrounding patient care in clinical or community-based institutions. There has been strong support for this concept from those who recognize the amount of knowledge required to go beyond the traditional treatment of crime victims and fill a greater role through forensic expertise in health care.

Forensic Science in Nursing

The majority of health care professionals in the United States misinterpret the meaning of the term forensic. According to *Taber's Cyclopedic Medical Dictionary,* the term forensic (Latin forensis: a forum) is defined simply as pertaining to the law, specifically related to public debate in courts of law. Therefore, any subdiscipline of science that practices its specialty within the arena of the law is practicing the principle of forensic science. Anywhere the world of law and the world of medicine collide, a medicolegal (meaning legal-medicine) or forensic case occurs. Traditionally, the term forensic carried with it a connotation of death, homicide, or murder. This association is due to the fact that until recently only one kind of forensic science in North America, forensic pathology, had received widespread attention. The forensic pathology subspecialty is concerned mainly with the scientific investigation of death, as opposed to clinical forensic practice, which is primarily concerned with the survivor of violent crimes or liability-related trauma. There is a new trend in clinical and community health care that involves the awareness and recognition of unidentified or previously unrecognized trauma and the collection of evidence from living patients. Survivors of trauma requiring the investigation of injuries are the concern of the clinician, not the pathologist, although well-trained and experienced forensic pathologists are often willing to assist. Clinical forensic practice is becoming recognized as an essential component of health care in the United States and Canada. Indeed, it has been a respected discipline in public health for 200 years in other parts of the world, including the United Kingdom, South America, East Asia, and Russia.

Defining Clinical Forensic Practice and Its Components

In a comprehensive approach to the unmet needs of forensic victims who survive violent crimes and traumatic injuries, enhanced involvement in assisting the living is being explored through new roles for the emerging clinical forensic medical and nursing specialist.[8, 11, 15, 17, 27] Previously, a patient had to die under extraordinary circumstances to be examined by an expert in forensic issues. New forensic specialists will become the designated clinicians who will evaluate and assess surviving victims of rape, drug and alcohol addiction, domestic violence (including abuse of spouse, children, elderly), assaults, automobile/pedestrian accidents, suicide attempts, occupationally related injuries, incest, medical malpractice and the injuries sustained therefrom, and food and drug tampering. Their injuries are the concern of society as a whole and require a combination of social systems interfacing with health care and the law to provide solutions. Contemporary roles require new responsibilities, including the determination of the circumstances surrounding trauma and the mechanism of injury, the identification of human rights violations (e.g., physical torture as well as neglect while in custody, during institutionalized/ protective care, or in private homes), and determination of unsafe conditions and products (e.g., workplace hazards, injuries from toys, exposure to toxins, vehicular accidents).

Any patient admitted to the hospital with liability-related traumatic injuries is considered a clinical forensic patient. The case must be reported to a legal agency to ensure that proper investigation and follow-up action will ensue. The hospital staff most often comes in contact with police, victims, and perpetrators of violence and crime in the emergency department. Protection of the patient's rights remains the common goal of police officers and trauma nurses. Every hospital, regardless of its size and location, must eventually address problems of conflict with law enforcement agencies. Most often, these conflicts concern patients in legal custody and perpetrators of crime, as well as the confidentiality of victims' medical records. Policies that increase mutual understanding, define responsibilities, and promote coordination contribute to multidisciplinary, multiagency cooperation. The nurse's role as a clinical investigator provides a vital liaison between the investigative process and courts of law.[15]

Forensic Science: Impact on Nursing

The introduction and expansion of new roles in clinical forensic nursing are bringing about constructive changes in management, education, and practice. These new roles may overlap existing roles, which often provided only fragmented or ineffective organization of treatment to crime victims. With formal and informal education in forensic nursing, more expert clinicians are available to provide services to patients that will help protect their legal rights. To establish the foundation upon which forensic nursing is designed, it is necessary to examine the history of clinical forensic medicine, or living forensics, as it is sometimes called. This is a new field of inquiry brought to the attention of clinical nursing through an integrative practice model that unites the disciplines of nursing science, forensic science, and criminal justice in the common goal of protection of the victim's legal, civil and human rights. As greater numbers of nurses are involved in the investigation process requiring the application of forensic science to nursing practice, increased collaboration with the criminal justice system is required.[15,16,17] Forensic nursing's scientific knowledge base emerges from theories of nursing, forensic science, criminal justice, police science, and legal studies. The relative isolation of these disciplines has contributed to the complex tasks and social climate facing emergency care. Commitment and insight will be required to improve these conditions.

The theoretical model of forensic nursing[14] evolved from the role of the police surgeon or police medical officer of the United Kingdom and European countries. This practitioner of clinical forensic medicine is hired by the police department and is responsible for facilitating the management of the crime victim from the scene of the incident through the legal process.

Forensic nursing, a clinical subspecialty, is complementary to clinical forensic medicine as it evolves in response to society's changing demands. In the past, medicine has had a working relationship with nursing, except in forensic medicine. The time has come to extend the interdisciplinary support and assistance to include the forensic physician and forensic nurse as a cooperative unit.[9]

Forensic nursing is the application of the nursing process to public or legal proceedings: the application of the forensic aspects of health care to the scientific investigation of trauma. Clinical forensic nursing is defined as the application of clinical nursing practice to trauma survivors or to those whose death is pronounced in the clinical environs, involving the identification of unrecognized, unidentified injuries and the proper processing of forensic evidence. A serious gap in the criminal justice system has either been left open or partially filled by health (nurses, hospital physicians, emergency medical technicians, paramedics) and justice practitioners (police officials and attorneys) who essentially lack a forensic background. These individuals must be able to recognize problems in the existing system and raise the awareness of potential solutions.[20] As a public service profession, nursing has a responsibility to maintain standards of practice while processing victims of human violence. Owing to the vast number of crime victims who present to the emergency department, the need for a forensic specialist has finally been recognized.[7] A historic lack of interagency cooperation involving law and nursing issues combined with the absence of forensic education available to nurses has often threatened the patient's legal rights. There is growing support for the role of forensic nurses by those who understand the significant contribution of the clinical forensic specialist in the advocacy and ministration to this plight. The National Victim's Center has introduced forensic nursing as the most recent advance in victim advocacy.

Forensic Nursing and Trauma Care

Trauma is recognized worldwide as a major public health problem. The needs and demands of each society constantly change with the escalation of violence. Trauma is advancing at an alarming rate, and the recognition of medicolegal cases resulting from human violence requires new knowledge.

Although each culture may present its own unique drama in types of crime, weapons, and drugs, no age, race, religion, or socioeconomic group is spared from the devastating effect of the trauma it produces, both physical and emotional. Trauma ranks higher than AIDS, heart disease, and cancer as a cause of hospitalization. Each year, millions of women, children, and the elderly are victims of interpersonal violence. More than 1.1 million incidents of violence against women, including murder, rape, and aggravated assault, are reported to the police each year. These cases are generally reported from the hospital emergency department. One reason that trauma care is of concern is that for all the reported crimes of human violence, there may be three times as many unreported crimes. Failure by health care providers to recognize the subtle signs and symptoms of abuse and neglect in the early warning stages, and failure to report to an investigating agency can contribute to further injury or death. Statistics indicate that trauma associated with violence is the leading killer of young Americans between 1 and 44 years of age. These premature deaths cause the loss of approximately 2.2 million potential years of lives.

Trauma nurses perform an important role in the investigation of crime and the legal process in terms of victims of violence, both living and deceased. For example, questions related to trauma that may be of later relevance in a court of law may remain unanswered because of an emergency department nurse's ignorance of forensic issues. Frequently, cases are won or lost based on the handling of evidence. If health care professionals fail to incorporate forensic guidelines, misinterpretation or omission of evidence may result in a miscarriage of justice.

Clinical forensic nursing is designed to provide a solution to medi-colegal-related problems in trauma departments. In addition to medi-colegal issues, sensitivity to victims and families has historically been an exclusive concern of victim advocates from the perspective of basic human rights. As a patient advocate, it is a concern for the clinical forensic nurse.

Specific Responsibilities of the Forensic Specialist in Trauma

Investigation of Trauma

Nurses have a unique opportunity to contribute to forensic science as they manage problems commonly encountered trauma care. Law enforcement officers struggle to safeguard evidence during medical interventions, and resultant conflicts of priority may ensue.

Medical-legal interface is critical among multidisciplinary teams investigating traumatic injuries, whether accidental, criminal, self-inflicted, or from unknown causes. Interface can be damaged, with serious consequences, when no forensic protocol exist. This occurs when police officers and hospital staff are not familiar with procedures that each is supposed to follow. The appointment of a designated hospital liaison to network with police and the coroner and/or medical examiner can provide a systematic approach to communication and coordination. This liaison should be knowledgeable of forensic concepts, legal responsibilities, and victim's issues. The forensic clinical nurse specialist is prepared to fill this role ideally.

Preservation of Evidence

Emergency nurses become involved when a patient is admitted for trauma care as a result of suspicious injuries that may be crime related or self-inflicted. These patients require nurses to be aware of the manner in which the assessment of injury, forensic evidence, and critical data are documented with law enforcement and crime scene officers.

The problem of gathering evidence in the emergency department is compounded by failure to develop and implement forensic guidelines for nurses. A classic problem is the lack of an acceptable method for preserving evidence from crimes that are discovered long after the patient has been admitted or has died. This situation is further complicated when the forensic pathologist becomes involved after the destruction of the evidence, or the condition of the body has been altered by surgical intervention.

Hospital emergency departments are regularly in contact with essential evidence in criminal cases. The most common types of evidence are clothing, bullets, blood stains, hairs, fibers, and small pieces of material such as fragments of metal, glass, paint, and wood.

Physical Evidence

Trace and physical evidence are concerns of the criminalist (crime laboratory examiner) and are used to establish the facts of a crime. If, however, proper precautions are not taken to ensure an unaltered condition when collecting specimens, the forensic examination is compromised. When crime victims are treated by emergency department staff, forensic evidence is often lost because medical personnel are not aware of its presence or potential value. Problems in gathering evidence in the emergency department, surgical suite, or any department in the hospital are not restricted to the failure to recognize or collect forensic evidence; often, there is failure to properly preserve fragile or perishable evidence. Documentation must reflect the accurate identification, description, and security of medicolegal evidence.

When to Collect Evidence

The dilemma of gathering evidence in the emergency department is a serious cause of concern in traumatic injury patients. The emergency staff should recognize the importance of recovering possible items of evidence in a legally acceptable manner in the following situations:

- Medicolegal cases: A medicolegal case is defined as a treatment situation with legal implications.[23]

- Suspicious deaths or crime-related injuries: Suspicious deaths and crime-related injures are classified as medicolegal cases.

- Accidents: It is not always possible to predict if an accident will have medicolegal implications. Nonetheless, almost all accidents result in some type of litigation, either civil or criminal.

Processing of Clothing

It is imperative that nurses in the clinical environment be taught to recognize and preserve vital fragments of trace evidence by careful handling of the patient's clothing and personal property. This is one of the most important actions nurses provide to aid the investigation process. Clothing worn at the time of the incident may contain trace evidence useful in linking the victim with the assailant or crime scene.

Observation

Careful examination of defects in clothes can be compared to wounds of the victim, and often clothes provide insight as to the type of weapon or wounding instrument used. Clothing should be checked for blood, semen, gunshot residue, or trace materials such as hair or fibers: document, diagram, photograph, collect, preserve. The clothing may contain fragments from the assailant. If the assailant was injured, his or her blood may be on the victim's clothing. Garments from automobile/pedestrian accidents may display tire impressions or conceal trace evidence such as paint chips or broken glass that could identify the vehicle that struck the victim. Laundry markings may offer a clue to identification or origin of an unknown, unconscious, near-death, or deceased individual. Special attention should be given to the examination and security of clothing from a gunshot victim. Gunshot residues surrounding bullet holes in the clothes may determine the distance of the firearm from the victim at the time of firing (range of fire).

Documentation

Documentation of the condition of the patient's clothing should be carefully noted. Color, type, unusual markings, and tears or other damages should be recorded. Occasionally, fibers or foreign debris from the crime scene on the victim's clothing may be transferred to the vehicle or assailant. Clothing is often the first circumstantial evidence that may help to identify a missing person or collaborate an eye witness statement:

Example: As search warrants for the examination of the car and residence were being prepared, the District Attorney requested a description of the clothing Emily wore on the drive home after spending the night in the woods. The Chief of Police telephoned the medical center to find out what Emily had worn. The hospital nursing supervisor's subsequent actions and the information the police chief said was relayed to him, later became a point of contention between the prosecution and the defense.

154

Removal

Clothing should be carefully removed to protect any foreign fragments adhering to them. Do not shake the clothes. Clothing is frequently cut away during resuscitation attempts and is subject to loss of both the article itself and/or evidentiary materials. The cutting of clothing is unavoidable in many life threatening situations and is necessary to provide immediate access to treatment sites. When this occurs, try to avoid cutting through tears, rips, and holes that may have resulted from the weapon or the assault. Clothing should never be discarded or thrown on the floor, as this can result in cross-contamination of trace evidence with debris from the treatment environment. Because of time constraints during lifesaving intervention, a clean, white sheet can be placed on an empty trauma table, mayo stand, or on the floor in the corner of the room for clothing to be placed until time permits for effective packaging. If a victim can remove his or her clothes, this should be done standing on a clean sheet or a large sheet of paper. This will collect any microscopic evidence that may become dislodged during removal. The sheet must be placed in a separate paper bag for transfer to the crime laboratory.

Preservation

If possible, clothing should be hung up to dry in a secure area if moist. Police should be told if clothing they are to retrieve is in a damp condition. Clean white paper should be placed over stains to avoid cross-contamination. Each item of clothing should be stored in separate paper, not plastic, bags. Plastic bags are inappropriate because there is a tendency for condensation to accumulate, resulting in a degradation of the integrity of the evidence. Each bag should be sealed and clearly marked with the date, time, and signature or initials of the individual doing the sealing. Fortunately, a hospital is an excellent place to find all manners of containers (bags, bottles, boxes, and tubes) for properly storing evidence.

Custody

Secure custody of the clothing must be maintained until it is turned over to the appropriate law enforcement agency. Personal property must not be released to family members. These items should be held for police and they are generally not returned to the family. In cases in which police jurisdiction is doubtful and/ or where family members are demanding return of the clothing, a legal opinion may be warranted.

Chain of Custody

The chain of custody begins with the person who collects the evidence. This refers to the identity of the individuals having control or custody over evidentiary or potentially evidentiary material or personal property. This chain of custody should be defined in the forensic protocol and generally requires a form of written documentation.

Rules of evidence require a chain of custody for each item recovered from the patient. This includes trace and physical evidence, laboratory specimens of blood/body fluids, clothing, and personal articles. The integrity of every specimen or piece of evidence seized must be ensured to protect the admissibility in a court of law. Failure to maintain the chain of custody renders potentially important evidence worthless if lost, damaged, or unaccountable from the hands of the nurse to the police officer.

Investigation of Wound Characteristics

The investigation of undiagnosed trauma often begins with the evaluation of wound pattern characteristics. Detailed documentation of the appearance of the wound may be the identifying factor in determining the type of weapon used to inflict the injury. Wound characteristics constitute evidence that may be obscured by emergency trauma care. Nurses who become involved in the investigation of traumatic injuries have a responsibility beyond the immediate treatment environment. These include issues related to the patient's right to know, the public's right to know, and the administration of justice. The nurse's documentation should include the location of the injury and approximate measurements of cuts, lacerations, and stab wounds. Diagrams, body maps, or photography are helpful in reconstructing injury patterns in subsequent investigations or at autopsy. For patients who survive, or whose wound is excised or extended surgically, later reconstruction of the injury is not possible. The specific importance of reconstruction is magnified when the patient lives for an indefinite period and later dies as a result of the injury. Treatment procedures and the natural healing process alter the condition of the wound, thus eliminating the possibility of determining if the wound was inflicted with a single or double edged blade knife, an entrance or exit gunshot wound and so forth.

Nurses should have an accurate knowledge of the types of injuries generally resulting in medicolegal patients and should be familiar with the appropriate terminology. Failure to recognize and describe injuries has confounded the testimony of victim and perpetrator as a defense strategy in the courtroom. The nurse not only appears unprofessional, but a serious crime may go unpunished. Medicolegal injuries are primarily categorized as

- Sharp injuries: Sharp force injuries include stab wounds and incised wounds resulting from penetration or cuts that can reflect patterns or characteristics consistent with the wounding object. It is important not to confuse a cut with a laceration. A laceration is not a sharp injury.

- Blunt injuries: Blunt force injuries usually result from assaults, abuse, accidents, or resuscitative intervention. Abrasions, contusions, lacerations, and fractures are blunt injuries resulting from crushing impact of a blunt object against the body. A laceration results only from blunt force impact.

- Dicing injuries: Generally small and numerous, dicing injuries are most often sustained from motor vehicle accidents. These injuries consist of multiple, minute cuts and lacerations caused by contact with shattering tempered glass.

- Bite mark injuries: Bite marks remain the patterned injury most frequently unrecognized or unidentified as evidence by nurses when assessing the patient. Human bite marks are indicative of abuse and are generally associated with sexual assault. Animal bite marks are usually accidental, but may incur civil or even criminal liability if an animal had been neglected, tortured, or trained to cause an injury and/or if a dangerous animal escaped captivity by negligence, a deliberate act, or other illegal action.

- Patterned injuries: Specific characteristics of an injury that reflects the identity of the wounding object or provides information about the nature of the weapon is referred to as a patterned injury.

- Defense wounds: Defensive injuries indicate the posturing of a victim in protection against attack. Defense wounds are most often found on the hands and arms, although they may be located on any part of the body used as a shield. These injuries can be either sharp or blunt depending upon the weapon used.

- Hesitation wounds: Usually superficial, sharp force wounds that are self-inflicted in the survivor of suicide and accompany a deeper, fatal incision in the decedent. Hesitation marks are generally straight wounds perpendicular to the lower extremities. They may be found at the wrist, elbow, or neck. Scars from hesitation marks indicate a previous attempt at suicide.

- Fast force injuries: Fast force injuries (usually gunshot) require nurses to be knowledgeable of the mechanics and specifics of gunshot and shotgun wounds to recognize the variations of patterns of injury produced by these weapons.

Investigation into the nature of gunshot wounds by nurses has been advanced by the awareness of forensic nursing specialists. "The nurse who understands (gunshot wound) factors can better assess the extent of injury, provide appropriate nursing care, and anticipate potential problems."[29] Nursing involvement in such investigations and associated responsibilities extends beyond the emergency department management of the patient. Responsibilities include collecting evidence, maintaining chain of custody, preventing alterations of evidence, and ensuring proper witnessing of various evidentiary procedures. The nurse involved in the initial management of a patient must make an assessment on the basis of the wound site, type of weapon involved, and length of time between the injury and emergency care. Cases involving gunshot wounds should be documented regarding the presence or absence of gunshot residue (powder, soot, particles, and/or small punctate hemorrhages) around the injury. Any bullet or fragments recovered during treatment should be properly packaged and turned over to the crime scene officer in an unaltered condition. Valuable notations, such as records of the names and addresses of witnesses, monitoring of the procedures or events prior to autopsy, and safeguarding of clothing and other personal effects should be documented.[22] Personal property may constitute forensic evidence and should never be released to the family without permission of the police. By implementing forensic protocol that emphasizes cooperation with the criminal justice sector, nurses are initiating a critical link in trauma systems that will provide for improved medicolegal outcomes.

Standards and Liability Issues

Accreditation Standards and Liability

Violent crime most often occurs against women, children, and the elderly. Violence is the exercise of power and control over more vulnerable individuals or groups; any unjust, unwarranted force or power to impose one's will, physical or verbal, upon another. It may involve the use of a weapon. Violence has a profound influence on the public health system and affects all areas of the health care institution. Identification of the most subtle signs of abuse and subsequent intervention are important responsibilities for nurses. Traditionally, these responsibilities were relegated specifically to law enforcement agencies. The support of preeminent nursing organizations such as the American Academy of Nursing (1993), the American Nurses Association (1992), the International Association of Forensic Nurses (1992), and the Nurses Networking on Violence Against Women (1993) provided an impetus that has served as a driving force to involve nurses in forensic roles.

Since 1992, the Joint Commission on Accreditation of Health Care Organizations (JCAHO) has published standards aimed at ensuring that all hospital staff be trained in the identification of crime victims and procedures needed to work with abuse survivors. These standards include criteria to identify possible abuse victims of physical assault, rape, or sexual molestation, including spouses, partners, and children. There is also guidance for patient evaluation procedures including patient consent, examination components, and treatment. A mandate that unequivocally provides for the role of the forensic clinician is set forth in the hospital's responsibility in collection, retention, and safeguarding of specimens, photography, and other trace and physical evidence. Medical record documentation, including examinations, treatment referrals to other care providers and community-based family violence agencies, and required notification of authorities, are among the responsibilities of the care provider. Nonetheless, the need to establish specific guidelines for the facilitation of both adult and child victims of suspected abuse or neglect has brought about little change in the majority of hospitals nationwide.

Research indicates that these issues remain a significant problem in California hospital emergency departments. In 1992,[13a] the Family Violence Prevention Fund in San Francisco and the San Francisco Injury Center for Research and Prevention conducted a study to evaluate the circumstances of victims of domestic violence admitted to California emergency departments. This survey, the first of its kind in the nation, found that only 5% of adult victims of domestic violence were identified. Reasons cited for the failure to meet JCAHO standards for dealing with this category of crime victims were (1) time constraints, (2) lack of training, and (3) reluctance by both the medical worker and the victim to talk about domestic violence. This landmark

1992 survey of 397 emergency departments revealed that as few as one in five are meeting the national hospital accreditation requirements on this issue. Only 59 had specific forensic policies, and only eight were adequately addressing identification, treatment, and intervention. Although response rate indicated that health care professionals were enthusiastic about helping these victims, few had developed programs to do so. California is not alone in facing violence and its associated trauma. If time constraints interfere with the ideal clinical intervention in such cases, the presence of forensic specialists in nursing can ease the workload of the physician and better meet the needs of the victim of domestic violence, the criminal justice system, and other medicolegal agencies.

Implementation of the role of clinical forensic nurse would provide a uniquely skilled and qualified forensic professional whose responsibilities would be (1) to develop the appropriate forensic protocols in compliance with accreditation standards, (2) triage patients at risk for forensic injuries, (3) report to proper legal agencies, (4) document, collect, and preserve evidence, (5) secure evidence and maintain the chain of custody, and (6) serve as liaison between the health care institution, law enforcement agencies, and the medical examiner/coroner and make referrals when medical treatment and/or crisis intervention is required. This essential component of a network of medical, nursing, law, and social services could initiate significant constructive changes. Forensic standards also serve as a means to transmit developing knowledge in technical and social interventions. The implementation of regular in-service programs on the Forensic Aspects of Health Care would be a primary responsibility of the forensic nurse specialist. She or he would advise the medical and nursing staff and other first responders on the legal requirements of trauma care. Those who are among the first to come in contact with victims of suspected abuse must understand the application of forensic policies to emergency medical services. Health care personnel are mandated reporters and must be vigilant about suspected abuse. According to the American Trauma Society,[30a] victims of domestic violence present to the hospital emergency department six times more often than the general population. Failure to report suspicious cases can result in criminal or civil liability. Ligation is a current professional concern; thus, recommendations for the inclusion of the role of the forensic nurse would not only help to protect the patient's rights but also would serve the best interest of the health care institution and their employees against liability claims.

Sudden and Unexpected Deaths in the Clinical Area

Death in the Emergency Department

Sudden and violent deaths most frequently represent the initial interface between the hospital staff and police in the emergency department.

Considering the number of sudden and unexpected deaths that occur in the clinical setting, nurses have a critical role to play in providing answers in questionable death situations. Deaths occur in the hospital environment on a regular basis: dead on arrival, during trauma treatment, in the operating room, delivery room, nursery, surgical intensive care, or postanesthesia room, among others. Deaths that occur as a result of trauma or unknown causes require investigation. Generally, any death that occurs during the first 24 hours after admission is reportable to the medical examiner/coroner system regardless of the history.

If death occurs in the trauma room, the trauma room suddenly becomes a scene of legal inquiry and is listed as the place of death on the death certificate regardless of where the initial incident occurred. The death scene must be protected until the body and evidence have been removed at the completion of the medicolegal investigation. Patients who die as a result of abuse or an accident must be reported; there must be investigation; and evidence must be retained. Current research indicates that one in six pregnant women are victims of abuse and an estimated 25% to 45% of women who are battered are battered during pregnancy. The delivery room is a frequent scene of death. Trauma during pregnancy provides direct correlation to the increase in stillbirths and the death of the mother.[19] Anesthesia-related deaths also may create a crime scene scenario. Who is responsible for preserving the scene, interviewing the witnesses, collecting evidence and managing forensic issues until the investigation is turned over to the proper authority? The presence of a nurse skilled in forensic technique and appropriate medicolegal procedures may be essential in each of these situations.

Maintaining an index of suspicion is essential when considering criminal activity as a cause of sudden and unexpected death. Preservation of evidence, careful documentation of the circumstances surrounding the death, and the decedent's social and medical history may form the basis for deducing the cause of death when it is not obvious. Often overlooked is the proper handling of items that might subsequently be considered evidence. Full documentation of the appearance of the victim on arrival at the hospital is also often neglected. Nurses are among the first to come in contact with the patient, interview family members, and handle the patient's property and laboratory specimens. They serve as a vital link between the victim, police, and medical examiner or coroner. Generally, the nurse elicits information that may clarify important points related to the cause or manner of death, and the nurse is often the first person to have access to evidence of a criminal nature in the medicolegal sense.

The critical factor in sudden and unexpected death is whether the initiating cause is natural or unnatural. It is not uncommon for physicians to incorrectly identify the cause of death because of failure to differentiate between cause, manner, and mechanism of death. Increasingly, states are passing nurse pronouncement laws, and nurses are pronouncing death. With the extent of greater involvement in death pronouncement, a clear understanding of these terms must become an essential component of nursing education. Although the nurse may not be filling out the death certificate, the data recorded in the chart is often copied by less knowledgeable people; therefore, it is vital that the entry be appropriate.

Cause of death is the injury, disease, or combination of the two responsible for initiating the sequence of disturbances that produce the fatal termination. The important word is "initiating"; note that causes may not be immediately fatal, such as carcinoma or a stab wound. *Manner of death* is the fashion or circumstance in which the cause of death arose. In the United States, there are five: natural, accident, homicide, suicide, or undetermined. *Mechanism of death* is the physiologic derangement or biochemical disturbance incompatible with life initiated by the cause of death. Clearly, if the mechanism is initiated by a cause, these two cannot be the same. They are, in effect, final common pathways out of life. Mechanisms include cardiac arrest, respiratory arrest, cardiopulmonary arrest, and so forth. Forensic pathologists characterize cardiac arrest as "the diagnosis of the diagnostically destitute!" (Besant-Matthews, personal communication, 1994). Many physicians and nurses fail to distinguish between cause and mechanism. A classic instance of this is when a patient brought into the hospital dies shortly thereafter and the physician on duty indicates that the cause of death is cardiac arrest. This is not a cause, however, and has no place on a death certificate. Coronary artery disease is a reasonable cause of death, whereas cardiac arrest is not a cause at all but a mechanism. In fact, the latest death certificates specifically state *"do not enter cause of death as cardiac or respiratory arrest, shock or heart failure,"* but this continues to be done.

Most deaths that occur in hospitals or long-term care facilities (e.g., nursing homes) are explained or expected because of age and/or disease and are classified as natural deaths. These deaths are exempt from investigation by a legal agency and are routinely handled by the attending physician, who is willing to certify the death due to natural causes. Often deaths that are expected may be unexplained by pathology and remain inconclusive in the investigation of the medical diagnosis. By definition, sudden death implies that death was not expected. Sudden natural death primarily involves three vital systems: cardiovascular, respiratory, and the central nervous system. The term *sudden death* commonly means deaths occurring in less than 5 minutes, frequently with instantaneous immobility.[6] In the absence of suspicion, unexpected deaths should fall within the jurisdiction of the medical examiner/coroner if no recent medical attention for a natural disease is documented. In contrast, unexpected deaths that are unnatural may include trauma, either intentional or unintentional; suicide, self-inflicted injury with the intention of taking one's own life; and homicide (injury inflicted by another with intention to kill); these require reporting to a legal agency. If death occurs during medical treatment attended by a physician, these cases are still notifiable because of the circumstances of the death. Sudden and unexpected death inevitably brings with it victims by extension—the decedents' family, partners, friends, and colleagues. When an act of random violence suddenly and unexpectedly takes an innocent life, the family is in a state of shock and denial and may look to the nurse to identify and define reality. An autopsy is generally unavoidable in these cases. The law requires the medical examiner to take charge of the body. Forensic nurses serving as medical examiner investigators at the scene of death help facilitate the correlation between the investigative agencies, health care evaluation, and the community at large.

Anatomic Gifts: A Vital Link to Life

Death is difficult under any circumstances for the family of a potential donor. There is a need for the survivors (the victims by extension) to transform a tragic loss into a positive outcome through the anatomic gift of life. Multiple organ and tissue recovery for transplantation is recognized as a vital aspect of trauma care. Knowledge of the legal framework of organ donation, familiarity with brain death criteria, and confident skills in required consent request are areas in which the forensic nurse can make a significant difference. When the

163

patient dies, death is impending, or brain death is impending or declared, the donor candidacy status must be considered and evaluated. In determining eligibility for organ/tissue donation (solid organs, eyes, bone, skin), the legal disposition of the body must first be defined, and consent for donation by the family must be obtained. Determining the *legal* status of the case, as well as obtaining consent, is generally the responsibility of the nursing staff. This can become a difficult situation for most nurses who may feel that this task is an intrusion during a period of great personal turmoil and crisis. The immediate postdeath period in cases of sudden death are stressful both for the grieving family and for the nurse involved in direct communication regarding anatomic gifts. This situation calls for expertise in both crisis counseling and medicolegal issues. The nurse must meet the legal requirements and at the same time provide emotional support to the grieving family.

Nationwide, over 31,000 people await lifesaving or life-enhancing organ transplants. According to recent studies, only 14,000 organs from 4,500 donors are available annually.[25a] A significant proportion of states now require hospital staffs to ask for organ-tissue donations when a patient dies under certain circumstances. Nurses often find the immediate postdeath period a mentally strenuous and emotionally charged situation, not only for the family but also for themselves, because it is their responsibility to seek anatomical consent. Many nurses have ambivalent feelings about the appropriateness of this intrusion on the family during a period of great personal grief. Many have personal misgivings about dealing with the turmoil of death and lack confidence in their ability to tactfully communicate the appropriate information. In systems where regional Organ Procurement Organizations (OPO) are designated by law to work with specific hospitals, the agency provides a transplant coordinator who assumes full responsibility for requesting and coordinating the anatomical recovery. The Organ Transplant Coordinator (OTC) is a nurse skilled in specific areas, such as determination of candidacy for organ donation, restrictions, cultural or religious beliefs, and the legality of administrative procedures. Legal requirements in a case of sudden and unexpected death provide the state or county medical examiner/ coroner with the ultimate jurisdiction over the body. With the increased emphasis on procurement of tissue and organs, however, a conflict between the officiator of death and the organ/ tissue transplant coordinator is emerging. Previously, no forensic death case could be processed without going through the proper channels, which detail necessary medicolegal protocol. Recently, laws have been passed that give the organ transplant coordinator greater access to patients who are potential candidates for procuring tissue and solid organs. This identified conflict has created a lack of coordination, resulting in a breakdown in the system. A comparative analysis of the medical examiner/coroner cases that were denied release for procurement indicated that as many as 2,979 people were denied transplants from 1990 to 1992.

To avoid any potential conflicts of interest and meet the needs of the grieving and bereaved, the indoctrination of the OTC in forensic nursing will allow for the designation of a forensic transplantation specialist. This liaison will be skilled in the scientific investigation of injury and death, and the collection and preservation of evidence, and could act as clinical investigator, representing the medical examiner/coroner in much the same way that hospice nurses in certain jurisdictions are deputized and act as investigators at the time of an anticipated death. The Joint Commission on Accreditation for Health Care Organization's guidelines have specific standards for specially trained members of the bioethics staff to act as counselors for the families of potential donors and to interact with the appropriate agencies. Many health care facilities are ill-equipped to establish the appropriate criteria and to address the educational needs of the staff. A forensic nurse transplantation specialist will be an ideally qualified clinician to ensure compliance with these requirements. This specialist, in an advanced nursing practice role at the administrative level, will be in a position to coordinate the legality of organ donor matters. As an expert in legal issues and with sensitivity to the deceased's family, a forensic nurse can be used (1) to provide consultation as necessary, (2) to foster staff education, and (3) to perform immediate interventions in the emergency department setting. As a nurse manager, the forensic nurse position can provide an opportunity to create or to advance existing protocol with greater emphasis on the coordination and cooperation between organ/tissue procurement and the medical examiner/coroner system.

If the system is properly organized, everyone will benefit. The medical examiner/coroner will acquire more diagnostic information and will no longer have reason to fear loss of evidence through the removal of tissues and organs. In an ideal system, forensic documentation begins before the official pronouncement of death, when features of injury are being recorded that otherwise would have been overlooked or lost. As a result, more tissue and organs will be released by the medicolegal authorities. With the growing need for anatomic gifts to meet the demands of medical science, recipients and legal protocol require mutual consideration. The forensic nurse liaison represents a comprehensive action plan that will build an effective alliance between the regional OPO and local officiators of death. This plan will protect forensically significant evidence, provide more complete clinical data, and establish collaborative strategies that can increase the availability of transplantable organs.

Managing the Psychological Impact of Death

With increasing frequency, the nurse is the one who must tell the family that their loved one has died. In this area, forensic nurses have made a significant contribution, often out of necessity, as grief counselors and crisis intervenors acting in the absence of designated professionals.[14-17] Forensic nursing education and experience provide a level of confidence in the nurse who becomes responsible for notification of death. The principles and philosophies of forensic nursing focus on the extended family, providing an empathic approach to catastrophic death trauma.

The murder of a child is probably the most tragic crime in our society. The psychological wounds inflicted on survivors often leave indelible marks. When the shock of death of one's child is compounded by murder, the parental reaction to the notification of death is frequently to be overwhelmed; the scenario often remains the focus of nightmares and flashbacks. Murder brings involvement with the medical examiner, police, district attorney, judicial system, and media into the lives of ordinary people. As professionals in the field of death investigation, we have a responsibility to try to minimize emotional trauma.

Prevention as an Antiviolence Strategy

A major principle of forensic nursing that parallels that of generic nursing is prevention. By educating nurses to think more about the legal issues surrounding patient care and to have a working knowledge of forensic responsibilities, the health care system will be able to provide a proactive approach. By implementing health care policies and practices that address forensic issues in nursing education, critical differences will be effected in the prevention of a vast number of cases of child abuse and crimes against women and the elderly. These will assist law enforcement in meeting the objectives of criminal investigation. Forensic nurses endorse and participate in public education programs that focus on preventable injuries that impose an unnecessary burden on the system involving trauma care and the law, such as liability-related injuries resulting from domestic violence, drunk driving, and inadequate automobile and bicycle safety. These cases generally involve a variety of specialists to interpret the law, identify the trauma, define a treatment plan, analyze the evidence, and determine the outcome of the trial. Forensic nurses' responsibility to the law and legal agencies, as well as to the crime laboratory technicians and the public at large, include contributions to the prevention of similar injuries, illness, and death in the future. Establishing formal education programs in this advanced nursing practice role will help to confront violence in our society and to alleviate human suffering resulting from this national health problem.

Pilot programs to educate nurses and other health care professionals to work in synthesis with law enforcement and forensic sciences experts must continue to be developed and implemented. To provide adequate education and scope of practice for the forensic nursing specialists, we must first recognize the combination of knowledge required to go beyond the treatment of symptoms and injuries and to fill a greater role in medicolegal expertise. The first residency-based clinical forensic medical training program and fellowship has been established in the United States.[27] The University of Louisville School of Medicine in Louisville, Kentucky, has made a commitment to provide a resource in these medicolegal issues. A course in clinical forensic medicine will result in a specialist jointly trained in forensic medicine and emergency medicine. This forensic specialist in clinical medicine will become the designated physician in the treatment of crime victims and/or perpetrators of criminal acts and all liability-related cases in emergency medicine.

The clinical forensic nurse is a vital component of clinical forensic practice because of the small number of physicians currently involved in this new medical program, which is to provide health care's first line of defense against violence. The physicians who developed this program support and encourage the development of the role of forensic nurse. This approach makes intuitive sense considering that the nurse is most frequently the first person to see the patient (often the first to identify the patient as a crime victim), come in contact with the evidence, make the documentation that will be used in a court of law, and contact the grieving family. It is important both to the professional development of nursing and to enhancement of the care of our society's most vulnerable citizens to continually update and validate the knowledge and skills required for quality trauma care. Legislation is currently being implemented in several states that provides registered nurses with the legal authority to pronounce death and provide sexual assault examinations. Owing to the vast number of nurses required to provide expert witness testimony in court, nurses are seeking out sources for education and experience that will provide them with the essential skills necessary to assist them in meeting these new challenges and demands on their expertise.

A proactive protocol for preventive practice emphasizes the importance of establishing and training a professional staff in the philosophy of clinical forensic practice. This should begin with emergency interventions. Clinical forensic education for emergency department nurses encompasses the following subjects: forensic photography; jurisprudence; interpretation of blunt, sharp, or fast (e.g., gunshot) trauma; bite mark interpretation and analysis; psychological abuse of the elderly and of children; sexual abuse and rape; physical child abuse and neglect; drug abuse; psychological and physiologic abuse from occult and/or religious practices; and tissue and organ donation.

Future Horizons in Clinical Forensic Nursing

Challenges for nurses in the clinical arena provide unique opportunities to make valuable contributions to forensic practice as they manage problems commonly encountered in the investigation of trauma. Areas of major importance include those that require specific nursing assessment and evaluation; such as social changes affecting public health and safety; manufacture of unsafe products; environmental hazards; negligence in diagnosis and failure to refer; adequate records; informed consent; legal obligations; methods of evidence recovery and preservation; chain of custody or possession; and definition of professional responsibility in forensic cases.

As we enter the next decade of nursing practice, forensic nursing will be well-established. With the increasing emphasis on the forensic nursing paradigm as one strategic step to break the pattern of cyclical, interpersonal violence, it is perceived that forensic nursing will become equally important to other standard specialties. Those who understand the need for a forensic specialist in nursing believe that it is realistic to expect that JCAHO will eventually lead to every hospital of a certain trauma level to have a forensically educated nurse on staff to ensure that mandates and needs are met with reasonable certainty.

New Responsibilities

Sexual violence is an area in which occupational opportunities and new roles are rapidly developing in clinical forensic nursing. As long as interpersonal violence continues to be defined as a contemporary health crisis, the need for broader solutions, intervention, and identification of these victims requires a team approach. Constructive action involving nursing, law, and forensic science provides an innovative approach to the investigation of both fatal and nonfatal trauma. Recent studies identify interpersonal violence, often involving sexual assault, as a prevalent crime against women and children. The National Victim Center recently released the results of a major study on sexual assault victimization conducted through interview and survey research. This study, summarized in a report entitled *Rape in America*,[12a] indicated that the actual rape rate in the United States may be four to five times higher than the National Crime Survey victimization reports, and over six and a half times higher than the Uniform Crime Reports disclosure of rapes reported to police. Rapes reported to the police are increasing steadily (from 22.3 per 100,000 population in 1972 to 42.8 in 1992), and indications are that this upward reporting trend will continue. Owing to increased workload on hospital emergency departments and downsizing of staff, forensic nurses, as independent contractors, are providing essential services. Forensic specialists in nursing provide sexual assault examinations for adult and pediatric victims, suspect examinations, evaluation of physical battery and neglect in children, battered women, elder abuse, wellness examinations for juvenile courts, and gynecologic consultations in suspected abuse cases. Currently, forensic nurse examiners have expanded these services to include postmortem examination of deceased persons in suspected sexual assault cases under the direction of a forensic pathologist.

Forensic nurses also provide enhanced services in sexual assault investigations that previously were unavailable by traditional means in the clinical setting, at the scene, or at autopsy. These services includes technical advances in the use of colposcopic examination, chemical markers, alternative light sources, and other modern techniques in forensic gynecologic examination and evidence collection. Expert witness testimony by forensic nurse specialists has become generally accepted and contributes to the overall team effort to identify and minimize interpersonal violence. The precedence for the inclusion of nurses in postmortem evaluation and investigation has been established and recognized by child death review committees across the United States.

Recent trends in the investigation of rape/ homicide cases indicates a movement among law enforcement agencies and forensic pathologists to support the role of nurse sexual assault examiners in assisting with forensic investigation at the crime scene and examination in the autopsy laboratory prior to postmortem procedures.[18] Postmortem findings indicative of force in victims who die under suspicious circumstances continue to be problematic for prosecutors when no magnification, chemical application, and/or alternative light sources are used to identify and interpret microtrauma at autopsy. For example, the use of toluidine blue, a dye that will stain the nucleated squamous cells in deep layers of exposed epidermis to document microtrauma resulting from forced sexual activity, is being recognized as a valuable tool in helping to rule out or confirm evidence of sexual abuse.[3] Forensic nurses providing postmortem sexual assault examinations need to remain aware of the most recent studies in the detection of genital, perineal, and anal lacerations in the deceased victim at autopsy. Examiners must be knowledgeable of postmortem conditions that may be confused with sexual trauma. The effective examination of sexual assault trauma in both living and deceased patients is a complex process that requires the combined expertise of a variety of professionals, including forensic pathologists, experienced law enforcement investigators, forensic nurse specialists, toxicologists, and criminalists. It is imperative that these professionals cooperate and coordinate their efforts as they work together in the service of social justice.

New Roles

A contemporary role in forensic nursing that is being recognized as a new occupational opportunity is that of independent contractor in forensic services. Western Nurse Specialists, Inc. (WNS)[2] is an example of this innovative approach. WNS is a privately owned corporation formed by nurses who serve law enforcement agencies in gathering forensic evidence. WNS also helps to advance nursing science in the forensic arena through their Institute of Forensic Studies in Nursing Education and Research. The WNS center, a research and evidence collection facility, contracts with police agencies to gather genetic evidence (biomedical specimens; such as blood, semen, tissue, hair, saliva) and other trace and physical evidence in cases of crime-related interpersonal violence.

WNS operates five Sexual Assault Response Team (SART) sites in California and recently opened the first privately owned sexual assault examination center in the United States. WNS has been based in Redlands, California, since 1990, is an independent contractor of forensic services provided by nurses to 70 law enforcement agencies. These services include the collection of blood-alcohol samples and urine drug screen materials, removal of taser darts, conduction of prebooking examinations, collection of reference samples from sexual assault suspects, and provision of on-call service 24 hours a day to document and preserve evidence from victims and perpetrators of sexual assault and domestic violence. When contacted by the police, WNS sends out a team of phlebotomists (blood extraction specialists) to the scene to collect the evidence from suspects in custody. The victims are transported to the examination center.

Each site has the equipment and supplies necessary to complete a detailed evidentiary examination of patients associated with sexual assault, battering, and abuse. These facilities employ 75 forensic technicians and nurses specifically skilled in the evaluation of trauma associated with forced sexual contact and maintain the state-of-the-art equipment necessary to document and preserve necessary evidence. These SART sites provide a one-stop specialized, dedicated center for rapid, sensitive examination and treatment of the client, prescription of medication, and collection of evidence. Each sexual assault examiner is a registered nurse educated in the forensic sciences, skilled in forensic techniques, and qualified as an expert witness in court. Forensic nurse examiners are responsible for case management of sexual abuse victims in coordination with police and rape crisis centers.

WNS maintains a comprehensive quality assurance program and is continually exploring avenues of advancement in contemporary technology. WNS forensic nursing specialists practice under the guidelines established by the Office of Criminal Justice Planning for the State of California. The center employs a Director of Clinical Forensic Medicine, who validates the nurse's forensic technique for quality assurance, consults when complex medical management problems occur, and provides direct patient care, when appropriate. The comprehensive preparation of each WNS nurse requires an intensive curriculum in medicolegal examination and instruction and competency in the use of the colposcope (a binocular microscope with variable magnification and photographic capability used to document microscopic genital abrasions).

The WNS research center is equipped with state-of-the-art technology, including a colposcope that can transmit images onto a color monitor, a camera, or via telephone lines to a monitor in a courtroom or even a hospital in another state. The new facility also has a lightstaining microscope designed to enhance the image of sperm and make it easier to detect. Studies published in the *Annals of Emergency Medicine* noted a significant correlation between successful prosecution and presence of physical findings, making colposcopic photo-documentation an essential component of effective examinations.[25] This center for research and education in forensic studies will provide the foundation for scientific advancement through nursing. The Institute will provide a renowned faculty of national and international forensic experts to teach the most current advances in the investigation of crime-related trauma and human behavior, as well as to demonstrate the latest technological developments in science that will help insure total quality management of victims and perpetrators of interpersonal violence. This facility will also serve as a research center for nurses and other forensic specialists to implement studies using the WNS database to create recommendations for changes in outdated or inadequate protocols involving health care and the law.

A private facility permits victims and law enforcement officers to circumvent the hospital emergency department, thus avoiding the hassles and delays often encountered in that setting. Furthermore, most emergency personnel often lack the time, equipment, or training to gather evidence necessary for a consultation. An added benefit is that physicians and emergency department staff, who are faced with increasing numbers of acute medical problems, are spared the additional burden of a lengthy evaluation and continuing responsibility of litigation associated with forensic cases. Police officers are out of circulation for a shorter period and can usually avoid the hospital emergency altogether. A private facility provides timely and sensitive examinations, which decrease the stress and humiliation of the experience for the victim. Thus, this comprehensive method contributes not only to the efficiency and effectiveness of forensic science but also encourages victims to report sexual offenses with confidence that they will be accorded justice through a thorough and empathic system.

Counties that subscribe to forensic nurse examiners find that public prosecutors advocate the use of forensic nurses to facilitate sexual assault prosecution.[2] Physical evidence that is unequivocally documented and clearly presented is generally not contested in court and results in a plea of guilt and an average annual savings of $40,000 per case in court cost to the prosecution.[2] Currently, WNS also operates in specially designated spaces at four other sites in Southern California. These SARTs and the preceptorship programs with didactic and internship components provide a model program that will be replicated throughout the United States, as well as internationally.

The traditional lack of comprehensive forensic instruction in schools of nursing has contributed significantly to the current situation in which there are large numbers of hospitals in which cases of liability-related injuries and deaths are inadequately and improperly investigated and treated. This is evident from recent headlines in the news media and has resulted in increased awareness of the need for the application of forensic science to the investigation of trauma associated with violence. In clinical cases as well as in the community arena, the subtle indications of pernicious human behavior require an investigation of the kind and depth necessary in an increasingly complex society. Today, large trauma centers are placing a major emphasis on professional skills in forensic issues and work in direct coordination with the Medical Examiner's office in establishing forensic protocol and procedures. Ryder Trauma Center in Miami, Florida, has an exemplar relationship with the Dade County Medical Examiner Department (Joseph Davis, personal communication, 1994). They have implemented a conjoint program between clinical cases and questioned deaths. With increasing focus on the forensic aspects of trauma, schools of nursing are responding with formal and informal arrangements for education and clinical experiences that incorporate forensic science, death investigation, criminal law, court procedures, and testimony, as well as an exploration of new roles, new responsibilities, and new occupational opportunities for nurses in these violent times. Professional knowledge that qualifies nurses to undertake medicolegal work continues to expand the boundaries of nursing beyond tradition.

Summary

The loss of human life and function due to violence constitutes a phenomenon that affects millions of patients annually. Society demands an investigation of trauma associated with criminal activity. No longer is it acceptable for health care professionals to operate in isolation of forensic philosophies and principles. It is assumed that the individuals responsible for the performance of the examination of forensic victims have the necessary basic education, experience, and skills. Health care professionals involved in the initial response to these victims, either at the scene or in the emergency department, are faced with unique problems as social changes require continual reevaluation of standards and professional responsibility.

As we enter a new era of nursing practice, forensic nursing is recognized as the most significant contemporary phase of nursing education, practice, and research as we prepare for critical issues in health care in the twenty-first century. Increasingly, nurses have an expanded role to play in the investigation of trauma, deaths, and crimes. In areas of the country where no medical examiner system exists and the clinical forensic physician has not yet been established, the forensic nurse may be the only medicolegal professional available and may be called upon by a variety of legal agencies to consult in cases of child abuse, sexual assault, elder abuse, and suspicious deaths. It must be emphasized that the objectives of the forensic nurse are not necessarily the same as those of law enforcement personnel but parallel them in a common perspective from a multidisciplinary approach. The nurse, physician, police, attorneys, and social services, therefore, should work together as a team and combine expertise to observe, document, and record all pertinent findings and ensure the acquisition and retention of all specimens in cooperation with the wider network of experts necessary to the resolution of the case in question.

The forensic nursing role has been expressly designed to provide solutions to some of the most urgent concerns in our society. Forensic nursing focuses on the areas in which medicine, nursing, and human behavior interface with the law. Existing problems are great and multifaceted and call for new solutions. The application of forensic science to contemporary nursing practice reveals a wider role in the investigation of crime and the legal process that contributes to public health and safety. The responsibility of the forensic nurse is to provide continuity of care from the health care institution or the crime scene to courts of law . . . from trauma to trial.

References

1. J. Barber, "Frontiers and Challenges in Critical Care: Foreword," *Critical Care Nursing Quarterly* 14: 3 (1991).

2. F. Battiste-Otto, "Aiding Justice: Forensic RNs Combine Nursing and Criminal Sciences," (abstr D 42). In Proceedings of the 47th Annual Meeting of the American Academy of Forensic Sciences, Seattle, 1995.

3. J. Bays and L. Lewman, "Toluidine Blue in the Detection of Autopsy of Perineal and Anal Lacerations in Victims of Sexual Abuses," *Archives of Pathology Laboratory Medicine* 11 (6): 620-1 (1992).

4. S. Birk, "Emerging Specialties: Expanded Opportunities," *American Nurse* 24: 7-9 (1992).

5. Brigham and Women's Hospital, *Know What the Insiders Know—Domestic Violence: A Manual for Healthcare Providers* (Boston: Brigham and Women's Hospital, 1994).

6. J. Butt, *Sudden Death and Police Investigation,* 2nd ed. (Calgary, 1993).

7. J. Duval, "Role of the Forensic Nursing Specialist in an Urban Trauma Center" (abstr D 44). In Proceedings of the 47th Annual Meeting of the American Academy of Forensic Sciences, Seattle, 1995.

8. W. Eckert, et al., "Clinical Forensic Medicine," *American Journal of Forensic Medical Pathology* 7: 182-5 (1986).

9. D. Filer and L. Filer, "Whither or Wither Forensic in the United Kingdom," (abstr 33). Programs and Abstracts of the 3rd World Meeting of Police Medical Officers, Harrogate, England, 1993.

10. A. Freeman, "Gunshot Wounds: Initial Assessment and Management," *Australian Nurses Journal* 10: 40-5 (1980).

11. M. Jezierski, "Abuse of Women by Male Partners: Basic Knowledge for Emergency Nurses," *Journal of Emergency Nursing* 20: 5 (1994).

12. Joint Commission on Accreditation of Health Care Organizations (JCAHO), *AMH Accreditation Manual for Hospitals* (Oakbrook Terrace, IL: JCAHO, 1995).

12a. D. Kirkpatrick, N. Edmunds, and A. Seymour, *Rape in America: A Report to the Nation,* [April 1992, National Victims Center, Arlington] (Charleston, SC: Crime Victims Research and Treatment Center, 1992).

12b. C. Koop, "President and Surgeon General Condemn Violence against Women, Call for New Attitudes, Programs," *National Organization Victims' Assistance Newsletter* 13 (1989).

13. K. Kopser, et al., "Successful Collaboration within an Integrative Practice Model," *Journal for Advanced Nursing Practice* 8: 6 (1994).

13a. D. Lee, et al., *California Hospital Emergency Department Response to Domestic Violence Survey Report* (San Francisco: Family Violence Prevention Fund, 1993).

14. V. Lynch, "Biomedical Investigation as a Mental Health Nursing Role," In *Adult Psychiatric Nursing,* 3rd ed., edited by J. Lancaster (New Hyde Park, NY: Medical Examination Publishing Co., 1988).

15. ———, "Forensic Nursing in the Emergency Department: A New Role for the 1990s," *Critical Care Nursing Quarterly* 14: 3 (1991).

16. ———, "Forensic Nursing: Diversity in Education and Practice." *Journal of Psychosocial Nursing and Mental Health Services* 31: 11 (1993).

17. ———, "Forensic Aspects of Health Care: New Roles, New Responsibilities." *Journal of Psychosocial Nursing and Mental Health Services* 31: 11 (1993).

18. ———, "Role of the Forensic Nurse Specialist in the Identification of Sexual Assault Trauma," (abstr D 43). In Proceedings of the 47th Annual Meeting of the American Academy of Forensic Sciences, Seattle, 1995.

19. F. McFarland, et al., "Assessing for Abuse during Pregnancy," *Journal of the American Medical Association* 261: 3176-8 (1993).

20. H. MacNamara, *Living Forensics* (seminar pamphlet) (Ulster County, NY: Office of the Medical Examiner, 1986).

21. J. Manon, "The Nurse Entrepreneur: How to Innovate from Within," *American Journal of Nursing* 1: 1 (1994).

22. T. Marsh, "A Nurse's Guide to Sleuthing (Or, How to Collect Evidence, Hospital Style)," *RN* 41: 48-50 (1978).

23. R. Mittleman, H. Goldberg, and D. Waksman, "Preserving Evidence in the Emergency Department," *American Journal of Nursing* 83: 1652-6 (1983).

24. J. Neff and P. Kidd, *Trauma Nursing: The Art and the Science* (Chicago: Mosby-Year Book, 1993).

25. B. Rambo, "Female Sexual Assault: Medical and Legal Implications," *Annals of Emergency Medicine* 21: 727 (1992).

25a. T. Shafer, et al., "Impact of Medical Examiner/Coroner Practices on Organ Recovery in the United States," *Journal of the American Medical Association* 261: 23-30 (1994).

26. C. Schramm, "Forensic Medicine: What the Perioperative Nurse Needs to Know," *American Operating Room Nursing Journal* 53: 3 (1991).

27. W. Smock, G. Nichols, and P. Fuller, "Development and Implementation of the First Clinical Forensic Medicine Training Program," *Journal of Forensic Sciences* 38: 4 (1993).

28. W. Smock, C. Ross, and F. Hamilton, "Clinical Forensic Medicine: How ED Physicians Can Help with the Sleuthing," *American Health Consultants* 5: 1 (1994).

29. C. Stewart, "Nursing Management of Gunshot Wounds to the Head," *Journal of Neurosurgical Nursing* 15: 5 (1983).

30. C. Swanson, N. Chamelin, and L. Territo, *Criminal Investigation,* 6th ed. (New York: McGraw-Hill, 1995).

30a. The American Trauma Society, *Domestic Violence: Battered Women, Children, and Elders* [booklet] (Upper Marlboro, MD: The American Trauma Society, 1993).

31. K. White, "Clinical and Medico-Legal Considerations in the Management of Gunshot Wounds," *Critical Care Update* 7: 12 (1980).

—by Virginia A. Lynch, M.S.N., R.N., FAAFS

Chapter 18

Forensic Anthropology

Introduction

Forensic anthropology, a subdiscipline of Physical Anthropology, applies a foundation of physical anthropology and, specifically, skeletal anatomy to medicolegal death investigation. The forensic anthropologist brings together an appreciation for human variation at the population and individual levels, a knowledge of skeletal trauma and practical experience in methods of identification as they relate to death investigation. A practicing forensic anthropologist should have an advanced degree in anthropology and practical case experience. Forensic anthropologists who have met certain requirements and have passed an exam are certified as Diplomates of the American Board of Forensic Anthropology. Although not necessary to practice in this field, this certification helps to give credibility, especially for cases in which testifying before a jury is necessary.

Medical examiners, coroners, and law enforcement utilize the forensic anthropologist for cases involving skeletal, mummified, decomposed, burned, and unidentified human remains. The forensic anthropologist is called upon to generate a biological profile of the decedent, establish positive identification through comparative radiography, estimate postmortem interval, and determine the extent of

From "Forensic Anthropology," October 1998. Produced by Carrie M. Weiler, B.A., and Katherine M. Taylor, M.A., King County Medical Examiner's Office, 325 9th Ave., Seattle, WA 98104. For complete contact information, please refer to Chapter 56, "Resources." Reprinted with permission.

179

skeletal trauma as it relates to the cause of death. In addition, their expertise in recognition of human remains and factors affecting decomposition make them an invaluable asset to a search and recovery effort.

Biological Profile

The forensic anthropologist is most called upon to develop a biological profile for unidentified remains. First and foremost is to determine whether the remains are human or nonhuman. Many skeletal remains reported to law enforcement agencies turn out to be of non-human origin. Once the forensic anthropologist has established that the remains are human, a biological profile can be developed. This profile can then be compared to records of missing persons to establish or confirm identification.

A biological profile includes the age, sex, race, stature, and osseous anomalies or pathologies of the human remains. Each of these characteristics is determined by recording both metric measurements and nonmetric (discrete) traits observed during examination of the human skeleton. Determination of characteristics such as age, sex, race, and stature is based on previous studies of known individuals. These studies allow the forensic anthropologist to make predictions regarding an unknown individual. However, systematic characteristics do not make for a positive identification. Individual identification will be based on idiosyncratic traits of the skeleton such as osseous anomalies and pathologies resulting from the effects of disease, trauma, and factors effecting growth and nutrition.

Predictions made while developing a biological profile can not take into account random, unknown factors that may have influenced the development of an individual. Therefore, many traits such as age and stature require that a certain amount of error be taken into account. By giving an appropriate range, the forensic anthropologist takes into account the variation within a population and avoids excluding individuals who may be potential candidates for comparison and positive identification. In addition to providing ranges, error can be minimized by using many different traits and methods to support a prediction.

When human remains are brought in for analysis, it is necessary to have as complete a skeleton as possible. Certain elements of the skeleton are more diagnostic depending on which characteristic is being predicted. Skeletal differences between males and females (sexual dimorphism) are most apparent in the structure of the pelvis. Cranial characteristics can also lend themselves to determination of sex, but are not as reliable as differences in pelvic morphology for making predictions. In addition, differences in the size of long bones exist and reflect the basic premise that males are larger in body mass than females. All of the characteristics used to determine sex are secondary sex characteristics and are thus not present until after puberty. It is therefore, impossible to determine the sex of immature skeletal material.

While sex is indeterminate in immature skeletal material, determining age at death for a child is more precise due to the known timing and sequence of growth events. Bones of the body complete growth at different but known times throughout their development. Similarly, eruption patterns have been determined for both permanent and deciduous human dentition through previous scientific studies. Thus, assessment of the stage of growth for different skeletal elements and documentation of dental development facilitate a fairly accurate prediction of age at death of a child.

Aging the adult human skeleton is more difficult due to the lack of systematic and successive changes taking place once we stop growing. Degenerative changes at joint surfaces can provide a rough idea of the age at death of an individual. Examination of the pelvic, cranial, and rib bones can also lead to an estimate of age. However, due to the enormous variation caused by different lifestyles, disease, nutrition, and environmental factors, age at death for adults is usually given in a wide range. A median age may be assigned, but the larger range assures that no one possibly fitting the description is mistakenly excluded. In cases when the most diagnostic bones are missing, age may be categorized as simply young adult, middle adult, and older adult.

Determination of race or ancestry is the most problematic task undertaken by the forensic anthropologist. For the purposes of death investigation, four groups are recognized by the forensic anthropologist and correspond to Native American, European, Asian, and African ancestry. The traits used, predominantly cranial characteristics, are recognized to occur in greatest frequency among individuals of similar ancestral continental origin. These traits, however, are not exclusive to individuals of specific ancestral continental origin, and therefore determination of race is most reliable when based on a large number of characteristics. In truth, there are more similarities between these populations than there are differences. Conventionally, anthropologists do not attempt to divide the human global population into distinct racial groups. However, in order to reconcile the tenants of anthropology with the demands of law enforcement, the forensic anthropologist must recognize skeletal race.

The purpose of the biological profile is to narrow the search for the identity of an unknown individual. Once a likely candidate is unearthed, either through investigation or missing persons, antemortem (before death) records must be found to facilitate positive identification.

Identification

Traditional methods of positive identification include visual identification, photographic comparison, and fingerprint analysis. Although fingerprint analysis is by far the most scientific, the method relies upon the deceased individual having been fingerprinted while alive. This is not always the case, and hence necessitates additional means of identification. Similarly, the condition of the body may negate the use of photographic or visual identification. In cases in which the traditional means of identification are unavailable, a coroner or medical examiner relies upon a radiographic (x-ray) comparison, either dental or medical, to identify a deceased individual.

Comparative dental radiography, often performed by a forensic odontologist, involves a comparison of antemortem to postmortem (after death) dental radiographs. Features that are used to make identification include dental restorations (fillings, crowns, root canals), crown and root morphology, and the overall positioning of the teeth relative to one another. While the presence of dental work provides the most obvious and useful markers of comparison, positive identification can be obtained from dental radiographic analysis in the absence of any dental restorations. Dental radiographic comparison is an accurate and scientific means of positive identification.

Often, dental radiographs are not available, either because the deceased individual did not have recent dental care or because no one associated with the decedent is able to provide the name of a dentist. In these cases, medical radiographs are sought. These may include radiographs of any part of the body that is also present postmortem. Cranial x-rays, for example, may feature the frontal sinus, a space in the frontal bone above the eyes which is as unique in size and shape as a fingerprint. Radiographs of the hands and feet are also particularly useful as roughly one quarter of the bones in the adult body are in the hands and one quarter are in the feet. This provides abundant opportunity to observe unique skeletal traits within a single radiograph. Other skeletal indicators include overall bone morphology, size and shape of joint surfaces, stress lines within the bone, osseous anomalies, and osseous pathologies.

Osseous anomalies are unusual bony developments that are present in a fraction of the population and include such things as a sternal foramina (a hole in the breast bone), bifurcated rib ends, or an extra rib, vertebra or tooth. Osseous pathologies include healed fractures and alterations to the bone resulting from disease processes which may include but are not limited to osteoporosis, arthritis, endocrine disorders, and nutritional deficiencies.

In addition to dental and medical radiography, DNA analysis provides a scientific method of positive identification. DNA extracted from the remains of the decedent can either be compared to antemortem samples of the decedent or to samples obtained from living family members. The use of DNA in the identification process is currently restricted by cost and availability of labs that can perform the analysis in a timely manner. The hope is that this method of identification will become more practical and widely used in the future.

Comparative radiography and DNA analysis provide positive identification. However, when antemortem radiographs cannot be located or do not exist, and DNA analysis is impractical, investigators may choose to utilize a method referred to as skull-photo superimposition. This involves superimposing a life size, front on, antemortem photograph of the decedent (preferably smiling) on the skull of the unidentified individual. This is accomplished utilizing computers or audiovisual equipment. Numerous points on the face and cranium are compared to verify correspondence between the photograph and the skull. At best, this method provides circumstantial rather than positive identification, but is useful when all methods of positive identification have been exhausted.

Perhaps the most popularly recognized investigative technique, due to its appearance in television and film, is that of facial reconstruction. In cases in which the identity of skeletal remains is completely unknown and all leads have been pursued, the investigative agency may choose to employ the services of a facial reconstructionist. Facial reconstruction combines scientific and artistic methods to create a visual representation of the decedent. This visual representation is then distributed with the aid of the media in the hope that someone who knew the decedent will recognize the likeness. Although potentially useful, facial reconstruction is an investigative tool, not a means of identification.

Trauma Analysis

A routine aspect of forensic skeletal examination involves trauma analysis; an identification and evaluation of trauma as it relates to the cause of death. Recognition and accurate diagnosis of trauma depends upon a familiarity with osseous defects resulting from gunshots, sharp implements, or blunt force trauma as well as the ability to differentiate such defects from naturally occurring osseous anomalies. For example, on occasion, individuals unfamiliar with skeletal variation have incorrectly identified a sternal foramina as a gunshot wound. Such a mistake yields substantial legal and investigative consequences. In addition, trauma must also be distinguished from postmortem changes.

Perhaps the most diagnostic trauma observed on bone results from the perforation or impact of a high-speed projectile (i.e., a bullet). In flat bones of the cranium, projectiles create a predictable pattern of beveling upon entrance and exit. Entrance wounds are typically internally beveled while exit wounds are externally beveled. This difference allows for the determination of projectile number and direction. In other flat bones of the skeleton such as the sternum, scapula, ilium, and ribs, the same principle applies. The entrance side will usually be smaller in diameter than the exit side of the defect. In addition, the anatomical location of gunshot wounds may indicate the position of the body at the time of the incident. This can be of enormous importance when corroborating witness statements or differentiating between homicide and suicide.

Sharp implement trauma such as that inflicted by knives, swords, axes, and saws can leave distinctive marks on the skeleton. Many times these marks can be very subtle and must be looked for carefully. Carnivore damage can mimic sharp implement trauma and thus microscopic analysis may be necessary to differentiate the two. In addition, microscopic analysis of a cut surface may yield clues as to the type of blade inflicting the trauma. Sharp implement marks can be identified on bone when advanced decomposition has rendered such defects undetectable on soft tissue. Therefore, consultation with a forensic anthropologist is particularly important when the body is decomposed and the cause of death not readily apparent.

Many weapons can be used to inflict blunt force trauma, from a baseball bat, to a hammer, to the handle end of a knife. Bone, more so than soft tissue, provides a resistant surface and therefore, blunt force trauma may be patterned with the size and shape of the defect reflecting the instrument used to inflict it. Evaluation of blunt force trauma to the cranium, for example, can determine the minimum number of blows and may indicate the direction of the blow as well as the type of instrument used. If and when a weapon is recovered, it can be compared to the defect to either rule out or substantiate its use as a possible murder weapon.

Fractures can also be helpful in reconstructing events surrounding death. If skeletal remains are found at the base of a cliff, for example, the obvious question is whether the cause of death is related to a fall. Thus, examination of the bones for trauma consistent with high-speed impact would serve to clarify the cause of death. In addition, it would be necessary to differentiate such trauma from postmortem artifact; damage to the bone after death resulting from environmental forces or animal activity.

When damage to bone is severe, reconstruction of the area of trauma may be necessary to get a full picture of the damage inflicted. This is particularly true for the cranium where small fragments and distortion of the bone may make it difficult to analyze blunt force trauma. A shotgun blast to the head will also fragment the cranium into many pieces making reconstruction necessary to determine entrance and exit. In addition, cases involving multiple traumas may require reconstruction to determine the type and extent of trauma present.

Reconstruction is accomplished by removing all soft tissue from the bone fragments and allowing them to dry. Each piece is then glued together in what is similar to constructing a bony jigsaw puzzle. The cranium is reconstructed most often, but any bone of the skeleton that has suffered trauma may be reconstructed in the same fashion. Although a time-consuming process, reconstruction provides the invaluable ability to reconstruct patterned trauma and can be an essential component of trauma analysis in fresh as well as skeletonized remains.

Determination of Postmortem Interval

The determination of time of death is an essential component of any death investigation. Contrary to what is frequently seen on television, the determination of time of death is not a precise exercise when a death is unattended. The longer the interval between death and the discovery of the body, the more difficult the determination becomes. A forensic anthropologist, familiar with the process of decomposition, can assist a pathologist in determining the approximate time of death. Rates of decomposition can vary depending on environmental factors such as temperature, setting, and whether the body has been wrapped or buried. In skeletal cases, a forensic anthropologist will consider a number of factors including the condition of the bone, evidence of insect activity, extent of soft tissue remaining, and the odor of decomposition to estimate the postmortem interval. Consultation with a forensic entomologist regarding analysis of insect evidence greatly enhances the ability to determine time period since death. The investigating agency is typically very interested in the approximate time of death for several reasons. First and foremost, it provides a search perimeter for utilizing missing person reports in an effort to establish the identification of the decedent. Secondly, in the case of a homicide, knowing the time frame involved allows investigators to better scrutinize a suspect's alibi or whereabouts at the time of the crime. Finally, it allows investigators to piece together the events leading up to the decedent's death.

Search and Recovery

Processing an outdoor crime scene involving the recovery of human remains, either buried or deposited on the surface, presents a unique challenge to law enforcement personnel. The forensic anthropologist can offer law enforcement his or her skills in archaeological methods to maximize the efficiency of the scene investigation and body recovery. For buried remains, this may include locating clandestine graves and the subsequent systematic excavation of the body. Using archaeological methods to excavate allows for the recovery of any and all evidence associated with the burial. In addition, the recognition of tool marks can be useful for identifying the types of tools that may have been used to dig the grave.

In instances of surface deposition, the forensic anthropologist may be the only one capable of recognizing human skeletal remains following decomposition and animal activity. Animal activity may include modification of the bone by chewing, crunching, scraping, or gnawing. Small animals, most notably rodents, will use human hair as nesting material and pull smaller bones into their dens. Large carnivores including cougars, bears, or coyotes will remove parts of the body and distribute them across the landscape. Carnivore activity is further evidenced by the discovery of bone fragments, hair, and clothing appearing in animal feces. Recognizing this animal activity and noting the distribution of skeletal remains is essential in developing an overall picture of what happened to the body after death.

It is worth noting that the forensic anthropologist, although essential, is but one of many specialists necessary for the thorough processing of an outdoor crime scene. These types of cases require a multidisciplinary approach and should include the expertise of an entomologist, botanist, and cadaver dog handler. In some cases, it may be necessary to utilize ground-penetrating radar which can contribute to locating subsurface disturbances.

The skills of the forensic anthropologist that lend themselves so well to outdoor scene investigation are equally beneficial in the processing of the mass disaster scene. Field methodology, ability to recognize human remains in all stages of decomposition, proficiency in trauma analysis, and skills in identification necessitate the inclusion of a forensic anthropologist on any mass disaster team.

Tools of the Trade

The forensic anthropologist has many tools at his or her disposal for observing and measuring traits of human skeletal remains. The most basic of these is the use of standard laboratory procedures when handling human remains. Human skeletal remains should be handled with care, and stored in a wooden box or something similar where they may be kept dry and allowed plenty of circulated air. They should never be left out where they can be damaged or modified. When handling human crania, the forensic anthropologist will often use a bean bag to cradle the skull during analysis. This simple device can prevent accidental rolling or falling from a height and provides stability while measurements are being taken.

Metric measurements are taken using a number of different devices depending on which part of the skeleton is being analyzed. Some measurements of long bones and pelvic bones are taken using an osteometric board. Other metric measurements of all bones are taken using sliding calipers. Measurements of the cranium are taken using spreading calipers which allow for the round shape of the cranium. Dial calipers are used for small measurements of tooth crown and alveolar shapes, and particular measurements of the mandible are done with a mandibulometer.

Statistical analysis is a powerful tool for the forensic anthropologist to use when developing the biological profile. Many scientific studies have been done on all areas of the human skeleton to develop formulas that may be used to predict characteristics such as sex, stature and ancestry. We now have vast collections of bone measurements that have been found to correlate with those attributes needed for the biological profile. These have been developed into tables to which we can compare measurements of an unknown individual. Thus, predictions can be made based on the results of these previous studies.

In the field, the forensic anthropologist uses materials and tools reminiscent of an archaeological excavation. The personal field kit might include rain gear, boots, gloves, trowel, scissors, branch clippers, colored string, small dowels, brushes, tape measure, line level, plumb bob, and various large and small digging implements. Larger hardware might include screens for sifting large amounts of dirt, shovels, stakes, and tarps for protecting scenes in inclement weather. The forensic anthropologist is usually ready to mobilize this equipment with little notice. Being active at the scene creates more opportunity for the recovery of all evidence and efficient closure of the case.

Conclusion

Despite the need for the expertise of a forensic anthropologist in death investigation, there are very few full-time positions in the United States. This discrepancy is due to the varying caseloads across the country and the fact that some law enforcement agencies have yet to recognize the need for this type of specialist. This notwithstanding, practicing forensic anthropologists can be found in four different areas. The most common employment is an academic appointment in a department of anthropology with forensic consultation either privately or through the academic institution. A number of forensic anthropologists can be found in physical anthropology positions at museums where they also consult on cases for law enforcement. Forensic anthropologists employed by military identification laboratories do much of their work overseas recovering and identifying United States military casualties. Recent years have seen an increase in the number of forensic anthropologists found working in medical examiner's offices. This is most likely due to the increased awareness by pathologists of the expertise a forensic anthropologist can bring to death investigation.

Legal council has also recognized the importance of forensic anthropologists, frequently calling upon them to testify in criminal and civil cases. Law enforcement has become more aware of the contribution that can be made by the forensic anthropologist and has increased efforts to consult with one when necessary. Lastly, The American Academy of Forensic Sciences recognizes Physical Anthropology as one of the ten professional disciplines within the academy.

Once thought to be only useful in cases of skeletal remains, the forensic anthropologist is now recognized to be a beneficial resource for determination of postmortem interval, trauma analysis, search and recovery, and the identification of human remains in any and all states of preservation.

—by Carrie M. Weiler, B.A., and Katherine M. Taylor, M.A.

Carrie Weiler received a Bachelor of Arts degree in Anthropology from the University of Washington and plans to pursue a graduate degree in Human Biology. She is currently employed as an Autopsy Assistant at the King County Medical Examiner's Office in Seattle, Washington. She is a student member of the American Academy of Forensic Sciences and editor of the *Young Forensic Scientists Forum* newsletter.

Katherine Taylor received a Master of Arts degree in Anthropology from the University of Arizona and is writing a dissertation to fulfill requirements for a Ph.D. She is currently employed as a Medical Investigator and Forensic Anthropologist at the King County Medical Examiner's Office in Seattle, Washington. She is a member of the American Academy of Forensic Sciences.

Chapter 19

Forensic Toxicology

History of Toxicology

The traditional definition of **toxicology** is "the science of poisons." As our understanding [has grown] of how various agents can cause harm to humans and other organisms, a more descriptive definition of toxicology is "the study of the adverse effects of chemicals or physical agents on living organisms."

These adverse effects may occur in many forms, ranging from immediate death to subtle changes not realized until months or years later. They may occur at various levels within the body, such as an organ, a type of cell, or a specific biochemical. Knowledge of how toxic agents damage the body has progressed along with medical knowledge. It is now known that various observable changes in anatomy or body functions actually result from previously unrecognized changes in specific biochemicals in the body.

The historical development of toxicology began with early cave dwellers who recognized poisonous plants and animals and used their extracts for hunting or in warfare. By 1500 B.C., written recordings indicated that hemlock, opium, arrow poisons, and certain metals were used to poison enemies or for state executions.

From "Toxicology Tutor I," [Online] undated. Available: http://sis.nlm.gov/toxtutr1; produced by the National Library of Medicine; and "The Forensic Sciences Foundation, Inc., Career Brochure," [Online] undated. Available: http://www.aafs.org/career/CareerBroch.html; produced by the Forensic Sciences Foundation, Inc., P.O. Box 669, Colorado Springs, CO 80901-0669. For complete contact information, please refer to Chapter 56, "Resources." Reprinted with permission.

With time, poisons became widely used and with great sophistication. Notable poisoning victims include Socrates, Cleopatra, and [the Roman emperor] Claudius. By the time of the Renaissance and Age of Enlightenment, certain concepts fundamental to toxicology began to take shape. Noteworthy in this regard were the studies of Paracelsus (1500 A.D.) and Orfila (1800 A.D.).

Paracelsus determined that specific chemicals were actually responsible for the toxicity of a plant or animal poison. He also documented that the body's response to those chemicals depended on the dose received. His studies revealed that small doses of a substance might be harmless or beneficial whereas larger doses could be toxic. This is now known as the dose-response relationship, a major concept of toxicology. Paracelsus is often quoted for his statement: "All substances are poisons; there is none which is not a poison. The right dose differentiates a poison and a remedy."

Orfila, a Spanish physician, is often referred to as the founder of toxicology. It was Orfila who first prepared a systematic correlation between the chemical and biological properties of poisons of the time. He demonstrated effects of poisons on specific organs by analyzing autopsy materials for poisons and their associated tissue damage.

The twentieth century is marked by an advanced level of understanding of toxicology. DNA (the molecule of life) and various biochemicals that maintain body functions were discovered. Our level of knowledge of toxic effects on organs and cells is now being revealed at the molecular level. It is recognized that virtually all toxic effects are caused by changes in specific cellular molecules and biochemicals.

Xenobiotic is the general term that is used for a foreign substance taken into the body. It is derived from the Greek term *xeno* which means "foreigner." Xenobiotics may produce beneficial effects (such as a pharmaceutical) or they may be toxic (such as lead).

As Paracelsus proposed centuries ago, dose differentiates whether a substance will be a remedy or a poison. A xenobiotic in small amounts may be nontoxic and even beneficial, but when the dose is increased, toxic and lethal effects may result.

Some examples that illustrate this concept are [shown in Table 19.1.]:

Forensic Toxicology

Forensic toxicology is concerned with the interpretation of analytical, clinical, and environmental data as it applies to law and medicine, often assisting the court (judge/jury) in a truthful decision (Forensic Sciences Foundation, Inc.).

The sophistication of medicine and its ability to cure disease with a "magic drug," combined with the recreational use of alcohol, sets the stage for the practice of polypharmacy by the general population. The toxicologist is often asked to assist emergency room physicians in determining the etiology of the comatose patient, to assist law enforcement officers in determining the cause of unsafe driving (DWI), or to assist the medical examiner in determining the cause of death in chemical/drug related cases.

The first challenge presented to the toxicologist is often the rapid identification of a toxic chemical in a limited sample of blood, urine, or gastric contents. The possibilities appear to be enormous, but with the artful combination of analytical methods, historical knowledge of the patient (often minimal), and knowledge of biological specimens, the dilemma frequently unfolds to resolution within a short time.

Basic Toxicology Terminology

Terminology and definitions for materials that cause toxic effects are not always consistently used in the literature. The most common terms are **toxicant, toxin, poison, toxic agent, toxic substance,** and **toxic chemical.**

Table 19.1. Principles of Clinical Toxicology (T. Gossel and J. Bricker, eds.)

Substance	Nontoxic or Beneficial Dose	Toxic Dose	Lethal Dose
Alcohol *Ethanol Blood Levels*	0.05%	0.1%	0.5%
Carbon Monoxide *% Hemoglobin Bound*	<10%	20-30%	>60%
Secobarbitol *(sleep aid)* *Blood Levels*	0.1mg/dL	0.7mg/dL	>1mg/dL
Aspirin	0.65gm *(2 tablets)*	9.75gm *(30 tablets)*	34gm *(60 tablets)*
Ibuprofin *e.g., Advil & Motrin*	400mg *(2 tablets)*	1,400mg *(7 tablets)*	12,000mg *(60 tablets)*

Toxicant, toxin, and **poison** are often used interchangeably in the literature; however, there are subtle differences as indicated below:

- **Toxicants:** substances that produce adverse biological effects; may be chemical or physical in nature; may be of various types (acute, chronic, etc.)

- **Toxins:** specific proteins produced by living organisms (mushroom toxin or tetanus toxin) most exhibit immediate effects

- **Poisons:** toxicants that cause immediate death or illness when experienced in very small amounts

A **toxic agent** is anything that can produce an adverse biological effect. It may be chemical, physical, or biological in form. For example, **toxic agents** may be chemical (such as cyanide), physical (such as radiation), and biological (such as snake venom).

A distinction is made for diseases due to biological organisms. Those organisms that invade and multiply within the organism and produce their effects by biological activity are not classified as toxic agents. An example of this is a virus that damages cell membranes resulting in cell death.

If the invading organisms excrete chemicals which is the basis for toxicity, the excreted substances are known as **biological toxins.** The organisms in this case are referred to as **toxic organisms.** An example is tetanus. Tetanus is caused by a bacterium, *Clostridium tetani.* The bacteria *C. tetani* itself does not cause disease by invading and destroying cells. Rather, it is a toxin that is excreted by the bacteria that travels to the nervous system (a neurotoxin) that produces the disease.

A **toxic substance** is simply a material which has toxic properties. It may be a discrete toxic chemical or a mixture of toxic chemicals. For example, lead chromate, asbestos, and gasoline are all toxic substances. Lead chromate is a discrete **toxic chemical.** Asbestos is a **toxic material** that does not consist of an exact chemical composition but a variety of fibers and minerals. Gasoline is also a **toxic substance** rather than a toxic chemical in that it contains a mixture of many chemicals. Toxic substances may not always have a constant composition. For example, the composition of gasoline varies with octane level, manufacturer, time of season, etc.

Toxic substances may be organic or inorganic in composition:

- **Organic toxins:** substances that were originally derived from living organisms (thus named organic) contain carbon and often are large molecules can be synthesized (that is, man-made) as well as be obtained from natural sources

- **Inorganic toxins:** specific chemicals that are not derived from living organisms (minerals) generally small molecules consisting of only a few atoms (such as nitrogen dioxide)

Toxic substances may be **systemic toxins** or **organ toxins.**

A **systemic toxin** is one that affects the entire body or many organs rather than a specific site. For example, potassium cyanide is a systemic toxicant in that it affects virtually every cell and organ in the body by interfering with the cell's ability to utilize oxygen.

Toxicants may also affect only specific tissues or organs while not producing damage to the body as a whole. These specific sites are known as the **target organs** or **target tissues:**

- Benzene is a **specific organ toxin** in that it is primarily toxic to the blood-forming tissues.

- Lead is also a specific organ toxin; however, it has three **target organs** (central nervous system, kidney, and hematopoietic system).

A toxicant may affect a specific type of tissue (such as connective tissue) that is present in several organs. The toxic site is then referred to as the **target tissue.**

There are many types of cells in the body and they can be classified in several ways: basic structure (e.g., cuboidal cells); tissue type (e.g, hepatocytes of the liver); germinal cells (e.g., ova and sperm); and somatic cells (e.g., nonreproductive cells of the body).

Germ cells are those cells that are involved in the reproductive process and can give rise to a new organism. They have only a single set of chromosomes peculiar to a specific sex. Male germ cells give rise to sperm and female germ cells develop into ova. Toxicity to germ cells can cause effects on the developing fetus (such as birth defects, abortions).

Somatic cells are all body cells except the reproductive germ cells. They have two sets (or pairs) of chromosomes. Toxicity to somatic cells causes a variety of toxic effects to the exposed individual (such as dermatitis, death, and cancer).

Toxic Effects

Toxicity is complex with many influencing factors; dosage is the most important. Xenobiotics cause many types of toxicity by a variety of mechanisms. Some chemicals are themselves toxic. Others must be metabolized (chemically changed within the body) before they cause toxicity.

Many xenobiotics distribute in the body and often affect only specific **target organs.** Others, however, can damage any cell or tissue that they contact. The target organs that are affected may vary depending on dosage and route of exposure. For example, the target for a chemical after acute exposure may be the nervous system, but after chronic exposure the liver.

Toxicity can result from adverse cellular, biochemical, or macromolecular changes. Examples are:

- cell replacement, such as fibrosis
- damage to an enzyme system
- disruption of protein synthesis
- production of reactive chemicals in cells
- DNA damage

Some xenobiotics may also act indirectly by:

- modification of an essential biochemical function
- interference with nutrition
- alteration of a physiological mechanism

Factors Influencing Toxicity

The toxicity of a substance depends on the following:

- form and innate chemical activity
- dosage, especially dose-time relationship
- exposure route
- species
- age
- sex
- ability to be absorbed
- metabolism
- distribution within the body
- excretion
- presence of other chemicals

The **form** of a substance may have a profound impact on its toxicity especially for metallic elements. For example, the toxicity of mercury vapor differs greatly from methyl mercury. Another example is chromium. Cr^{3+} is relatively nontoxic whereas Cr^{6+} causes skin or nasal corrosion and lung cancer.

The **innate chemical activity** of substances also varies greatly. Some can quickly damage cells causing immediate cell death. Others slowly interfere only with a cell's function. For example:

- hydrogen cyanide binds to cytochrome oxidase resulting in cellular hypoxia and rapid death

- nicotine binds to cholinergic receptors in the central nervous system altering nerve conduction and inducing gradual onset of paralysis

The **dosage** is the most important and critical factor in determining if a substance will be an acute or a chronic toxicant. Virtually all chemicals can be acute toxicants if sufficiently large doses are administered. Often the toxic mechanisms and target organs are different for acute and chronic toxicity. Examples are [shown in Table 19.2.]:

Table 19.2. Toxic Mechanisms/Target Organs

Toxicant	Acute Toxicity	Chronic Toxicity
Ethanol	Central Nervous System Depression	Liver Cirrhosis
Arsenic	Gastrointestinal Damage	Skin/Liver Cancer

Exposure route is important in determining toxicity. Some chemicals may be highly toxic by one route but not by others. Two major reasons are differences in absorption and distribution within the body. For example:

- ingested chemicals, when absorbed from the intestine, distribute first to the liver and may be immediately detoxified

- inhaled toxicants immediately enter the general blood circulation and can distribute throughout the body prior to being detoxified by the liver

Frequently there are different target organs for different routes of exposure.

197

Toxic responses can vary substantially depending on the species. Most species differences are attributable to differences in metabolism. Others may be due to anatomical or physiological differences. For example, rats cannot vomit and expel toxicants before they are absorbed or cause severe irritation, whereas humans and dogs are capable of vomiting.

Selective toxicity refers to species differences in toxicity between two species simultaneously exposed. This is the basis for the effectiveness of pesticides and drugs. Examples are:

- an insecticide is lethal to insects but relatively nontoxic to animals

- antibiotics are selectively toxic to microorganisms while virtually nontoxic to humans

Age may be important in determining the response to toxicants. Some chemicals are more toxic to infants or the elderly than to young adults. For example:

- parathion is more toxic to young animals

- nitrosamines are more carcinogenic to newborn or young animals

Although uncommon, toxic responses can vary depending on **sex.** Examples are:

- male rats are 10 times more sensitive than females to liver damage from DDT

- female rats are twice as sensitive to parathion as male rats

The **ability to be absorbed** is essential for systemic toxicity to occur. Some chemicals are readily absorbed and others poorly absorbed. For example, nearly all alcohols are readily absorbed when ingested, whereas there is virtually no absorption for most polymers. The rates and extent of absorption may vary greatly depending on the form of the chemical and the route of exposure. For example:

- ethanol is readily absorbed from the gastrointestinal tract but poorly absorbed through the skin

- organic mercury is readily absorbed from the gastrointestinal tract; inorganic lead sulfate is not

Metabolism, also known as biotransformation, is a major factor in determining toxicity. The products of metabolism are known as metabolites. There are two types of metabolism—**detoxification** and **bioactivation.** Detoxification is the process by which a xenobiotic is converted to a less toxic form. This is a natural defense mechanism of the organism. Generally the detoxification process converts lipid-soluble compounds to polar compounds. Bioactivation is the process by which a xenobiotic may be converted to more reactive or toxic forms.

The **distribution** of toxicants and toxic metabolites throughout the body ultimately determines the sites where toxicity occurs. A major determinant of whether or not a toxicant will damage cells is its lipid solubility. If a toxicant is lipid-soluble it readily penetrates cell membranes. Many toxicants are stored in the body. Fat tissue, liver, kidney, and bone are the most common storage depots. Blood serves as the main avenue for distribution. Lymph also distributes some materials.

The site and rate of **excretion** is another major factor affecting the toxicity of a xenobiotic. The kidney is the primary excretory organ, followed by the gastrointestinal tract, and the lungs (for gases). Xenobiotics may also be excreted in sweat, tears, and milk.

A large volume of blood serum is filtered through the kidney. Lipid-soluble toxicants are reabsorbed and concentrated in kidney cells. Impaired kidney function causes slower elimination of toxicants and increases their toxic potential.

The **presence of other chemicals** may decrease toxicity **(antagonism)**, add to toxicity **(additivity)**, or increase toxicity **(synergism or potentiation)** of some xenobiotics. For example:

- alcohol may enhance the effect of many antihistamines and sedatives

- antidotes function by antagonizing the toxicity of a poison (atropine counteracts poisoning by organophosphate insecticides)

Toxicity Testing Methods

Knowledge of toxicity is primarily obtained in three ways:

- by the study and observation of people during normal use of a substance or from accidental exposures

- by experimental studies using animals

- by studies using cells (human, animal, plant)

[Refer to Chapter 14 ("Analytical Tools") for information on analytical instruments.]

Interpretation of the results often requires a team effort by combined expertise of a physician, the medical examiner, and a criminalist, or an adversarial judicial process with all opinions based on reasonable scientific probability.

The Role of Government Regulatory Agencies

Most chemicals are now subject to stringent government requirements for safety testing before they can be marketed. This is especially true for pharmaceuticals, food additives, pesticides, and industrial chemicals.

Exposure of the public to inadequately tested drugs or environmental agents has resulted in several notable disasters. Examples include:

- severe toxicity from the use of arsenic to treat syphilis

- deaths from a solvent (ethylene glycol) used in sulfanilamide preparations (one of the first antibiotics)

- thousands of children born with severe birth defects resulting from pregnant women using thalidomide, an anti-nausea medicine

By the mid-twentieth century, disasters were becoming commonplace with the increasing rate of development of new synthetic chemicals. Knowledge of potential toxicity was absent prior to exposures of the general public.

The following federal regulatory agencies were established to assure public safety:

- Food and Drug Administration: for pharmaceuticals, food additives, and medical devices

- Environmental Protection Agency: for agricultural and industrial chemicals released to the environment

- Consumer Product Safety Commission: for toxins present in consumer products

- Department of Transportation: for the shipment of toxic chemicals

- Occupational Safety and Health Administration: for exposure to chemicals in the workplace

Exposure Standards and Guidelines

Exposure standards and guidelines are developed by governments to protect the public from harmful substances and activities that can cause serious health problems.

Exposure standards and guidelines are the products of risk management decisions. Risk assessments provide regulatory agencies with estimates of numbers of persons potentially harmed under specific exposure conditions. Regulatory agencies then propose exposure standards and guidelines which will protect the public from unacceptable risk.

Exposure standards and guidelines usually provide numerical exposure levels for various media (such as food, consumer products, water and air) that cannot be exceeded. Alternatively, these standards may be preventive measures to reduce exposure (such as labeling, special ventilation, protective clothing and equipment, and medical monitoring).

Exposure standards and guidelines are of two types:

- **Standards:** these are legal acceptable exposure levels or controls issued as the result of Congressional or Executive mandate. They result from formal rulemaking and are legally enforceable. Violators are subject to punishment, including fines and imprisonment.

- **Guidelines:** these are recommended maximum exposure levels which are voluntary and not legally enforceable. Guidelines may be developed by regulatory and nonregulatory agencies, or by some professional societies.

Federal and state regulatory agencies have the authority to issue permissible exposure standards and guidelines. They include the following categories:

- Consumer Product Exposure Standards and Guidelines

- Environmental Exposure Standards and Guidelines

- Occupational Exposure Standards and Guidelines

Cases in Forensic Toxicology

The Mickey Finn[1] (Old Story/New Drugs)

An international entrepreneur, after a successful week, visits a local bar in an exclusive hotel in Dallas. He sports a Rolex watch from

Switzerland, a diamond ring from Amsterdam, and an Italian-made suit. After a few drinks, he strikes up a conversation with an attractive woman. The next morning he is found by a hotel employee in the garage of the hotel in a state of confusion, without his watch, ring, or billfold. He is escorted to the local hospital emergency room for evaluation where blood and urine are routinely collected, and a drug screen and alcohol determination are requested. A small amount of ethanol is found in the blood, and a routine urine drug screen via Thin Layer Chromatography (TLC) and immunoassay are negative. Since a robbery was reported, the police found a glass from the hotel in his car. Analysis by TLC and gas chromatography/mass spectrometry revealed the presence of lorazepam (Ativan) in the drink. Further analysis of the blood via capillary chromatography with an electron capture detector revealed the presence of nanogram quantities of lorazepam. Lorazepam in combination with ethanol may produce short term amnesia and enhance the effects of ethanol. That is, the etiology of the drug induced state (Mickey Finn) was explained via a combination of forensic sciences and analytical toxicology.

Therapeutic Misadventure

The unexplained death of a 34-year-old female led to the investigation of cause of death by a medical examiner's office. An extensive autopsy investigation was essentially unremarkable except for the finding of pulmonary and hepatic congestion. Toxicology studies revealed the presence of amitriptyline (a tricyclic antidepressant) and a very large amount of its major metabolite nortriptyline. In addition, therapeutic amounts of chlorpromazine (a tranquilizer) also were found in the blood.

The medical examiner's report indicated that the cause of death was drug related. This resulted in an angry response from the husband and parents of the woman. The physician explained that he had carefully prescribed only small amounts of amitriptyline, thus making it impossible for her to commit suicide. In addition, the chlorpromazine was justifiably prescribed based on the physician's clinical opinion of her unique depression.

Further investigation revealed that the phenothiazine (chlorpromazine) inhibits the metabolism of nortriptyline (the metabolite of amitriptyline), allowing it to accumulate to toxic concentrations while receiving therapeutic doses of amitriptyline. Thus, the cause of death was accurately determined via a combined effort of the medical examiner and toxicologist. Any death is tragic, but the knowledge gained may prevent future therapeutic drug interactions (therapeutic misadventures).

Notes

1. Mickey Finn: Drug(s) added to an alcohol drink to produce short term unconsciousness allowing an opportunity for an uncontested robbery. Historically, this drug was chloral hydrate (or "knock-out drops").

Chapter 20

Forensic Odontology

Forensic dentistry (odontology) is a branch of dentistry which deals with the collection, evaluation, and proper handling of dental evidence in order to assist law enforcement officers and to assist in civil and criminal proceedings. There are three general areas in which the services of a forensic dentist are required:

- Identification of deceased persons through dental remains.

- Bite mark analysis; determining or ruling out possible suspects in crimes in which bite marks are left on a victim or other object.

- Examination of oral-facial structures for determination of injury, possible malpractice, or insurance fraud.

Most of a forensic dentist's caseload is the identification of deceased people. A forensic dentist is called upon to determine identity when a person is an unknown victim of an accident or homicide, or is one of many victims in a mass disaster such as a flood, an earthquake, or an airline crash. A forensic dentist may also be called as a "friend of the court" to give expert testimony concerning scientific investigation, or to provide professional opinions about evidence introduced into a trial.

Excerpted from "The Forensic Sciences Foundation, Inc., Career Brochure," [Online] undated. Available: http://www.aafs.org/career/CareerBroch.html. Produced by the Forensic Sciences Foundation, Inc., P.O. Box 669, Colorado Springs, CO 80901-0669. For complete contact information, please refer to Chapter 56, "Resources." Reprinted with permission.

Education and Training

The prerequisites for this field include an educational background in dentistry (preferably a doctorate degree). However, there are many others, such as dental hygienists and assistants, who make up an integral part of the forensic dental team. A dental education provides the fundamentals required for the tasks encountered during forensic work. Skills required in order to succeed include the ability to recognize each tooth in and out of the mouth, different tooth surfaces, types of filling materials, racial and sociological differences in dentition, and a knowledge of oral pathology and closeup photography. Beyond this, specialized postgraduate training in the field of forensic dentistry should be obtained. There are currently several courses offered in North America and in Europe. Many of these courses teach the fundamentals of evidence collection and handling, charting systems, autopsy protocol, etc.

Usually, courses in forensic dentistry are taught through a dental school at a major university. The dental schools of Loma Linda University, University of Texas, Louisiana State University, Northwestern University, University of Louisville, New York University, and University of Southern California are some which offer undergraduate and postgraduate training in forensic dentistry. The Armed Forces Institute of Pathology in Washington, D.C., offers a course annually.

Employment Opportunities

Employment opportunities exist either at a dental school or on an individual contract basis with a law enforcement agency. Affiliation with a dental school provides the opportunity to teach forensic dentistry and to conduct research projects, in addition to involvement in actual case work. However, the majority of forensic dentists today are in private practice. They are usually affiliated with the law enforcement agencies of the county in which they live or work, and provide forensic services by contract or on a "fee-for-service" basis.

A forensic dental consultant never knows when he or she will be called upon. Accidents and crimes are unpredictable, and frequently will occur at times which are not convenient for postponing investigation. For this reason, the forensic dentist must have a tolerant attitude about day-to-day schedules, and there must be a genuine interest in assisting whatever agency requests his or her services.

Forensic dentists are encouraged to maintain current, up-to-date knowledge of the state of science by attending regular meetings and courses given for and by colleagues. A good example of this is the annual meeting of the American Academy of Forensic Sciences (AAFS). During this week-long meeting, numerous papers are presented in the forensic sciences showing the latest techniques and advances in the field.

In addition to the Odontology Section of the AAFS, there are two organizations whose members are only forensic dentists: the American Society of Forensic Odontology (ASFO) and the American Board of Forensic Odontology (ABFO). The ASFO meets annually at the AAFS meeting and distributes a newsletter quarterly to its members.

To become certified by the ABFO, one must be able to document a reasonable amount of "hands-on" experience to demonstrate qualifications and then pass a two-day written examination. Recertification occurs every five years, and active participation in forensic dentistry must be demonstrated to the ABFO through submission of cases.

Forensic odontology is an exciting and challenging field which is becoming more sophisticated and scientifically oriented. The future will bring more utilization of complex investigative equipment such as electron microscopes, ultraviolet light photography, laser scanners, and computerized solutions to identifications in mass disasters.

Chapter 21

Forensic Entomology

Introduction

This [chapter] was created in order to assist in the education of crime scene technicians, homicide investigators, coroners, medical examiners, and others involved in the death investigation process. A basic knowledge of what forensically important insects look like and the proper method for their collection will allow investigators to make more accurate and representative collections from the death scene. Enhanced basic knowledge on the behalf of law enforcement officials will provide for better communication between the police and the forensic entomologist. Improved communication will promote more frequent use of entomological resources and more accurate collection of entomological evidence. This will allow forensic entomologists to be more precise in their statements and determinations, particularly in the area of postmortem interval estimations.

What Is Forensic Entomology?

Forensic Entomology is the use of the insects, and their arthropod relatives that inhabit decomposing remains to aid legal investigations. The broad field of forensic entomology is commonly broken down into

From "Forensic Entomology," [Online]. Available: http://www.forensic-entomology.com. © 1998 by Jason H. Byrd, Ph.D., Dept. of Entomology and Nematology, P.O. Box 110620, Bldg. 970, University of Florida, Gainesville, FL 32611. For complete contact information, please refer to Chapter 56, "Resources." Reprinted with permission.

three general areas: medicolegal, urban, and stored product pests. The medicolegal section focuses on the criminal component of the legal system and deals with the necrophagous (or carrion) feeding insects that typically infest human remains. The urban aspect deals with the insects that affect man and his immediate environment. This area has both criminal and civil components as urban pests may feed on both the living and the dead. The damage caused by their mandibles (or mouthparts) as they feed can produce markings and wounds on the skin that may be misinterpreted as prior abuse. Urban pests are of great economic importance and the forensic entomologist may become involved in civil proceedings over monetary damages. Lastly, stored product insects are commonly found in foodstuffs and the forensic entomologist may serve as an expert witness during both criminal and civil proceedings involving food contamination.

Life Cycles

Here is some information about the development and appearance of some common forensically important insects.

Insects have existed on earth for about 250 million years; comparatively humans have existed for about 300,000 years. Such an enormous amount of time has allowed insects to attain a wide diversity in both form and development. There are currently about 700,000 described species and it is estimated that there may be more than 10 million species of insects. Some insects have evolved a gradual or "paurometabolous" development in which there is an egg that hatches into an immature [form] or "nymph", which resembles the adult form, but is smaller and lacks wings. In the forensically important insects, this [is] best represented by the cockroaches. However, most forensically important insects undergo a complete or "holometabolous" development. There is an egg stage (except for a few insects such as the flesh flies that deposit living larvae) which hatch into a larval form and undergoes a stepwise or incremental growth. This pattern is caused by the successive molts (shedding of the outer skin that has become too small) that the larva must undergo before it finally enters the inactive pupal stage. The pupa is simply the hardened outer skin of the last larval stage and the adult will develop inside of this protective skin.

Blow Flies

In the insects that undergo complete development, the larval stages appear quite different from the adult form. The larvae of flies (order

Diptera) that are commonly recovered from decomposing human remains lack functional legs, and the body of many species appears cream colored, soft-bodied, and quite "maggot-like". Once the larva or "maggot" is through feeding, it will migrate away from the corpse in order to find a suitable site to form the pupal stage. The pupae of blow flies are often overlooked, as they closely resemble rat droppings or the egg case of cockroaches. The pupal stage is an extremely important stage to the forensic entomologist and a thorough search should be made for the presence of pupae at any death scene. If the adult insect has not emerged, the pupa will appear featureless and rounded on both ends. If the adult insect has emerged, one end will appear as if it has been cut off, and the hollow interior will be revealed. Most adult blow flies appear a metallic green or blue and are easily recognizable.

Beetles

The beetles (order Coleoptera) are one of the largest groups of animals and they also undergo complete development. Because of their development, the larvae appear very different from the adult form. Although the larvae or "maggots" of a large number of blow fly species may look almost identical, the larvae of beetles may look very different from one species to the next. Beetle larvae recovered from corpses can be easily differentiated from maggots as they have three pairs of legs and the maggots found on decomposing remains will not have any legs. Once a larva as been identified as that of a beetle, further field identification can be accomplished because of the wide diversity of larval forms. The bodies of beetle larvae may range from almost white, robust, and hairless to dark brown, slender, and quite hairy. Others may appear almost black and have armored plates on their back.

What Information Can a Forensic Entomologist Provide at the Death Scene?

Forensic entomologists are most commonly called upon to determine the postmortem interval or "time since death" in homicide investigations. The forensic entomologist can use a number of different techniques including species succession, larval weight, larval length, and a more technical method known as the accumulated degree hour technique which can be very precise if the necessary data are available. A qualified forensic entomologist can also make inferences as to possible postmortem movement of a corpse. Some flies prefer specific habitats such as a distinct preference for laying their eggs in an out-door or indoor environment. Flies can also exhibit preferences for carcasses in shade or sunlit conditions of the outdoor environment. Therefore, a corpse that is recovered indoors with the eggs or larvae of flies that typically inhabit sunny outdoor locations would indicate that someone returned to the scene of the crime to move and attempt to conceal the body.

Similarly, freezing or wrapping of the body may be indicated by an altered species succession of insects on the body. Anything that may have prevented the insects from laying eggs in their normal time frame will alter both the sequence of species and their typical coloni-zation time. This alteration of the normal insect succession and fauna should be noticeable to the forensic entomologists if they are famil-iar with what would normally be recovered from a body in a particu-lar environmental habitat or geographical location. The complete absence of insects would suggest clues as to the sequence of postmor-tem events as the body was probably either frozen, sealed in a tightly closed container, or buried very deeply.

Entomological evidence can also help determine the circumstances of abuse and rape. Victims that are incapacitated (bound, drugged, or otherwise helpless) often have associated fecal and urine soaked clothes or bed dressings. Such material will attract certain species of flies that otherwise would not be recovered. Their presence can yield many clues to both antemortem and postmortem circumstances of the crime. Currently, it is now possible to use DNA technology not only to help determine insect species, but to recover and identify the blood meals taken by blood feeding insects. The DNA of human blood can be recovered from the digestive tract of an insect that has fed on an individual. The presence of their DNA within the insect can place suspects at a known location within a definable period of time and recovery of the victims' blood can also create a link between perpe-trator and suspect.

The insects recovered from decomposing human remains can be a valuable tool for toxicological analysis. The voracious appetite of the insects on corpses can quickly skeletonize the remains. In a short period of time the fluids (blood and urine) and soft tissues needed for toxicological analysis disappear. However, it is possible to recover the insect larvae and run standard toxicological analyses on them as you would human tissue. Toxicological analysis can be successful on in-sect larvae because their tissues assimilate drugs and toxins that accumulated in human tissue prior to death.

Death Scene Procedures

It is important to note that the collection of insects and other arthropods from a death scene may disturb the remains. Therefore, the entomologist (or the crime scene personnel charged with making the collection) should contact the primary investigator and make plans for the collection of entomological evidence. Once a course of action has been determined, utmost care should be taken during insect collection so that the remains are disturbed as little as possible. Before collections are made, notes should be taken as to the general habitat, ambient weather conditions, and location of the body. Observations should also be made to describe the microhabitat immediately surrounding the body.

Scene Observations and Weather Data

Entomological investigation of the death scene can be broken down into the following steps (detailed in *Entomology and Death: A Procedural Guide,* E. P. Catts and N. H. Haskell [ed.]).

1. Observations of the scene should note the general habitat and location of the body in reference to vegetation, sun or shade conditions, and its proximity to any open doors or windows if recovered within a structure. Locations of insect infestations on the body should be documented as well as noting what stages of insects are observed (such as eggs, larvae, pupae, or adults). It is also useful to document evidence of scavenging from vertebrate animals and predation of eggs and larvae by other insects such as fire ants. Observations such as these can be noted on [a] Death Scene Form.

2. Collection of climatological data at the scene. Such data should include:

    *   air temperature at the scene taken approximately at chest height with the thermometer in the shade. DO NOT EXPOSE THERMOMETER TO DIRECT SUNLIGHT!

    *   Maggot mass temperature (obtained by placing the thermometer directly into the larval mass center).

    *   Ground surface temperature.

    *   Temperature at the interface of the body and ground (simply place the thermometer between the two surfaces).

- Temperature of the soil directly under the body (taken immediately after body removal).

- Weather data that includes the maximum and minimum daily temperature and rainfall for a period spanning one to two weeks before the victims disappearance to three to five days after the body was discovered. Such information can be gathered by contacting the nearest national weather service office, or your state climatologist.

Collection of Insects from the Body at the Scene

The first insects that should be collected are the adult flies and beetles. These insects are fast moving and can leave the crime scene rapidly once disturbed. The adult flies can be trapped with an insect net available from most biological supply houses. They are inexpensive and readily obtainable. Once the adult flies have been netted, the closed end of the net (with the insects inside) can be placed in the mouth of a "killing jar" (which is a glass container with cotton balls or plaster soaked with ethyl acetate, or common fingernail polish remover). The jar is then capped and the insects will be immobilized within a few minutes. Once they are immobile they can be easily transferred to a vial of 75% ethyl alcohol. Beetles can be collected with forceps or gloved fingers and placed directly into 75% ethyl alcohol.

It is extremely important that the collected specimens are properly labeled. Labels should be made with a dark graphite pencil, NOT IN INK. The label should be placed in the alcohol along with the specimens, and alcohol can dissolve the ink from the paper! However, pencil is not affected by alcohol and should be used for labeling purposes. The collection label should contain the following information:

1. Geographical location
2. Date and hour of collection
3. Case number
4. Location on the body where removed
5. Name of collector

Note: A duplicate label should be made and affixed to the exterior of the vial.

Once the adults have been collected, the collection of larval specimens from the body can begin. First the investigator should search for the presence of eggs, which are easily overlooked. After this step, the larvae should be readily apparent on the body. Generally speaking, the largest larvae should be actively searched for and collected. Additionally, a representative sample of 50 to 60 larvae should be collected from the maggot mass. These insects can be placed directly into a killing solution or ethyl alcohol. However, the specimens are better preserved if they are placed in boiling water for about 30 seconds. Obtaining boiling water at a scene is difficult, so boiling of the larvae upon returning to the proper facility is satisfactory. If the larvae are boiled with about 48 hours of initial preservation, a good specimen should result. It is important to note that some forensic entomologists prefer not to have the submitted larvae boiled. Therefore, the investigator should discuss preservation techniques with their cooperating entomologist. In any case the exact preservation techniques should be documented and forwarded to the forensic entomologist. If the body has more than one area of colonization (more than one maggot mass), each site should be treated separately.

Once the preserved collections have been made, duplicate samples should be made for live shipment. Living specimens can be placed in specimen containers or Styrofoam cups with tight fitting lids along with some moist paper toweling, or most preferably a food substrate such as beef liver or pork meat. Tiny air holes should be poked in the lid using an ice pick or similar instrument. This cup should be placed into a slightly larger container that has about ½ inch of soil or vermiculite in the bottom to absorb any liquids that may accumulate and leak. This entire container should be enclosed in an appropriate shipping container and shipped overnight to a forensic entomologist.

Collection of Insects from Scene after Body Removal

Many of the insects that inhabit a corpse will remain on, or buried, in the ground after the body has been removed. The steps listed above should be followed when collecting insects from the soil (i.e., both a preserved and a living sample should be taken). Soil and litter samples should also be taken both immediately under where the body was positioned, and from the immediate surroundings. It is not necessary to dig deeply. A good technique is to collect the leaf litter and debris down to the exposed upper surface of the soil, and then make a separate collection from about the first two or three inches of topsoil. Each soil collection area should be about 4 to 6 inches square, and be taken from underneath the head, torso and extremities. All soil samples should be placed in a cardboard container for immediate shipment to a forensic entomologist. These collections should be labeled and forwarded to the forensic entomologist along with the insects collected from the body.

How Should Insects Be Shipped to a Forensic Entomologist?

Properly collected and preserved insects (see above) should be shipped using overnight express either via the United States Postal Service (U.S. Mail), or via the United Parcel Service (UPS). Federal Express will not ship living insects (and they don't like to ship preserved insects either).

Forensic Insect Field Identification Cards

Most crime scene investigators have no specialized entomological training and the result is that valuable evidence may be overlooked, ignored, or mishandled. As a step towards the education and training of investigators in the recovery of entomological evidence, the Forensic Sciences Foundation (American Academy of Forensic Sciences) has recently funded a grant for the development of a field reference tool and visual identification aid. This work will help investigators to determine which insects are of forensic importance, while also providing basic collection and preservation information.

Each card set consists of fifty 3" x 4" plastic coated cards with a color photograph of a forensically important insect on the front, and a brief statement about the biology of the insect on the back. Both scientific and accepted common names are provided whenever possible to improve communication between investigators and the cooperating forensic entomologist. A life-sized silhouette of each insect located in the lower margin tells users at a glance the actual size of the insect.

Although the cards are not a comprehensive record of all insects that may be found associated with human remains, they will familiarize the user with the most common species found throughout the United States and Canada. The result of this project is that a more informed selection and preservation of insect specimens from the death scene will be obtained, and a more accurate interpretation of insect evidence can be made for use in civil and criminal legal proceedings. The Forensic Insect Field Identification Cards may be ordered by contacting the Forensic Sciences Foundation (American Academy of Forensic Sciences), P.O. Box 669 Colorado Springs, CO 80901-0669, or by phoning (791) 636-1100 or by faxing (719) 636-1993.

—by Jason H. Byrd, Ph.D., University of Florida

Chapter 22

Forensic Palynology

What is it?

It is the science of using both modern and fossil palynomorphs (primarily spores and pollen) to help solve legal problems.

When was it first used?

It is not precisely known where and when it was first used, but the early 1950s is probably a good guess. The first well documented case was in Austria in 1959 involving a criminal case where a man on a journey down the Danube River disappeared near Vienna. His body was never found. A suspect, with a known motive for killing him, was later arrested and charged with the man's murder. With no body or confession the case was in jeopardy of default. The only real clue seemed to be a locally uncharacteristic mud found on the defendant's shoes. Identification (by Wilhelm Klaus of the University of Vienna) of the palynomorphs within the mud consisted of the trees—spruce, willow, and alder, as well as an extinct fossil hickory pollen twenty million years old. Only one small area along the Danube Valley had soils with the precise modern pollens in association with the rocks

217

containing the fossil pollen. When confronted with this information the defendant confessed and showed authorities precisely where he had buried the body.

When and where is it used today?

As in the past, it is rarely used; not because the science lacks validity, but because it is not widely known or understood. Doctors Vaughn Bryant, John Jones, and Dallas Mildenhall conducted surveys of major law enforcement agencies in the United States which indicated that little is known about this area of forensics (forensic palynology). Among the major countries of the world, only law enforcement agencies in New Zealand routinely collect and use forensic palynological studies in civil and criminal cases.

On or from what can it be used?

Palynomorphs can be recovered from almost any substance and any environment. Typical items from which palynomorphs are recovered for forensics research range from dirt, clothing, hair, rope, packing, and baskets to even include blood from a crime scene. These "materials" can yield a possible geographic origin or can link an individual or item with the scene of a crime. Likewise, the palynomorphs found in illegal drugs, like marijuana and heroine, can link those drugs with their users or (according to Dr. Mildenhall of New Zealand) even their source area, and can show which shipments of drugs originated from the same, or from different, source areas.

Due to the ruggedness of the exterior of many palynomorphs (which is also the reason for their excellent fossilization), they can be recovered from baked goods, canned goods and even the stomach contents of a murdered victim. This last fact may sound gruesome, but it may aid in a victim's identification by indicating what or where that person ate their last meal. This is especially useful with partially decomposed or neo-mummified bodies.

Precedent for forensic palynology in the United States?

Probably the most noted mention of forensic palynology in the United States occurred on a television show popular in the 1970s— *Hawaii Five-O*. In that series plot a group of thieves in Hawaii were tracked to their "hideout" by examining the pollen trapped in their abandoned car's air filter. The examined pollen was deemed by the palynologist to be representative of plants found only in a particular part of the island—the "hideout." In truth, this may in fact be one application of forensic palynology.

The Case of the Corn Pollen. An individual in the late 1970s in rural Illinois was kidnapped, assaulted, and killed with an ax, and his car was subsequently stolen. Later, transients were arrested for "breaking and entering" in a town close to where the car was abandoned (after it ran out of gas). Suspicious of the transients' story, but with no real clues to link them with the murder, the Illinois Bureau of Investigation turned to forensic palynology for possible help. Pollen analysis of a transient's shirt revealed it was covered with fresh corn pollen, especially in the area of the shoulders. To the palynologist, Dr. James King, this palynological information indicated that the transients had recently walked/run through a corn field. The only large corn field in the area was located between where the murder victim's car was abandoned and the town where the transients were arrested. Yet, the transients stated that the location in question was an area they had never been close to. Subsequent to the palynology report, people living near the large cornfield were contacted by authorities to possibly identify the transients. Later, several positive identifications (by area neighbors), as well as the corn pollen identification, led to the conviction of the transients for murder (Case #77CF65, *Illinois* vs. *Bobby Cole and Arthur Wilson,* Macoupin County, Illinois, Date of Trial—1979). The above case was relayed by Dr. James King who is presently Director of the Carnegie Museum in Pittsburgh, Pennsylvania.

Until recently, the New York City Police Department Crime Lab maintained a palynologist on staff by the name of Dr. Edward A. Stanley. It was reported that Dr. Stanley was a key person in the solving of several criminal cases. One such case involved a shipment of cocaine hydrochloride that was seized in a New York City drug raid. Though the suspects were not caught, the raid and subsequent cocaine seizure yielded important trafficking information. Palynological analysis of the cocaine hydrochloride revealed a number of different pollen suites that indicated the cocaine was processed in South America (probably Bolivia or Colombia), sent to a locale in northeastern North America where it was "cut and packaged," and finally on to New York where it was "cut" again and in the process of being prepared for distribution when it was seized.

Documented forensic palynology cases with "legal precedent" are few and far between in the United States. Presently the only country that seems to have fully tapped the enormous potential of forensic palynology is New Zealand, with Australia and Malaysia starting to catch up. In the United States, the only "agency" where forensic pollen studies are conducted on a fairly regular basis is the palynology laboratory of Dr. Vaughn Bryant in the Anthropology Department of Texas A&M University.

— by Dr. Terry J. Hutter, Palynological Specialist

Dr. Terry J. Hutter is the president and owner of TH Geological Services, Inc.

Chapter 23

Forensic Geology

Purpose of Soil Analysis

By far the most common examination conducted by a forensic geologist is the analysis and comparison of soil samples. This type of examination is requested in order to establish a relationship between soils from different sources. A typical soil case involves the comparison of two or more soils; one or more usually from persons or objects associated with a criminal offence and the others, comparison soil samples submitted from known locations. Investigators wish to know whether or not the soil samples they have collected may have common origins. It is the job of the forensic geologist to answer this question by analysing and comparing certain soil properties.

Introduction

Soil consists of loose aggregates of rocks, minerals, and organic matter. Due to its widespread occurrence and its tendency to adhere to most materials, soil is frequently present on items of physical evidence. Common sources include cultivated fields, construction sites, banks of streams and rivers, paths, roadways, and gardens.

From "Procedure For Soil Analysis," [Online] undated. Available: http://www.erin.utoronto.ca/academic/FSC/FSC239Y_SOIL.htm. Produced by William J. Graves, Forensic Geology, Centre of Forensic Sciences, University of Toronto at Mississauga, 3359 Mississauga Rd., Mississauga, ON, Canada L5L 1C6. Reprinted with permission.

Soil in its natural state could be compared on the basis of a great number of properties. Some of these properties—degree of saturation, pH, density and porosity—are subject to change when soil is removed from its natural environment, as it is when transferred to shoes or clothing. Other soil properties, organic content and density gradients for example, appear to vary almost as much within small "footprint-size" areas as over considerably greater distances. Obviously these properties will not be appropriate for making forensic comparisons. To be useful to the forensic geologist, a soil property will ideally remain uniform within small areas and will vary considerably over larger distances. Just as importantly, it will not be subject to change upon removal from its natural setting. Experimental work with soil samples collected in Ontario has shown the following soil properties to meet these criteria:

1. Colour
2. Mineralogy
3. Range of Grain Size

The evidential value of soils derives from the large number of distinguishable soil types and the limited area covered by each. Based on studies carried out at the Centre of Forensic Sciences, the number of soils in Southern Ontario distinguishable on the basis of colour alone is conservatively estimated to be about 400. Similarly, published literature confirms our findings at the Centre that there is a great diversity of mineral and rock particles in the soils of Ontario. Further, it has been found that soil colour and mineralogy are largely independent of each other with soil colour determined to a great extent by such factors as iron content, the quantity and nature of organic constituents and the type and degree of weathering. For this reason these two soil properties, colour and mineralogy, serve to distinguish between thousands of soils. A soil may also be classified according to its range of grain size. Particle size within soils can vary from coarse gravel to finer grained silts and clays. Most soils consist of various intermixtures of two or more of these different size fractions.

Aside from comparing these three soil properties, the soil examiner is frequently required to identify and compare various substances contained in the soil samples. The more common of these include glass fragments, paint chips, metal spherules or fragments, fertilizers, cinders, asphalt, and brick, plaster, or concrete particles. Since the majority of soil cases relate to urban or industrial sites, these additional traces often contribute to the significance of the findings.

The usefulness of a soil comparison in any investigation may be limited by a number of factors:

- Size of soil sample
- Type of soil
- Wetness of soil
- Intermixing of different soils
- Collection and handling of comparison samples

Generally, the quantity of soil required for a soil comparison is quite small: an amount the size of a wooden match head is sufficient in most cases. In a small number of cases a greater quantity of soil is required in order to evaluate all three properties (colour, range of grain size, and mineralogy). When samples consisting primarily of coarse sand or gravel are received, the requisite sample size is considerably larger than for samples containing silty sands or sandy silts. The same is often true for samples consisting predominantly of clay or of organic matter, although an alternate approach can be used to assess the mineralogy of clay samples.

The type of soil sample can also limit the comparison of soil samples. Sand samples present the most problems for the soil examiner. As mentioned above, coarse sands necessitate a greater sample size, but sand samples also pose additional problems. In general, sands do not adhere as well to other materials as do finer-grained soils. Also, they tend to readily fall from clothing and footwear, especially as the sand grains and clothing become dry. This loss is weighted towards the coarser grains, such that any soil remaining on the clothing has a finer range of grain size than a comparison soil from the location of the transfer. Information relating to range of grain size is lost for such samples. Corresponding size fractions of such samples can still be compared in terms of colour and mineralogy. Finally, sand samples are also the most susceptible to the problem of intermixing; many sand samples represent an accumulation from multiple locations.

The degree of wetness of a soil will affect its adhesion to footwear and clothing. Dry or frozen soils will not readily adhere. Moist and wet soils will usually adhere to other materials, with clays demonstrating the greatest adhesion and sandy soils, the least. Saturated soils such as those located below water level do not adhere as well as moist soils.

Intermixing of soils can also cause problems. Once two or more different soils have been intimately intermixed, the resultant soil will differ from all of the initial soils. Consider an instance where soil from a given location is completely intermixed with a different soil previously or subsequently transferred to footwear. A forensic comparison of such soils will determine that they differ with respect to their forensic properties. (Note: This finding does not mean that none of the soil could have come from the location in question.)

All soil investigations depend on the ability of the investigator to select and properly handle the appropriate samples. Recommended procedures and precautions relating to collection of samples are detailed in the Centre's manual for investigators.

Apparatus and Reagents

- Drying oven
- Low power magnifying lens (with light source)
- Stereomicroscope (with fibre optic continuous-ring illumination)
- Petrographic microscope (with added oblique light source)
- Stainless steel sieves
- Buchner funnel (12 cm diameter)
- Ultrasonic bath
- HCl (10% solution)
- Hand magnet
- X-Ray diffractometer or Debye Scherrer cameras

Procedure

The following comparison procedure applies to most soils encountered as forensic samples, including naturally occurring soils, industrial products in fine particulate form and mixtures of the two. The procedure is based on comparisons of soils with respect to three useful forensic properties; colour, range of grain size, and mineralogy. Two soil samples are considered different if they are found to vary in any one of these properties. The efficiency of the procedure is maximized by comparing first, colour, followed by range of grain size, and, finally, mineral content. As these comparisons are successively more time-intensive, it is frequently possible to achieve substantial savings of time when samples can be distinguished during the first two steps.

Sample Preparation

1. Remove items of clothing (or other objects submitted) from their packaging, while holding the item and the packaging over a large sheet of paper.

2. Search the packaging for any remaining soil or debris, and place any such material in a separate container. Use this sample only if the quantity of soil remaining on the items is inadequate for one or more of the comparisons.

3. If any of the samples are damp or wet, allow them to air-dry in a warm place for 12 hours. (Generally, items will be dry when received.)

4. Dry comparison samples in an oven at 95° C for 4 hours. Before drying, break up any lumps larger than 2 cm in diameter.

Preliminary Examination of Items

1. Describe the location of soil deposits on clothing or other objects. Frequently, this is best accomplished by means of a sketch.

2. Describe the quantity and nature of these deposits (i.e., stains, dust deposits, smears, splatters).

3. Note direction of smearing, when possible, as well as any associated features such as tears or scuff marks.

4. Note the sequence of deposition when two or more soils are found in the same deposit (i.e., layered deposit on footwear).

5. Examine the shapes of soil lumps under a stereomicroscope. They may bear fabric impressions or could be casts of patterns from various objects (soles of shoes, grooves of tires, or even fingerprints).

6. As a general rule, do not remove soil from clothing or other items until it becomes necessary.

Colour and Texture Comparison

1. Lay out the dried comparison samples in a well and evenly illuminated place (daylight from a northern window or fluorescent lighting).

2. Detach a lump of soil from clothing or other object and position this test lump directly over and close to each of the comparison samples.

3. After the removal of soil from any object, check the soil for the presence of trace materials from the item to which it was

adhering. Remove any such traces from the soil as they could affect the colour comparison. (Fibres from clothing are a common contaminant of this type.)

4. Note the relative colour differences between the test sample and the comparison samples (in terms of hue, chroma, and value).

5. If one or more soils do not differ in colour from the test sample, examine the samples at a higher magnification using the stereomicroscope. Compare the textures of the samples (relative proportions of sand silt and clay). Note also the proportion of dark to light particles, the porosity of the samples, and any other notable features pertaining to the fabric of the sample.

6. Search for any soil contaminants such as cinders, fertilizers, paint chips, glass fragments, brick, concrete, or plaster fragments, and metal spherules, filings, or fragments.

7. When ample quantities of soil are available, add a drop of 10% HCl solution to a small subsample from each. Observe any reaction using the stereomicroscope.

Note: It may be necessary to alter the above procedure depending upon the nature of the soil samples. Given very small sample size, friable soil samples, or very thin deposits, the procedure is modified accordingly:

• When the quantity of soil adhering to an item is very small, there is a risk associated with its removal. The reliability of the colour comparison would suffer if it were to break up into smaller fragments. In these instances, the recommended procedure is to take lumps of soil from the comparison soils and position each, in turn, carefully on the item as near as possible to the soil deposit. This procedure requires that the background be of uniform colour.

• Friable soils, including most sand samples and some organic soils, cannot be compared in the usual way. These soils are not available in discrete lumps but rather as individual particles. Such samples must be removed from the items and transferred to a piece of white paper. Colour and texture comparisons are then made between these samples and subsamples from the comparison samples on separate pieces of paper.

- Very thin soil deposits whose colour is affected by the colour of the underlying material are common. If there is a large quantity of soil in such a stain or smear, the soil is removed carefully from the object, transferred to a piece of white paper, and compared to subsamples of the comparison samples as for the sand samples described above. If there is a limited quantity of soil in thin deposits, the soil is left on the item. Lumps of soil from a comparison sample can be used to make test smears on the item. The colours of the smears are then compared. A prerequisite of this test is that the soiled item must offer a uniformly consistent colour as a backdrop for the two smears. This is the least precise method of colour comparison and the significance of a colour match is much reduced compared to the other comparisons. A difference of colour between the smears, however, still serves to differentiate between the two soils.

Range of Grain Size and Colour

1. Place two nested stainless steel sieves (100 and 200 mesh, 3" diameter) over a Buchner funnel with a Whatman #4 filter inserted.

2. Place a subsample of soil in the upper 100 mesh sieve. With a wash bottle, wet the sample and disperse it until it is sorted by grain size in the appropriate sieves. Use gentle pressure with a finger to help break up any remaining lumps.

3. Clean the fine sand fraction (100 to 200 mesh) by partially immersing the 200 mesh sieve in an ultrasonic bath for 15 minutes. The water level should be about 1 cm below the upper rim of the sieve.

4. Dry the three separated fractions in an oven at 95° C.

5. Repeat the above steps for all soils to be compared.

6. Place the separated and dried fractions on appropriately labeled sheets of white paper.

7. Note the range of grain size for each subsample. (This step complements the texture comparison of the previous section.)

8. Compare the colours of corresponding size fractions between different soil samples, especially that of the fine and coarse sand fractions (100 to 200 mesh fractions and >100 mesh fractions).

9. Using the stereomicroscope, look for any extraneous trace materials within the separated fractions.

10. Proceed with a mineralogical analysis if two or more soils are not distinguishable on the basis of the comparison procedure to this point.

Note: Additional sieve sizes are used when working with medium-to coarse-grained sand samples (typically 20, 40, and 80 mesh).

Mineralogy

A) The following mineralogical procedure describes the comparison of two samples that contain an appreciable mineral content in the fine sand fraction. As such, it applies to most soil samples received at the Centre. (For comparisons involving more than two samples, the procedure varies accordingly.)

1. For each soil, mount about 1500 grains (~3 mg) of the fine sand fraction in 3 drops of silicone oil on a microscope slide. The refractive index of the oil should be in the range of 1.53 to 1.54. The same oil must be used for each of the soils to be compared.

2. Thoroughly mix the grains and disperse them evenly in the oil using a wooden applicator stick. Use a separate applicator stick for each slide.

3. Complete each slide by placing a cover slip over the oil.

4. Compare the qualitative mineralogy of the samples using a petrographic microscope. If the two slides contain different types of mineral species, the samples are different and the comparison ends.

5. If the two slides are qualitatively similar, note the relative proportions of the various minerals and rock particles in the samples. If there are significant differences between the slides, the analysis ends with the conclusion that the samples are distinguishable. If no such differences in mineralogy are found, the samples are found to be indistinguishable with respect to colour, range of grain size, and mineralogy.

6. For soils with complex mineralogies, it is useful to count and identify about 250 to 300 grains in order to establish their respective mineralogies in a semiquantitative sense.

7. When two soils are found to be similar with respect to the relative proportions of their mineral content, keep a record of the proportions of all categories of minerals and rock particles as established by the counting procedure.

8. Assign a name to each comparison sample using appropriate relative colour terminology which serves to distinguish between soils of different colour. The Munsell soil colour charts offer a useful guide to assigning soil colours.

B) Clay soils rarely contain sufficient material in the fine sand fraction. For these soils, an alternate approach is used to compare the mineral content, as described below. (Note that "clay" is used in the sense of grain size and not of mineral type.)

1. Using the -200 mesh sample (often the only fraction in a clay sample), prepare a sample for the X-ray diffraction camera or the X-ray diffractometer. Sample preparation is the same as that required for any finely powdered aggregate.

2. Compare the positions and intensities of the X-ray patterns obtained from the different soils. Soils similar in colour and range of grain size may be distinguished on the basis of their clay-size minerals.

Results and Discussion

The findings pursuant to soil comparisons are conveniently separated into two different categories. The primary results relate to the degree of similarity, or lack thereof, between the soil samples submitted for comparison. A secondary consideration, whose relevance is directly tied to the first issue, is the location and nature of soil deposits on clothing or other items. Some of the more common results stemming from the soil comparison procedure are listed below:

• Two soils are differentiated in any one of their properties; colour, range of grain size, or mineralogy.

• A very thin smear of soil on clothing or other item is found to be similar in colour to a test smear made with a comparison sample. (This procedure serves to distinguish fewer soils than other comparison procedures. It is useful in that it does serve to distinguish between the initial smear and smears made by most other soils.)

- A very small lump of soil adhering to an item is not distinguishable in colour from a comparison sample. The quantity of soil is not of sufficient size to compare texture or mineralogy.

- A small lump of soil adhering to an item is not distinguishable from a comparison sample with respect to colour or texture. The quantity of soil is not sufficiently large to permit a mineralogical comparison.

- A lump of soil taken from an item is not distinguishable from a comparison sample with respect to colour, range of grain size, or mineralogy.

- Soils found on two different items (i.e., clothing from a suspect and complainant) are not distinguishable with respect to colour, range of grain size, and mineralogy.

- Two or more soils associated with casework items are found to match corresponding comparison soils.

- Matching industrial contaminants are found in two soils that also match with respect to colour, range of grain size, and mineralogy.

Once the possibility of common origin for two samples has been established, other findings relating to the location and nature of the soil deposits on various items becomes significant. Some common findings are noted below:

- The location of soil found on clothing demonstrates which portions of the clothing were in contact with the ground or other soil source, and may strongly suggest the position of the person wearing the clothes at the time of soil transfer.

- The nature of the soil deposits (stains, dust deposits, smears, or mud splatters) can be indicative of the manner of soil deposition. Stains indicate deposition from a suspension of soil, usually in water, onto another material such as cloth. Dust deposits indicate transfer of soil grains in a dry state as occurs in contact with dry ground. Smears are formed when wet conditions prevail at the time of contact; information about relative movement between source and item is frequently found in these deposits. Splatters of mud, round or elliptical, indicate that soil transfer occurred without direct contact with the ground.

- A sequence of deposition may be established from layered soil deposits. This evidence may support, or detract from, a supposed or alleged sequence of events.

Conclusions

One of the most frequent findings in soil casework is that a soil associated with one or more of the submitted items matches a comparison sample with respect to colour, range of grain size, and mineralogy. In these cases, the opinion expressed in court is that the two soils samples could have come from the same location. Further, it has been established that two soil samples taken 100 metres or more apart in urban or industrial areas are unlikely to correspond with respect to these properties. This is based on analyses of casework soil samples submitted to the Centre from communities across Ontario.

Less conclusive opinions are expressed when smaller amounts of soil limit the comparison to one or two of the three forensic properties. In such instances, the conclusion drawn is similar to that expressed above, but the weight attached to this evidence is lessened as a consequence of the larger number of soils that could match the case samples. In effect, there is a higher probability that a randomly chosen sample would match any given soil sample with respect to one or two of its properties than with respect to all three of its forensic properties.

More conclusive results are sometimes established in soil cases. When two or more different soils from casework items are found to match corresponding comparison samples, the opinion expressed in court is that these samples could have come from the same location. Further, it can be stated that the possibility of finding two matching soils at some random location is very low.

Another factor leading to more conclusive results relates to the inclusion of industrial debris within soil samples. The number of soils that match with respect to their three forensic properties, and also contain matching debris, is much reduced over the number of soils that match on the basis of colour, range of grain size, and mineralogy, alone. Sometimes the evidential value of the debris may outweigh that of the soil evidence. The combination of these two types of evidence provides very useful circumstantial evidence.

Aside from the issue of common origin, the location and nature of soil deposits on clothing or other items may provide additional evidence. The value of this information is suggested in the previous section. As the nature of this evidence is usually readily apparent to most people, it is usually left to the jury to draw their own conclusions.

References

Berry, L. G., and B. Mason. *Mineralogy.* San Francisco: W. H. Freeman and Co., 1959.

Brewer, R. *Fabric and Mineral Analysis of Soils.* New York: Wiley, 1964.

Brown, G. *X-Ray Identification and Crystal Structures of Clay Minerals.* London: Mineralogical Society, 1961.

Chapman, L. J., and D. F. Putnam. *The physiography of Southern Ontario,* 3rd ed. Toronto: Ontario Geological Survey, 1984.

Dell, C. I. "Methods of Study of Sand and Silt from Soils," *Canadian Mineralogist* 75 (3): 363-71 (1959).

―――."A Study of the Mineralogical Composition of Sand in Southern Ontario," *Canadian Journal of Soil Sciences* 39: 185-96 (1959).

Journal of Soil Sciences 43 (2): 189-200 (1963).

Dreimanis, A. "Heavy Mineral Studies in Tills of Ontario and Adjacent Areas," *Journal of Sedimentary Petrology* 27 (2): 148-61 (1957).

Dryden, A. L. "Accuracy in the Representation of Heavy Mineral Frequencies," *Proceedings of the National Academy of Sciences* 5: 233-8 (1931).

Flint, R. F. *Glacial and Pleistocene Geology.* New York: John Wiley and Sons Inc., 1957.

Graves, W. J., "A Mineralogical Soil Classification Technique for the Forensic Scientist," *Journal of Forensic Sciences* 24 (2): 323-38 (1979).

Graves, W. J. and D. M. Lucas. "The Evidential Value of Soil," *Crowns' Newsletter* - Ontario Crown Attorneys' Association: 1-5 (May 1974).

Hewitt, D. F., and P. F. Karrow. *Sand and Gravel in Southern Ontario.* Toronto: Queen's Printer, 1963.

Hough, J. L. *Geology of the Great Lakes.* Urbana, Ill.: University of Illinois Press, 1958.

Judd, D. B., and K. L. Kelly. *Color: Universal Language and Dictionary of Names.* Washington, D.C.: NBS Special Publication 440, 1976.

Kornerup, A., and J. H. Warscher. *Methuen Handbook of Colour,* 3rd ed. London: Eyre Methuen Ltd., 1978.

Krumbein, W. C., and F. J. Pettijohn. *Manual of Sedimentary Petrography.* New York: Appleton-Century-Crofts, 1938.

Laboratory Aids for the Investigator, 4th ed. Toronto: The Centre of Forensic Sciences, 1984.

Larsen, E. S., and H. Berman. *The Microscopical Determination of the Non-Opaque Minerals,* 2nd ed. Washington, D. C.: U.S. Geological Survey Bulletin 848, 1934.

McCrone, W. C., and J. G. Delly. *The Particle Atlas,* 2nd ed. 6 vols. Ann Arbor, Mich.: Ann Arbor Science Publishers, 1973-1979.

Milner, H. B. *Sedimentary Petrography.* Vol. 2. New York: MacMillan, 1962.

Munsell, A. H. *A Color Notation,* 11th ed. Baltimore: Munsell Color Co., 1961.

———.*A Grammar of Color.* Toronto:Van Nostrand Reinhold Company, 1969.

Munsell Soil Color Charts. Baltimore: Munsell Color Co., 1954.

Murray, R. C., and J. C. F. Tedrow. *Forensic Geology.* New Brunswick, N. J.: Rutgers University Press, 1975. 2nd ed, 1992.

Ontario Geological Survey Special Volume 4, Geology of Ontario, Parts 1 and 2. Ontario: Ministry of Northern Development & Mines, 1992.

Rogers, A. F., and P. F. Kerr. *Optical Mineralogy,* 2nd ed. New York: McGraw-Hill, 1942.

Winchell, A. N., and H. Winchell. *The Microscopic Characters of Artificial Inorganic Solid Substances.* New York: Academic Press, 1964.

—by William J. Graves, Forensic Geology,
The Centre of Forensic Sciences, Toronto

Chapter 24

Forensic Engineering

Definition

Forensic Engineering is the application of the art and science of
engineering in the jurisprudence system, requiring the services
of legally qualified professional engineers. Forensic engineering
may include investigation of the physical causes of accidents and
other sources of claims and litigation, preparation of engineering reports, testimony at hearings and trials in administrative
or judicial proceedings, and the rendition of advisory opinions
to assist the resolution of disputes affecting life or property.
(Milton F. Lunch, former General Counsel to the National Society of Professional Engineers (NSPE).

Forensic engineering generally relates to the following.

Industrial accidents:

- determination of the physical cause of events leading up to a financial loss, accident, or the death or injury of a worker.

From "Forensic Engineering," [Online] undated. Available: http://www.erin.
utoronto.ca/academic/FSC/FSC239Y_FORENSIC_ENGINEERING.htm. Produced by John Mustard, Centre of Forensic Sciences, University of Toronto at
Mississauga, 3359 Mississauga Rd., Mississauga, ON, Canada L5L 1C6. For
complete contact information, please refer to Chapter 56, "Resources." Reprinted with permission.

- often required as part of an inquest investigation when a death is involved.

- civil liability actions usually involve independent investigations by various interested parties.

- conclusions may simply be used within the organization to avoid future similar losses.

Motor vehicle accidents:

- determination of the sequence of events leading up to a collision.

- often referred to as "accident reconstruction."

- may help direct a police investigation or substantiate criminal charges.

- routinely required by each party involved in civil litigation.

- government agencies perform limited analysis to gather accident statistics and improve road safety.

Fire investigations:

- determination of the cause of fires or explosions.

- analysis to improve fire safety or minimize fire impact in future events.

- can involve civil, mechanical, electrical, chemical, and other specialties.

- a broad knowledge of fire dynamics is also required.

- may substantiate a criminal charge such as arson or may be important in assigning civil liability.

Civil engineering investigations:

- determination of the cause of failure of large structures.

- failure is most often not catastrophic but can be very costly to remedy.

- often involve inappropriate or hazardous cracking of concrete structures or leaking and deterioration of roofs, walls, floors, and basements.

- often a catastrophic structure collapse results from a failure of a much smaller component or improper design or construction.

- conclusions may assist in civil litigation or in eliminating future costs for the property owner.

Some Specific Types of Analysis

A) Mechanical Failures

"Failure is an unacceptable difference between expected and observed performance" (Technical Counsel on Forensic Engineering).

Typical questions to be answered:

- Did component fail and cause the accident or did the failure result from the accident?

- How much force was required to cause the failure?

- What was the direction and manner of force application?

- Do the answers to the above indicate unusual or inappropriate use of the equipment?

- If a defect exists, is the manufacturer or some other party liable?

Modes of Failure

Brittle:

- sudden.
- low energy absorption.
- granular surface texture.
- may or may not be acceptable.

Ductile:

- provides warning of impending failure.
- safest kind of failure.
- high energy absorption.
- more fibrous surface texture, often at about 45 degrees to direction of force.
- usually due to extreme overload.

Fatigue:

- part loses load capacity over time due to cyclic loading.
- no warning of impending failure.
- energy absorption.
- occurs under normal operating conditions.
- two distinct surface textures—fatigue area is smooth, often rusted, perpendicular to stress.
- never an acceptable type of failure.

Corrosion:

- part loses load capacity over time due to environmental attack.
- may or may not be readily visible.
- may or may not provide a warning of impending failure.
- usually results from an inappropriate metal or unexpected environmental condition.

B) Lamp Examinations

Typical questions to be answered:

- Were a vehicle's lights on or off at the time of the accident?
- Which filament, if any, was illuminated?

Filaments:

- coil of fine tungsten wire connected to a filament post at each end.
- properties of tungsten change dramatically between "hot" and "cold" conditions.
- when cold, tungsten is brittle, shatters on impact and remains shiny in the presence of air.
- when hot, above about 300° C, tungsten is ductile, stretches on impact and oxidizes rapidly in air.
- normal incandescent temperature is about 2500° C.
- if the glass envelope shatters, small particles of glass will fuse to a hot filament.

Glass envelope:

- maintains filaments in a low pressure, inert gas atmosphere— usually a combination of argon and nitrogen.

- quartz-halogen lamp inserts contain high pressure bromine gas around the tungsten filament.

C) Tire Examinations

Typical questions to be answered:

- Did the tire(s) fail and possibly cause the vehicle to lose control or was the tire damaged as a result of the collision?

- Are any defects a result of manufacturing, sabotage, misuse, or collision?

- Could improper combination of tires have caused control problems?

- All examinations are based on the premise that sound tires do not spontaneously fail; examination centers around identifying a pre-existing weakness.

D) Speed Determination

Usually an approximate range of speeds for an involved vehicle can be determined.

Calculations are based on:

- laws of physics.
- distance the vehicles skid before and after impact.
- coefficient of friction of the road surfaces.
- vehicle weights, number of wheels skidding, road irregularities.
- vehicle or object airborne trajectories.
- 'yaw' marks.
- road markings such as gouges, scrapes, scuffs, etc.
- not generally based on vehicle damage alone for court purposes.

> *— by John Mustard, Forensic Scientist, Engineering,*
> *Centre of Forensic Sciences, University of Toronto*

Chapter 25

Firearms Identification

Firearms identification is a discipline of Forensic Science that has as its primary concern to determine if a bullet, cartridge case, or other ammunition component was fired from a specific firearm.

Whenever a shooting occurs, the firearms evidence is collected and evaluated as to its importance to the case. The evidence submitted to a lab's Firearms Section will typically include a firearm or firearms, fired bullets, spent cartridge cases, spent shotshells, shot, shotshell wadding, live ammunition, [and] clothing. . . . The role of the firearms examiner is to perform specific scientific examinations upon the evidence submitted using various tools and instruments.

Probably the most common examinations conducted by the firearms examiner involve trying to determine if a submitted firearm fired the bullet removed from the body of a shooting victim or fired spent cartridge cases found at the scene of a shooting incident. . . .

Firearms identification involves a great deal of comparative analysis. The firearms examiner will compare ammunition components to each other for common characteristics or similarities. When making such comparisons the firearms examiner will initially look for similarities in what are called *class characteristics.*

Excerpted from "An Introduction to Forensic Firearms Identification," [Online]. Available: http://www.geocities.com/~jsdoyle. © 1996-97 by Jeffrey Scott Doyle, Firearms and Tool Mark Examiner, Jefferson Regional Forensic Laboratory, 3600 Chamberlain Lane, Ste. 410, Louisville, KY 40241. For complete contact information, please refer to Chapter 56, "Resources." Reprinted with permission.

Class Characteristics

The first step in any comparison is to determine if the items you are comparing have any similar class characteristics.

Class characteristics are those that would be common to a particular group or characteristics that were designed into the make-up of a group of items.

A very basic example would be that several no. 2 pencils in a box are yellow and have pink erasers. The color and eraser type is a common class characteristic to all of the pencils. When it comes to firearms and ammunition, it is not quite so simple.

To determine if a particular bullet was fired from a specific firearm you must first determine if the questioned bullet exhibits class characteristics consistent with those that would be produced by the suspect firearm.

Class characteristics of firearms that relate to the bullets fired from them include the *caliber* of the firearm and the rifling pattern contained in the barrel of the firearm.

Caliber

When a bullet is submitted for examination, one of the first examinations conducted will be to determine the bullet's caliber. If you don't know a whole lot about firearms this part may get a little confusing.

Caliber is a term used to indicate the diameter of a bullet in "hundredths of an inch".

A bullet that is 32 hundredths of an inch (.32) in diameter is called a 32 *caliber* bullet. The term caliber is of English origin and is a term commonly used by arms manufacturers in the United States. Firearms and ammunition of European origin use the metric system and would refer to a 32 caliber bullet as an 8mm bullet.

Now, the 32 caliber bullet can vary in length, weight, and appearance. These factors as well as the type of cartridge case used with the bullet help determine what the *cartridge* designation will be. Examples of different 32 caliber cartridges are 32 Long Colt, 32 Smith & Wesson, and 32 AUTO.

[Some of the] cartridges . . . in the 22 caliber "family" . . . [include the] 22 Blank, 22 Short, 22 Long, 22 Long Rifle Shot, 22 Viper, 22 Long Rifle, 22 Stinger, 22 Magnum, and 22 Maximum.

If the caliber of the bullet submitted for examination matches the caliber of the submitted firearm, the firearms examiner will look for additional class characteristics in the form of rifling.

Rifling

Most handguns and rifles have rifled barrels. Rifling consists of grooves cut or formed in a spiral nature, lengthwise down the barrel of a firearm. . . . The rifling in a barrel will grip bullets as they travel down the barrel. The spiral or twist to these grooves will impart a spin on the bullet. Because bullets are oblong projectiles they must spin (like a thrown football) in their flight to remain accurate.

The whole point to this is that different firearms can have different patterns to their rifling. One firearm may have a six-grooved barrel with the grooves twisting to the left where another firearm's barrel may have eight grooves that twist to the right. As a bullet travels down the barrel of a firearm, the rifling will impart its negative impression on the sides of the bullet.

When a bullet is submitted for comparison to a firearm, it must not only match in caliber but the rifling impressions on the bullet must match the rifling pattern found in the barrel of the firearm. If both of these class characteristics match between the bullet and firearm, then the firearms examiner will look for what are called *individual characteristics.*

Individual Characteristics

Individual characteristics are those characteristics that are unique to an item. They can also be referred to as accidental characteristics.

[It is] the ability for one item to transfer individual characteristics to another that makes firearms identification possible. Firearms identification is based on the principle that any two objects that come into contact with each other can cause the softer of the two objects to be marked by the harder object. When a bullet . . . travels down the barrel of a firearm, the barrel typically marks the outer surfaces of the bullet, the barrel being made of a harder material than the bullet. Also, cartridge cases that pass through the action, or are fired in a firearm can be marked in the process by the harder materials that make up the internal parts of the firearm. These marks are the individual characteristics that a firearms examiner will look for to make a positive identification.

You may now be thinking, "what makes one gun different from another?". . .

The inner surfaces of the barrel may appear very smooth to the eye but when enlarged under a microscope, these surfaces contain imperfections that can leave a unique mark on a bullet. This mark is sometimes referred to as a "mechanical fingerprint".

When a firearm is manufactured, the individual parts (barrel, chamber, etc.) are made with tools that are in a constant state of change. The surfaces of the various parts of a firearm, when shaped with these tools, can be left with an irregular surface. Additional imperfections and irregularities can occur from use and neglect. As a result, no two guns will leave the same marks on the ammunition components. Because the parts of the firearm are made out of a hard material, they do not change very rapidly and they have the potential to mark every bullet or cartridge case fired in them the same way.

The firearms examiner will attempt to reproduce the marks being transferred to the ammunition components through test firing a suspect firearm and making comparisons between test *standards* and evidence bullets and/or cartridge cases. Most firearms sections use a water tank like the one below to test fire the firearms. The muzzle of the firearm is placed in the opening at the end of the tank and the firearm is fired. Bullets from the firearm strike the water in the tank and friction from the water slows the bullets down. The bullets end up on the bottom of the tank and usually about half-way down the length of the tank. The tank is only about 3 feet deep, 3 feet wide, and 10 feet long.

Standards are examined first to determine what marks are being transferred and how unique and consistent the marks are. Once a unique pattern to the marks is identified on standards, the standards are compared to the evidence bullets and cartridge cases to see if the same pattern of marks exists on the evidence. To make these comparisons, the firearms examiner will use a *comparison microscope*.

The comparison microscope is the most valuable instrument used by a firearms examiner. The comparison microscope is basically two microscopes mounted side by side that are connected by an optical bridge. The comparison microscope is used to compare one specimen to another. When looking into the comparison microscope the examiner sees a round image with the two exhibits being examined on the left and right sides of the image. The exhibits being examined can be rotated and moved around to see if any microscopic similarities are present.

Breech marks are located on the primers of cartridge cases. [They] are typically referred to as an impressed mark. The breech face of the firearm has left a negative impression of its surface irregularities on the cartridge case.

[When comparing] two bullets, [the] marks found around the sides of a fired bullet are referred to as *striated marks*. These are basically microscopic scratches on the surface of the bullet.

When comparisons are made between firearms and fired ammunition, the results can read as follows:

1. Exhibit 1 (bullet) was identified as having been fired from Exhibit 2 (revolver).

2. Exhibit 1 (bullet) was not fired from Exhibit 2 (revolver).

3. Exhibit 1 (bullet) could not be identified or eliminated as having been fired from Exhibit 2 (revolver). All comparisons were inconclusive.

As you can see from the results above, not all ammunition components can be identified back to a specific firearm. There are a lot of times when the bullets may be damaged to the point that little or no striations are visible. Also, some firearms just don't leave good individual characteristics on the ammunition fired from them.

There are times too when the investigators will submit a firearm that wasn't the one used to fire the submitted bullet. In this case there is often a distinct difference in class as well as individual characteristics.

Unknown Firearm Exam

Shootings frequently occur where no firearm is recovered. The only evidence of the shooting will be bullets and/or cartridge cases from the scene. To aid the investigators, the firearms examiner can examine these items of evidence and provide a list of possible manufacturers of the firearm from which the items were fired.

As described earlier under *Class Characteristics,* most firearms have *rifling* in their barrels. When a bullet travels down the barrel of a firearm it picks up the impression of the rifling on its outer surface. By examining a fired bullet the firearms examiner can use the rifling impressions to generate a list of firearm manufacturers that produce firearms with barrels rifled in a pattern that matches the impressions on the bullet. The rifling consists of a series of *grooves* cut lengthwise down the barrel. The space between two grooves is called a *land.*

There are a number of different rifling patterns used in the firearms industry. Some [typical] rifling patterns are 4/right, 5/right, 6/right, 6/left, 8/right, 10/right, 16/right, and 22/right.

The grooves in [a barrel may be] twice the diameter of the lands. These dimensions can vary between one firearm and another. When a bullet is examined, the diameters of the land and groove impressions are measured by the firearms examiner in thousandths of an inch (.000). By using the caliber of the bullet, the rifling pattern (i.e., 8/right), and the diameters of the individual lands and grooves, the firearms examiner can search through a database of known rifling parameters. The firearms examiner will usually search with a +/-.005 tolerance. The resulting search will help the investigator narrow down the search for the unknown firearm.

The database used by firearms examiners all over the world is one provided and maintained by the FBI. The FBI has been recording rifling data from firearms for over 20 years. As new firearms are manufactured the rifling data is included in the database. Updates to the database are mailed to firearms examiners on an annual basis.

A typical search would involve a 9mm Luger bullet, fired from a 6/right rifled barrel, with a land width of .055 and a groove width of .125. The results of the search might look like the following table.

Many years ago a double murder occurred in our community. An elderly couple was found shot to death in their home by their son. It appeared from the scene that there had been a break-in, but the son

Table 25.1. Luger Bullet Characteristics

Cartridge	Manufacturer	Twist	L&G	Land	Groove
9MM Luger	AA Arms Inc.	R	6	.055	.120
9MM Luger	Astra	R	6	.053	.128
9MM Luger	Beretta	R	6	.055	.130
9MM Luger	Hi-Point Firearms	R	6	.055	.120
9MM Luger	Interdynamic	R	6	.055	.124
9MM Luger	Llama	R	6	.054	.120
9MM Luger	Mauser	R	6	.054	.128
9MM Luger	Smith & Wesson	R	6	.056	.122
9MM Luger	Star	R	6	.054	.126
9MM Luger	SWD Inc.	R	6	.055	.120

was immediately a suspect. Investigators had a feeling that the son may have committed the crime but could not determine if he had owned or had access to a firearm. Bullets from the scene were examined and it was determined that they were of 38 caliber and were fired from an 8/right rifled barrel. A list of manufacturers was compiled and given to the investigators. Using this list the investigators searched a weekly "Bargain Mart" classified ad publication. By calling the ads for firearms included on the list of possibilities, the investigators found one individual who said he had sold his revolver to an individual who matched the description of the son. The son was then picked out of a police line-up by the individual who had sold him the gun. When confronted with the evidence, the son confessed to the killings and is now on Kentucky's death row.

Determining the manufacturer of a firearm that fired a questioned cartridge case is usually not nearly as specific as described above. Most firearms don't leave characteristics on the cartridge cases that are specific to a particular manufacturer. One notable exception is with the Glock and Smith & Wesson "Sigma" firearms. These have a fairly unusual oval firing pin nose. . . . When cartridge cases are submitted with characteristics like these it makes the job of the firearms examiner a bit easier. Otherwise, the examination of only cartridge cases will result in a very limited amount of information.

Firearm Function Exam

It is not too uncommon in shooting investigations for a suspect or victim to claim that a firearm accidentally discharged when it was dropped or otherwise mishandled. The accidental discharge of a firearm can occur, and most of the time the only harm done is a hole shot in Uncle Pete's pick-up truck. However, all too frequently, deaths and serious injuries result from the accidental discharge of a firearm.

[Such a case involved a vest containing] a derringer in its right front pocket. The wearer removed the vest and tossed it to a table. The derringer's hammer struck the table and the derringer discharged causing [a] large hole. The bullet struck the owner in the chest, killing her instantly.

The firearms examiner's job usually involves the inspection of submitted firearms to determine if there is any basis for a claim of accidental discharge.

When a firearm is submitted to the laboratory, there are a number of tests performed to determine if the firearm is functioning properly. The firearm is inspected for damaged, worn, or missing parts, and it is examined to determine what safeties, if any, are incorporated into the design of the firearm.

In the case mentioned above, the derringer was not found to have any mechanical deficiencies. However, the derringer had a safety that required the operator to manually cock its hammer back into a half-cocked position prior to loading. Without engaging the safety, the hammer would be resting directly against the firing pin of one of the derringer's chambers.

Most modern manufactured and a great number of antique firearms have some type of safety designed into the firearm to minimize the potential for accidental discharge.

Gunshot Residue Exam

Firearms examiners routinely examine clothing and other items from shooting incidents for the presence of gunshot residue. There are a number of examinations and chemical tests firearms examiners will perform to detect the concentration and size of the pattern of deposited residue. The firearms examiner can then test a submitted firearm and determine at what distance it will deposit a similar pattern of gunshot residue, and in turn, possibly prove or disprove the circumstances surrounding the shooting.

Several years ago, a shooting occurred in Louisville where a 14-year-old male was shot in the back. In what appeared to be a "drive-by" shooting, a friend of the victim stated that the shot was fired from a car some 50 feet from where the victim was standing. Investigators from both local and federal departments immediately started a massive search for the assailant. After about a week of unsuccessful searching, the victim's shirt was brought to the lab for examination. The shirt was analyzed and found to have a significant deposit of gunshot residue around the bullet hole in the back. The presence of the residue on the shirt directly conflicted with the scenario described by the only witness to the shooting. Gunshot residues emitted from a firearm do not travel in the distances described by the witness. The investigators were advised of the findings and using this new information confronted the victim's friend. The 16-year-old friend confessed to the shooting and admitted that he had *accidentally* shot his friend. He stated that he made up the story about the shot having been fired from a passing car. Had the evidence been submitted to the lab earlier, and if the investigators had not immediately assumed the witness was telling the truth, hundreds of man-hours would have been saved.

Gunshot residue is a combination of materials that are emitted from firearms during the firing process. This material includes, unburned gunpowder particles, burned gunpowder particulate, vaporous lead, and particulate lead.

When a firearm is fired, the burning gunpowder creates pressure, and this pressure forces the bullet down the barrel and down range. The pressure building behind the bullet is released as the bullet exits the muzzle and the gunshot residues are also blown out of the firearm's barrel at a high velocity. Because these particles are very small and lack mass, they lose their energy very [quickly] and typically will only travel a maximum of between 3 and 5 feet.

Examinations Conducted

There are basically three steps taken by the firearms examiner to process an item for the presence of gunshot residue. The first examination that the firearms examiner will conduct is to visually and microscopically examine the exhibit submitted. The firearms examiner will document the presence of any gunshot residues found around the bullet hole and note the shape and appearance of the hole. The next two steps involve chemically processing the exhibit to enhance the visibility of residues that are not visible to the eye.

The first chemical test is called the **Griess Test.** This is a test to detect the presence of *nitrite* residues. Nitrite residues are a particulate by-product of burned gunpowder. The Griess Test is performed by first treating a piece of 8" x 10" photographic paper with a chemical that makes it change color when contacted with nitrite residue. The exhibit is placed against the piece of photo paper with the bullet hole centered on the paper. The back of the exhibit being examined is then steam ironed using a dilute acetic acid solution to make the steam. The acetic acid vapors will penetrate the exhibit and react with any nitrite particles present on the exhibit to cause an orange dot to form on the photographic paper.

The next chemical test performed is sometimes referred to as the **Sodium Rhodizionate Test.** The exhibit being examined is first sprayed with a weak solution of a mixture of Sodium Rhodizionate and distilled water. The exhibit is then sprayed with a buffer solution. These chemicals will react with any lead that may be present and turn the lead a very bright pink. The pink color is only an indication of the presence of lead residue. To confirm the presence of lead residue, the area is then treated with a diluted Hydrochloric Acid solution. If the pink turns to a blue then the presence of lead is confirmed.

After processing a garment for gunshot residue, the suspect firearm can be fired at various distances into test cloth. These test cloths are processed in the same way the exhibit was processed, and the resulting residue patterns produced by the firearm are used to estimate the muzzle-to-target distance.

Results

By examining the target material, a firearms examiner may be able to determine the muzzle-to-target distance as 1. Contact/Near Contact, 2. Close range, 3. Intermediate range, or 4. Unknown:

1. Contact/Near contact: A contact or near contact gunshot will normally deposit a very intense ring of residue right around the margins of the bullet hole, higher velocity firearms can rip and tear clothing, and the heat and flame from the burning gunpowder can melt synthetic fibers.

2. Close range: Close range gunshots will typically result in a very concentrated deposit of residue around the bullet entrance hole and will include a sooty deposit of visible residue. A close range gunshot will typically be in the near contact to approximately 12-inch range of fire.

3. Intermediate range: An intermediate range gunshot usually will deposit a significant amount of particulate residue that is not easily seen with the eye but can be detected through a microscopic examination and through chemical enhancement. An intermediate range gunshot can range from just beyond 12 inches . . . to 24 to 36 inches. This depends greatly upon the caliber, barrel length, and powder type used in the ammunition.

4. Undetermined range: When no residues are found around the bullet hole, it can mean that the firearm was at a distance far enough away that the residues did not reach the garment or that there was possibly an intervening object between the firearm and target when fired. When firearms examiners are presented with this situation they will generally report that no muzzle-to-target distance could be determined.

—by Jeffrey Scott Doyle,
Firearms Examiner, Kentucky State Police

Chapter 26

Questioned Document Examination

Even though we are in an age of electronic communication, paper documents and handwritten signatures are still the way most business is transacted. Many civil and criminal legal cases, domestic disputes, and other controversies hinge on alleged irregularities in checks, wills, contracts, insurance policies, deeds, and other documents. When there are questions about a document, an expert is often called upon to examine said document and to give an opinion which answers the question.

Good Standards in Document Examination Cases

In cases involving questioned documents, lawyers can take certain steps to ensure that the document examiner has the necessary materials to perform a thorough and conclusive examination. A questioned document examiner examines documents in cases where foul play is suspected. Cases frequently involve handwriting comparisons, typewriting comparisons, physical alterations to a document, and many variations on these themes. Some document examiners are involved with chemical testing of documents, while others concentrate on physical and mechanical testing. The document examiner is often a qualified expert witness, accepted in court by a judge after being examined and cross-examined by counsel.

The most important factor in any document examination is the quality of the standards (the documents of known origin that are compared with the questioned documents). The questioned document is important too, but it is a "given." It defines the outer limits of the examination, but how far the examiner can go within those limits depends on the standards.

The important facts about standard documents are:

- There must be no doubt about the authenticity of the standards;

- The document examiner needs to be able to rely on the standards;

- The standards may need to be accepted as evidence in court.

Within the bounds of reason, there cannot be too many standards. Every handwriting shows natural variation. In cases where varying letter forms is an issue, if the examiner doesn't see enough standard writing, he or she will not have the information needed to form a good opinion. Typewriting cases often depend on identification of some individualizing defect of a machine. Defects can be sporadic, especially in their developmental stages. A few lines of typing or a quick run through the alphabet will not yield enough material to reveal the real character of the typing element.

The question arises, how much is enough? There is not an "across the board" answer. There are unusual cases where one or two signatures or a few typewritten lines will suffice. It all depends on the nature of the question. Be aware that in many cases the amount of standard material is an issue, and begin to amass samples early in the investigation. At the same time, realize that quantity is no substitute for quality, which will be discussed next.

There are two types of standards: collected and requested. Collected standards are those already in existence that the attorney or investigator collects. They may be bank records, letters, legal forms, and the like. Requested standards are those that the subject is requested to give to facilitate the document examination.

The best standards are those that most closely emulate the time frame, circumstances, materials and content of the questioned document. Therefore, look for collected standards executed close in time to the questioned document. This is especially critical in cases involving illness, death, accident, mental imbalance, substance abuse, or anything likely to cause a dramatic change in the subject's behavior.

Find out everything possible about the circumstances under which the questioned document was allegedly prepared. Was the subject lying sick in bed, standing at a counter, holding a clipboard in his or her lap? Try to obtain standards written under similar conditions.

Is the questioned document a check, letter, legal form, passport? Is it written on blank paper, lined paper, graph paper, cardboard? Was pencil, ballpoint, felt tip, or fountain pen used? If there was anything unusual about the materials of the questioned document, try to duplicate that uniqueness in the standards.

Content can be important in a document examination. Look for collected standards that share letter combinations, words, phrases, or numbers with the questioned document. When requesting standards, prepare a text that will include such similar content.

There is a method for obtaining good requested standards. In a handwriting case the material to be written should be dictated to the subject, rather than copied by the subject. Prepare the text and assemble the proper materials. Have on hand blank paper and any necessary forms and a selection of writing instruments. The subject may provide a pen or pencil and should be allowed to use it for the first writing sample.

Have the subject do some free writing to loosen up. Then dictate the material at a reasonable speed. Do not give any help with spelling or punctuation. Have the subject sign and date the sample. Take the sample and set it aside out of view. After some general conversation, ask the subject to repeat the task. This is a good time to request that the subject use a different paper or writing instrument if appropriate. Dictate a bit faster the second time. More repetitions may or may not be needed.

If you are especially interested in standard signatures, prepare several forms or blanks with the same layout as the questioned document for the subject to sign. Have the subject sign these forms one at a time. A column of signatures on a single sheet of paper may be useful if it appears in conjunction with several other types of standards, but by itself is not the best standard for examination. A column of ten signatures written this way tends to become ten copies of one signature rather than ten distinct signatures.

Depending on the questioned document, it may be important to request that the subject write in printed or cursive form. Also, it may be necessary to request samples written with the unaccustomed ("wrong") hand.

Number the samples so that the document examiner will be aware of the order of things, and keep a separate anecdotal record of anything unusual that happens during the session.

Handle all documents carefully. Do not fold documents—even those already folded. Repeated folding and unfolding of documents can cause damage and obscure that which needs to be examined. The best way to handle, transport, and store documents is unfolded and in archivally safe covers away from strong light and moisture. If any change is made to a document (staples removed, an accidental tear, etc.) a note should be made (but not on the document).

Document examinations often begin with, and even end with, photocopies. When possible, keep track of the generation of any copy made. With each successive copy, some loss of detail and addition of superfluous markings can occur. Sometimes a good opinion can be formed based on photocopies and sometimes it cannot. Of course, originals are always preferred.

Unless attorneys have been involved in a questioned document case they often have no reason to think of the necessary precautions. Each point made here can be expanded and taken in several directions. The best way to assure good results is to contact the document examiner early in the investigation and work with the examiner to plan an approach to the specific case.

Some Typical Document Examination Applications

By far the greatest number of questions I am asked about documents involve handwriting—especially signatures. Such as:

- Is the signature genuine?

- Is the document forged, and if so is it forged by a particular person?

- Is the same person the author of several documents?

- Which of a group of people wrote an anonymous letter?

- Did someone guide a person's hand as a will was signed?

- Did the doctor come back later and alter the medical records?

- Did the signer of the document also initial the changes?

- What is written under the crossed out portion of the writing?

- Was the document written on the date indicated?

There are also questions about typewriting:

- Are both documents typed on the same machine?

- Was the document removed from the typewriter and later reinserted during its preparation?

- Did a particular person do the typing?

Some questions are not concerned with handwriting or typewriting at all:

- Is the age of the paper or form consistent with the alleged date of the document?

- Are there erasures on the document?

- Are there perforations, folds, staple holes, or other physical clues on the document?

Depending on the nature and condition of the documents involved, these questions can be answered by the trained experienced questioned document examiner. The first group of questions, involving handwriting, requires a close side by side examination of the questioned and known (exemplar) documents. This examination is done with the unaided eye and with a microscope set at varying powers of magnification. The one question that can not be approached in this manner is that of the date of the document. Physical clues on the document may allow the examiner to reach some conclusions about time and sequence of preparation of the document, but to actually date the ink, an ink chemist is consulted.

Typewriting is becoming a relic of the past as more people use computers and word processors. A whole new area of document questions involving photocopies, facsimiles and computer printouts is evolving. In order to answer these questions, a questioned document examiner must study the characteristics of the whole class of machines, such as photocopiers, and then have access to detailed files which show the specific characteristics of the output of each specific brand of machine.

In regards to typewriting, individualizing characteristics often develop due to wear or damage to the typing element. This may result in a distinctive appearance to the document which the examiner can detect through careful observation and measurement. The question most difficult to answer is whether one individual typed a document, and only certain circumstances allow an answer to this question.

In a similar situation to the one above involving office machines, questions about paper require the examiner to know a great deal about the characteristics of paper, and to have a library of paper samples at his or her disposal if questions about paper are to be answered. And, just as in the case of ink dating, if paper is to be actually dated, a specialist is consulted.

Questions involving indentations, erasures, and alterations can be answered with careful use of lighting, photography, and simple, nondestructive chemicals in the document examination laboratory. Infrared and ultraviolet photography are used to answer questions that remain mysteries under normal lighting.

Frequently Asked Questions

Can you describe an individual's personality from examining handwriting?

There is a separate field of study called "Graphology" which deals with personality and handwriting. Questioned Document Examination is a forensic science, concerned with identification of handwriting and technical aspects of document preparation. In some countries during some time periods, document examination and graphology have been studied together and practiced by the same professionals. Today, in the United States, the two fields tend to be mutually exclusive.

Can right- or left-handedness be detected by examining handwriting?

Contrary to popular belief, there are three things that can not be reliably ascertained by examining handwriting. One of those is the "handedness" of the writer. The other two things are the author's gender and age.

Can you compare printed writing to cursive writing?

No. That is an "apples and oranges" situation. Although there are some writing traits that carry over between cursive and printing, you can not project from cursive how an individual's printing would look, and vice versa.

Can you examine documents in a foreign language?

Yes, it is possible, but the examiner must first learn about the characteristics of the written language and how that writing is taught.

For example, in some languages, placement of diacriticals (distinguishing strokes) is important, and in other languages, shading of handwritten strokes is significant. The actual methods of examination are the same, but factors are weighed differently when the structure of the writing varies among languages.

Can a document examiner work with photocopies of questioned documents?

This question must be answered on a case by case basis. If the copy is a good one and if there is enough information in the writing to allow an opinion, a copy is sufficient. But there are some situations where the opinion rests on a subtle aspect of the writing that might only be visible on an original viewed under the microscope. In such situations, examination of the original is critical.

Can a client fax documents to you for examination?

A fax of a questioned document is of very little use. The fax process digitizes the copy, obscures detail, and adds flaws to the document. Of course, there are document questions about faxed documents, but those are best handled by examination of the original faxes themselves.

Handwriting and Signatures—Some Basic Facts and Theory

Handwriting originates in the brain when a mental picture of letters and words is formed. The signal to try to duplicate the mental picture is sent to the arm and hand through the muscles and nervous system. The actual output is almost never an exact match of the original mental picture.

The Physiology of Handwriting Production

Let's look at how a human learns to use his or her brain and nervous system to write.

When a baby is born, it is equipped with certain basic, automatic abilities. It can breathe, cry, suck, move its limbs randomly. To accomplish more complex tasks, the baby must learn. Patterns must be formed and stored in the brain which then will trigger messages to travel through the nervous system to the muscles to produce movements (behavior). Smiling is a simple behavior that a baby learns early in life. At first, he

257

imitates his parents' smiles, and as this behavior is rewarded by more smiles and hugs from his parents (positive feedback), a pattern is built in the baby's brain. The baby learns to call upon that pattern to produce a smile. Soon, smiling becomes automatic, just like breathing.

In a similar way, the baby learns to reach, grasp, speak, and walk. More and more complex actions become possible as the baby builds the neural pathways that travel between the muscles and the brain via the nervous system. Handwriting is an extremely complex motor task, which is not usually learned until the child is five or six years old and has mastered simpler skills.

The motor system controls the movement and posture needed for handwriting by contraction and relaxation of muscles. Messages go to and from the muscles and brain via the nervous system. During the learning process, the senses and muscles send messages (feedback) back to the brain to let it know how the sequence, timing, and force applied worked out. The brain makes the adjustments needed to give a maximal outcome. Eventually a motor program is formed. This is a set of muscle commands that can be carried out with the correct timing and sequence automatically, without feedback, to give the best possible result.

Handwriting is the result of such stored motor knowledge. Handwriting is distal, meaning that it occurs at the extremities and involves fine motor activity as opposed to a skill like walking which is proximal—a large, or gross motor skill. One reason individuals find it difficult to simulate the handwriting of others is that to do so successfully requires understanding the essence of the writer's motor control program and executing that same program.

Now, let's do an experiment. Take a clean unlined sheet of paper and write your signature near the top. Next, hold your pen or pencil in your clenched fist and sign your name by moving your wrist and arm. Then bend your arm fully and hold the pencil in the crease at your elbow and sign your name with your elbow guiding the pen. While the second and third signatures do not have the fluency, size, and proportion of the first signature, you will see that the same overall pattern prevails. This is because the programs to perform the complex movements required to produce a written word are stored in the brain, not in the muscles. If you want to further prove this to yourself, try to write your first name in the air with your nose or your foot. You can do it, right? The basic information to do this came from your brain, not from the muscles of your shoulder, arm, fingers, or nose.

Once the basic pattern is established, the muscles and nerves of the shoulder, arm, hand, and fingers become important because they certainly affect the appearance of the written line. You can think of the body as a machine, a series of levers and fulcrums (pivot points) with each part influencing the working of the next part in the link. The strength and flexibility of the muscles, the position of the pen grip and the overall posture of the writer all affect the output.

Variety: The Natural Range of Handwriting

None of the factors that produce handwriting are rigid and unchanging. In addition to the organic factors (physical anatomy and health, mental acuity, etc.) there are environmental factors affecting the handwriting. These include the writing instrument itself, the writing surface and what lies beneath it, and other variables of the writing situation. Because the primary motor pattern is itself a fluid image and because there are so many organic and environmental variables that interact in the production of handwriting, it has become an accepted axiom that a person is unlikely to ever duplicate any signature exactly. Each person has a range of natural variation. But even with this range of variation, each person grows in his or her writing from the classic forms taught in childhood into an individual and identifiable form of written expression.

Handwriting is a free-form activity, and there are an infinite number of ways to write even the simplest letter combination. It is highly unlikely that any person will write his or her own name exactly the same way twice in an entire lifetime.

Actually, every person has a range of handwriting variation determined by his or her physical writing ability, training in "penmanship", and other factors. To the experienced expert, a study of known samples of writing reveals personal writing characteristics which can allow the expert to identify or exclude an individual as the author of some questioned writing.

Handwriting characteristics come in two categories—general, or class characteristics, and individual characteristics. Depending on the cultural setting (time and place) when writing is learned, entire groups of individuals are taught to write in the same way. When these individuals are first learning to write, there are differences in their ability to do the task, and the results are not all the same, but the true individualizing differences appear over time. As we grow and mature physically and personally, our handwriting becomes more of an individual product—through conscious changes made to fit a mental picture of how we want our writing to appear, or unconsciously.

Handwriting can also be affected by other factors—injury, illness, medication, drug or alcohol use, stress, the writing surface, the writing instrument, or attempted disguise. It is the job of the document examiner to understand these factors as they might relate to a specific situation.

Questioned Documents in the Spotlight

Questions about the legitimacy of documents are probably as old as documents themselves. [In this section,] I will discuss a few of the interesting cases in questioned document history, followed by a bibliography for interested readers.

In 1795, a Mr. Ireland brought forward what he claimed to be a new version of "Kynge Leare" which was allegedly written by William Shakespeare himself. In 1796, Edward Malone published a refutation of this document. Mr. Malone had discovered that the questioned manuscript contained pages with twenty different watermarks. He reasoned that an author of Shakespeare's caliber who was also famous and affluent at the time Lear was written, would have gone to a papermaker and secured as much paper of one type as was needed for his work. But someone who wanted to forge an Elizabethan play 200 years later would ferret out such scraps of old paper as he could—from the flyleaves and blank pages of old manuscripts. Indeed, in 1805, the forger wrote his confession and admitted that he had done exactly that. He had paid a bookseller to let him cut out blank pages from the older volumes in his shop.

Many questioned document cases are proven on evidence other than handwriting examination. For example, in 1928, there was a famous case known as the Duke "Lost Heirs Case" which was tried in Somerville, New Jersey. A family Bible was introduced inscribed with the birth dates of children of the family. The mother claimed that she wrote the dates in the Bible shortly after the birth of the children in 1887 and 1889. However, careful examination of the Bible itself showed that it was copyrighted in 1890, invalidating the timing claimed by the mother.

A document examiner must be relentlessly thorough in considering all aspects of a document. In the 1920s, the Oliver Will case was tried in White Plains, New York. The question revolved around the date on which the will was written. A legal form which had the date and name and address of its printer at the top was used for the will, but a piece of the document which showed the date had been torn away. There were two possibilities for the date of the form—January 8, 1924, or October 8, 1924. The date of the alleged will was September 20, 1924, so the only form that could have been used was the one printed earlier in the year. Upon close examination, it was found that in tearing away the dated portion of the form, the tail of the comma in the address was still visible, and the position on the paper of that comma tail proved that the form could not have been the January 8th form. The questioned will was therefore written on a form that did not exist on the date it was allegedly prepared.

Early in 1972, a Federal Grand Jury heard the testimony of a Questioned Document Examiner from the Crime Laboratory of the U.S. Postal Inspection Service regarding questioned documents allegedly written by Howard R. Hughes. In these documents, permission was granted for a biography of Mr. Hughes to be written by Clifford Irving. Mr. Irving had used these questioned documents to convince the editors of McGraw-Hill Book Co. and Life Magazine that he had a deal with Mr. Hughes—an allegation hotly contested by Howard Hughes when he learned of it.

The testimony of the experts from the Postal Inspection Service was that the questioned documents were not written by Mr. Hughes. Often in forgery cases it is possible to conclude that the alleged author of a document did not do the writing, but it is more difficult to conclude that a particular person did do it. This is because the writing habits of the forger will often be buried in the attempt to simulate the pictorial look and style of the "target" writing. However, in this case, there was a large amount of writing in question. Mr. Irving had even had "Mr. Hughes" write a letter to the editors of Mc-Graw Hill to validate his agreement with Mr. Irving. The volume of questioned writing was enough that Mr. Irving was not able to keep up his "disguise" and his own individual writing characteristics showed through the veneer of the simulated "Hughes" writing.

Another famous case involving questioned documents and Howard Hughes was the "Mormon Will" case which arose when Hughes died in 1976 leaving an estate estimated to be between two and three billion dollars, and no apparent will. While attorneys and executives of Hughes' corporations scrambled to find a will, speculation ran rampant through the country. One possibility was that Hughes had written a "holographic" will, which is a will written totally by hand—usually in the person's own words without benefit of the presence of an attorney. One Hughes attorney stated that Hughes had asked him twice about the legalities of a proper holographic will.

Shortly after this information was published, an alleged holographic will of Howard Hughes was found left anonymously on a desk in the office building of the Church of Jesus Christ of Latter Day Saints (the Mormon Church). With the will was a note saying that the document had been found near the home of Joseph Smith (founder of the Mormon Church) and that it should be delivered to the President of the Mormon Church. A questioned document examiner gave the preliminary opinion that the will might have been written by Howard Hughes, and the Mormon Church filed the will in the Las Vegas county court which is where jurisdiction of the estate had settled.

One provision of the will (which became known as "The Mormon Will") was that a 1/16th share of the estate ($156,000,000) would go to Melvin Dummar of Gabbs, Nevada. Melvin Dummar and his wife owned and operated a small gas station in Willard, Utah, at the time this information came to light. Mr. Dummar claimed that he had no knowledge of the will or how it ended up in the hands of the Mormon Church. He told reporters that years previous he had picked up a bum in the desert who claimed to be Howard Hughes and that he had given this man a ride into Las Vegas and dropped him off behind the Sands Hotel after giving the man what spare change he had in his own pocket.

From April through December of 1976, Melvin Dummar was under intense media scrutiny and public interest. He spoke everywhere, and always maintained that he knew nothing about the will, or the circumstances of its appearance in the Mormon Church offices. But while Mr. Dummar was dealing with his public, forensic examinations were going on behind the scenes. The will had been found in an outer envelope which was found to have a fingerprint matching that of Melvin Dummar. Also, Mr. Dummar was a part-time student at Webster State College at the time the will was discovered. In the college library was a copy of the book, *Hoax,* which was written about the Clifford Irving forgeries described above. This book had many examples of the writing of Howard Hughes and other anecdotal information. The book from the library also had a fingerprint on it that matched a print of Mr. Dummar.

The Mormon Will had been found with an inner envelope and an outer envelope and slip of paper which asked that the will be delivered to the head of the Church. A document examiner concluded that the writing on the outer envelope and the slip of paper was probably disguised writing of Melvin Dummar. When Mr. Dummar was confronted with the fingerprinting and handwriting evidence, he flatly denied all allegations of his involvement in any forgery of the document and insisted that the evidence was being faked in a conspiracy against him by the Hughes corporate executives.

In the face of constant questioning and clear evidence, after several intermediate changes of story, Mr. Dummar settled on an official version in which a mysterious man drove into his service station and gave him the will along with several pages of instructions. Mr. Dummar admitted that in following these instructions (which he had since burned), he had placed the will in the envelope, written the note on the slip of paper, and delivered the package to the Mormon Church offices.

This case was essentially a one issue case—whether the will was a forgery or not. At least four very prominent American questioned document examiners concluded that the will was forged. A definite conclusion was possible because there were three full pages of questioned writing to work with, as well as a large body of contemporaneous known writings by Howard Hughes. To make matters even more clear, Mr. Hughes had undergone an obvious change in some of his handwriting habits during a two year period just before the alleged will was written. Only someone with access to current writings of Mr. Hughes and sophisticated understanding of handwriting would have known how Mr. Hughes' writing should have looked on the date in question. All in all, the forgery was quite clumsy, both in the handwriting and in the attitudes expressed by its content. Although this case probably should have been settled early on, it had a momentum of its own and would not die. It culminated with a seven-month trial and millions of dollars expended by the estate of Howard Hughes. In the end, the court ruled the will a forgery and the billionaire, Howard Hughes died intestate.

My own brush with famous documents came with a case in 1992. I was asked to verify the authenticity of an alleged original copy of The Declaration of Independence. An elderly Southern gentleman had purchased an old trunk and found this document with its contents. He was quite insistent that I travel to his home to see the document and I prepared myself to do so. He was not willing to send me a photocopy, and I was not sure whether the answer to the problem would come from handwriting evidence, paper or ink analysis, or historical information, so I gathered information on all of the above. From the history department at a local university I learned about the various stages of preparation of the famous document. There were "broadsides" printed and posted before the actual document was signed, and various copies prepared on different dates were signed in stages by the Representatives. There were slight changes in wording in some editions of the document. There were also commemorative editions of the Declaration printed in various formats in the years just after the Revolution. Actually, there are still such editions printed today. I hoped that by understanding the history of the actual document, I could look at the questioned document and make some preliminary decisions about it.

I am neither an ink nor paper expert, and I did some networking to locate such experts who would be willing to work with me if my preliminary examination indicated that the document had a chance of being authentic. I also spoke with archivists who helped me secure additional comparison signatures of the people whose names I expected to see signed on the document. When the time for the trip came, I felt as prepared as possible to do at least a preliminary investigation and then to route the document to additional experts for nondestructive chemical testing.

I reached my destination via plane and rental car, checked into a hotel, and arranged to meet with my client. This document had become a focal point of the lives of this man and his family. If it were genuine it would have great value, and there was a question of pride involved as well. Unfortunately, it did not take long for me to shatter their fondest hopes. A careful look through the microscope revealed that the printing process used on the document was not available in the late 1700s. The signatures were not done individually in ink as the owner of the document had insisted they were. My final conclusion, which was later borne out by a paper expert, was that at best the document was one of many sets printed commemoratively in 1876 at the Centennial celebration of the Revolution. This would set its value at approximately $100.00 according to a consultant at a famous auction house. My client was very disappointed, but glad to have the matter resolved. I was also disappointed, but not surprised. I was glad to have had the impetus to learn more about American history and to feel close to it for a brief time.

References

Cabanne, R. A. "The Clifford Irving Hoax of the Howard Hughes Autobiography." *Journal of Forensic Sciences* 20: 5-17 (1975).

Freese, Paul L., J.D. "Howard Hughes and Melvin Dummar: Forensic Science Fact Versus Film Fiction." *Journal of Forensic Sciences* 31 (1): 342-59 (January 1986).

Harris, John J., B.S."The Document Evidence and Some Other Observations about the Howard R. Hughes 'Mormon Will' Contest." *Journal of Forensic Sciences* 31 (1): 365-75 (January 1986).

Hilton, Ordway. *Scientific Examination of Questioned Documents,* revised ed. New York: Elsevier Series in Forensic Science, 1984.

Osborn, Albert S. *Questioned Documents,* 2nd ed. Montclair, NJ: Patterson Smith, 1973.

— by Emily J. Will, Certified Document Examiner

Part Four

Emerging Forensic Subspecialties

Chapter 27

Automated DNA Typing

Although highly reliable in clinical or research applications, the standard technology used for DNA typing—known as RFLP-VNTR[1] analysis—has been less satisfactory in the forensic setting. RFLP-VNTR requires abundant and clean specimens; samples typically found at crime scenes, however, are both quantitatively and qualitatively inadequate—very small and often environmentally degraded from exposure to heat, light, and humidity. Further, police investigations call for a quicker turnaround time than is possible with the standard method, which can take months to complete.

An NIJ-sponsored project at Baylor University's College of Medicine sought a DNA typing system that overcomes the limitations of samples found at crime scenes. The project replicated the DNA sample (i.e., synthesized new DNA from existing DNA) to obtain sufficient quantities for analysis and then identified genetic markers[2] for DNA typing. That procedure, known as PCR-STR,[3] can produce reliable results with degraded specimens, is quick, and can be automated to permit the creation of a vastly improved database of DNA profiles of convicted offenders. PCR-STR promises to extend the application of DNA typing as a powerful criminal justice tool that helps to establish, with a high degree of certitude, the guilt or innocence of suspects.

From "Automated DNA Typing: Method of the Future?" in the U.S. Department of Justice, Office of Justice Programs Series, *NIJ Research Preview,* February 1997.

Basic Facts about DNA

Understanding the importance of DNA typing to criminal investigations requires knowledge of some fundamental facts. Each molecule of DNA, the primary carrier of genetic information in living organisms, consists of a very long spiral structure that has been likened to a "twisted ladder." The handrails of the ladder string together the ladder's "rungs," which are called bases. Bases, composed of four varieties of nucleic acid, combine in pairs called "nucleotides." The sequence of these base pairs constitutes the genetic coding of DNA.

DNA in humans is found in all cells that contain a nucleus (i.e., in all except red blood cells). Each nucleated cell (with the exception of sperm and egg cells) usually contains the full complement of an individual's DNA, called the "genome," that is unvarying from cell to cell. The genome consists of approximately 3 billion base pairs, of which about 3 million actually differ from person to person. However, the base pairs that vary represent a virtually incalculable number of possible combinations. Person-to-person differences within a particular segment of DNA sequence are referred to as "alleles."

DNA typing focuses on identifying and isolating discrete fragments of these alleles in a sample and comparing one sample with another. For example, a forensic scientist might compare a semen sample retrieved from a rape victim to a DNA sample taken from a suspect. If identical fragments appear in both samples, a match is declared. To determine the likelihood of a match being mere coincidence, a particular combination of alleles is compared to the frequency with which the combination appears in the statistical population.

PCR-STR Procedure

The replication process. Many of the frequently encountered and frustrating shortcomings of forensic specimens—i.e., contamination, environmental degradation, and the generally small quantity of testable material—are surmounted by PCR analysis. This technique involves extracting DNA from a small evidence sample and then replicating it through a complex operation of repeated heating and cooling cycles and exposure to an enzyme. Because each cycle doubles the quantity of DNA, the original extraction can be replicated several million times within a short period of time. By examining several locations (loci) where variation occurs, a typing profile can be produced.

Baylor researchers focused on isolating 13 STR (short tandem repeat) loci, each of which contains a short region where a sequence of three, four, or five nucleotides is repeated a different number of times in different people. Samples identified by a radioactively labeled, allele-specific probe are blotted onto a membrane, according to standard PCR protocol. Each dark spot that appears can be read as "yes" or "no" to the question of whether a particular individual possesses a given allele.

When comparing DNA samples from known individuals with evidence samples, a difference of a single allele can exclude someone as the donor of that evidence sample. The more locations that show the same allele pattern, the stronger the evidence that the two samples came from the same individual. PCR amplification techniques allow DNA typing results to be obtained from even badly degraded samples, and STR analysis permits exact allele designations. Thus, PCR-STR allows samples analyzed at different times to be easily compared.

Automation

STR analysis was initially developed as a manual process, but automated methods are becoming available. Key to this technology is the use of fluorescent chemicals during the PCR process. A laser-generated fluorescent signal from the STR alleles passes information to a computer, where the collected data are analyzed to produce DNA profile information. In addition, robotic workstations are available to process DNA samples and assist with other procedures. With automation, the entire process—from DNA extraction to data interpretation—could be accomplished with little human involvement or manipulation, thereby reducing the possibility of error.

Realization and acceptance of full automation will take some time. All the pieces, however, are currently available and can be integrated. Laboratories, companies, and individuals associated with the Human Genome Project, molecular biology, and forensic science could work together to bring the newest technology in molecular analysis to the crime laboratory. Every criminal case with relevant biological evidence could be analyzed—without the time, cost, and technical limitations that thwart the full potential of forensic DNA typing. Most importantly, accurate and rapid DNA typing capability advances the foremost criminal justice objective: to shield the innocent and convict the guilty.

Notes

1. RFPL-VNTR stands for restriction fragment length polymorphism-variable number of tandem repeats.

2. A marker is a gene with a known location on a chromosome and a clear-cut phenotype (physical appearance or functional expression of a trait) that is used as a point of reference in the mapping of other locations.

3. PCR stands for polymerase chain reaction and is the technique used to replicate DNA. STR (short tandem repeat) refers to the region on a DNA strand where a sequence of three, four, or five nucleotides is repeated a different number of times in different people—the so-called STR loci.

    —by Holly A. Hammond, M.A., and C. Thomas Caskey, M.D.

A summary of a research study conducted by the authors at the Baylor University College of Medicine.

Chapter 28

Criminal Profiling

In 1972, the FBI's newly formed Behavioral Science Unit developed and propagated some of the earliest psychological profiling techniques and training, which were first taught to students at the FBI National Academy by SA Howard Teten and SA Pat Mullany. They espoused the idea that constructing a criminal profile from the physical evidence in an unsolved case could effectively aid in the process of suspect development, and investigative strategy. The past three decades have been a continual exercise in demonstrating that they were right.

The *Crime Classification Manual*,[4] developed by the FBI's National Center for the Analysis of Violent Crime, describes the ideal process of developing a criminal profile, which it terms criminal investigative analysis:

"The FBI defines criminal investigative analysis as an investigative process that identifies the major personality and behavioral characteristics of the offender based on the crimes he or she has committed . . .:

1. Evaluation of the criminal act itself

2. Comprehensive evaluation of the specifics of the crime scene(s)

From "The Role of Criminal Profiling in the Development of Trial Strategy," [Online]. Available: http://www.corpus-delicti.com. © 1997 by Knowledge Solutions, LLC, for Brent Turvey, M.S., 1271 Washington Ave., # 274, San Leandro, CA 94577-3646; Phone: (510) 483-6739; Fax: (415) 840-0012; E-mail: bturvey@corpus-delicti.com. Reprinted with permission.

3. Comprehensive analysis of the victim

4. Evaluation of preliminary police reports

5. Evaluation of the medical examiner's autopsy protocol

6. Development of the profile, with critical offender characteristics

7. Investigative suggestions predicated on the construction of the profile"[4]

As mentioned, this concept is an ideal, and one that most modern day profilers fall woefully short of in actual practice. In fact, most of those who call themselves criminal profilers have all but abandoned the above deductive tenants in favor of statistical databasing from which inductive profiles are generated. The reason behind this shift seems to be the reality that most modern day investigators are not adequately trained to evaluate forensic evidence of any kind, and therefore are not prepared to engage the above steps.[7] It should be mentioned that this author does not advocate or even recommend the use of inductive profiles in criminal or non-criminal investigations for suspect development.

Work done by Hazelwood, et al.,[3] takes the FBI's concept of criminal investigative analysis to the next logical level, in terms of applying the information developed in the profile to courtroom proceedings. Hazelwood, et al.[3] demonstrates how a criminal profile can be used to help develop trial strategy. They[3] define a criminal profile as

the characteristics and traits of an unidentified offender that differentiate him from the general population. These characteristics are set forth in such a manner as to allow those who know and/or associate with the offender to readily recognize him.

They further define trial strategy in a general fashion as "analyzing a case to provide attorneys with recommendations to the strengths and weaknesses of the opposition's case, cross-examination techniques, and expert witnesses."

There is some agreement in the literature regarding the types of cases which can benefit the most from the profiling process.[2, 3, 4] The *Crime Classification Manual*[4] specifically addresses the crimes of murder, arson, and rape/sexual assault because they represent the most serious types of interpersonally violent criminal behavior. However, it has been demonstrated that cases which have benefited from the profiling process can include just about any case where the forensic evidence or crime scene presentation indicates mental, emotional, or personality aberrations.[3, 6]

The purpose of this paper, then, is to discuss the profiling process, and how it directly lends itself to the development of trial strategy. Specifically, it will address how the criminal profiling process can help attorneys understand the nature and quality of the forensic evidence in a case, offender fantasy behavior and/or motivation, offender state of mind during the commission of the crime, and help link cases by illuminating offender patterns in terms of Modus Operandi (MO) and signature behavior.

The Problem

Many agencies who request a criminal profile, whether they are law enforcement agencies, prosecutorial bodies, or defense attorneys of any kind, are unified by a misperception that the profiling process will somehow answer specific questions about criminal behavior while circumventing the work required to analyze the often complex physical evidence in a particular case (there are a number of people calling themselves profilers who think this way, too, just to add to the confusion). This is not surprising at all, given that most criminal cases do not involve the use of physical evidence of any kind, and, even when available, physical evidence is seldom seen by anyone involved as having any intrinsic value. In fact, a literature review conducted by Horvath and Meesig[7] determined that physical evidence is used in less than 25% of the cases prosecuted in the United States, with the percentage in some regions dipping to less than 5%.

As stated, the notion that physical evidence does not have intrinsic value is a popular misperception, but not one shared by the criminal profiler. For the competent profiler, physical evidence and its proper documentation in a given case are the very basis for any and all deductions about an offender's characteristics.

This points to the real issue that needs to be confronted in criminal investigations and subsequent judicial proceedings, which is that in crimes involving violent, aberrant, sexual, and/or predatory behavior, the physical evidence has generally not been fully examined by qualified investigators or forensic experts. The necessary result of this nearly pathological failure to recognize the intrinsic value of physical evidence is a failure to recognize the importance of, and even gross misinterpretations of, the nature and intent of even the most basic criminal behaviors. The use of competent criminal profilers, who are trained to examine physical evidence and exploit it to its fullest natural conclusion, can be an effective after-the-fact solution to this problem, even years after the crime has been committed.

Objectivity

One of the largest issues that any forensic examiner faces is the question of objectivity. The objective forensic investigator's role is that of a neutral, disinterested participant, never degenerating into that of an advocate. As forensic investigators of fact, criminal profilers are no different from other forensic examiners and are bound by the same ethical standards.

In cases where the offender is unknown, it is less difficult to navigate objectively than in cases where a suspect or a defendant is involved. To better maintain objectivity, a profiler should not conduct suspect interviews, and further should not have contact with case related defendants, at any time prior to the development of the final profile. This guideline helps to prevent the profiler from "tailoring" their conclusions to include or exclude a particular type of individual based on contact with a suspect or defendant. Adherence to this guideline keeps the final profile a product of crime scene behavior and victimological assessments deducted purely from forensic evidence and witness testimony, and truly enables a more objective rendering.

As Burgess, et al.[2] explicitly state in their treatise on the subject of sexual homicide analysis, regarding case material submissions by requesting agencies:

> Information the profiler does not want included in the case materials is that dealing with possible suspects. Such information may subconsciously prejudice the profiler and cause him or her to prepare a profile matching the suspect.

This author would go even further by stating that the influences of suspect or defendant information on subsequent profiles can be conscious as well as unconscious. Again, this is an ethical issue that each profiler must confront, but that can be avoided by adherence to the above guideline. However, a reality of the nature of profiling is that pure objectivity is an ideal and not always attainable. So whether the profiler is retained by the prosecution, the defense, or another interested party, the value of any interpretations or opinions rendered should ultimately be judged solely by how well they account for the facts of the case and nothing more.

Benefits

The criminal profiling process offers many benefits to the trial attorney. This section will overview some of the more salient benefits with general examples.

Recognizing Evidence

As discussed, the most effective criminal profilers tend to be those who have first been trained as competent forensic investigators, with an appreciation for the value of forensic evidence, and the ability to perform at least some level of wound pattern analysis. In as much as this is true, a profiler should first go through the process of analyzing the physical evidence in the case presented to them, in an effort to determine the actual nature of the interaction between the victim and the offender from all available documented sources. This includes first responder's reports, investigators' reports, autopsy reports, results of sexual assault examination, witness interviews, victim statements (when available), and all available photos and videos. The net result of this equivocal forensic analysis is that the profiler becomes better informed about the larger picture of the investigation, and better able to illuminate areas in the first stages of the investigation where weaknesses in evidence collection or recognition may have occurred, as well as potential errors in forensic interpretation, and even complete omissions in evidence recognition.

This author has worked on several capital cases where crucial evidence was not recognized or collected by investigating detectives, coroners, and even highly trained medical examiners. Yet the same evidence was clearly visible in the crime scene and autopsy photos, waiting for someone to look for it.

The type of physical evidence most commonly missed in the case experience of this author includes such highly probative evidence as petechiae in the eyes and nasal mucosa, bloodstain patterns of varying nature and origin, bite mark evidence misinterpreted as blunt force trauma, blunt force trauma misinterpreted as stab wounds, lacerations misinterpreted as stab wounds, victims' gaping anal sphincters misinterpreted as anal rape, and pattern injuries of varying origins. The major tenets of wound pattern analysis as they can be applied to criminal cases are explored in Geberth[6] and DiMaio, et al.[5]

The profiler's role in these instances, where crucial physical evidence has been overlooked, is not necessarily to interpret it, but to direct counsel to the appropriate forensic expert—i.e., if a bite mark appears evident on a victim's breast, then the profiler would recommend that counsel seek out a forensic odontologist.

Fantasy and Motivation

A common misconception on any side of the courtroom is that there is such a thing as a motiveless crime. As Geberth[6] states in his definitive treatise on homicide investigation, "No one acts without motivation." What is also true, however, is that very often the specific motivation for a particular crime may only be known to the offender.

It is the job of the profiler, in concert with criminalists, to reconstruct behavior from the physical evidence, then look for patterns in that behavior, and illuminate that behavior's meaning within the context of a specific crime or series of crimes, to a specific criminal offender. That is, the profiler interprets the psychological value and meaning of each crime behavior committed by an offender. Behaviors either serve the MO, and are necessary to complete the crime, or they serve a fantasy constructed by the offender. For descriptions of this process in great detail, readers can reference a number of highly respected learned treatises on the subject.[2, 3, 4, 6, 8]

State of Mind

One of the major contributions of a profiler to trial strategy is the interpretation of offender state of mind before, during, and after the commission of the crime. This is accomplished very effectively by the profiler because the only source of information used is the offender's crime scene behavior and interaction with the victim. Where forensic psychologists and other assessors may use post-apprehension interviews, polygraph examinations, or personality measures which have been duped countless times by offenders over the years, the profiler carefully examines what the offender did, and has little use for what the offender has to say about what they did.

Examples of behaviors that can give insight into offender state of mind include, but are not limited to: bringing a rape-kit to the crime to facilitate a victim's torture (indicating some level of pre-planning), as opposed to using available materials (indicating some level of spontaneity); using the victim's shirt to cover their face during the commission of the crime (indicating some level of spontaneity), as opposed to bringing a blindfold or tape to cover the victim's eyes (indicating some level of pre-planning); the presence of violent, frenzied slashing injuries to the victim's face (indicating some level of rage and familiarity, or perhaps a need to depersonalize), in contrast to careful, methodical exploratory stab wounds (inflicted either to torture a conscious victim, or to satisfy the offender's curiosity with an unconscious victim).

MO Behavior and Signature Behavior

As previously mentioned, MO behaviors are those committed by the offender during the commission of the crime which are necessary to complete the crime. MO behaviors are unstable across offenses, and may alter as the offender gains confidence or experience. Fantasy behaviors are committed to serve the offender's fantasies, and psychological and/or emotional needs. Fantasy behaviors are also called signature behaviors, are thematic in nature, and tend to be more stable over time. These concepts are thoroughly explored by Geberth[6] and Turvey.[8]

The profiler identifies signature behaviors and MO behaviors, and interprets their meaning for the purpose of linking two separate crimes together as having been potentially committed by the same offender, or for the purpose of demonstrating how two crimes may be psychologically different, indicating two separate offenders.

Conclusions

The objective, deductive process of criminal profiling as described in this paper, and the subsequent benefits as detailed, can directly lend themselves to the development of trial strategy. Specifically, the criminal profiling process can help attorneys understand the nature and quality of physical evidence, offender fantasy behavior and/or motivation, offender state of mind during the commission of the crime, and help link or exclude cases by illuminating offender patterns in terms of Modus Operandi (MO) and Signature Behavior.

It is further important to note that profiling will not implicate a specific individual in a specific crime, but can be used to implicate a specific type of individual, with specific psychological and emotional characteristics. As with any such process, it is subject to abuses by those who do not adhere to requisite ethical standards in their zeal to either seek conviction, or seek an acquittal. In competent hands, it can be a constructive and useful tool.

It is also important to recognize that the results of the profiling process are only as competent as the original investigative efforts and processes which provide (or in many cases fail to provide) the physical evidence from which criminal behavior is reconstructed. This is due to the reality that not only is it possible for investigators to misinterpret the physical evidence which has been recognized and collected, but it is also possible for investigators to fail to recognize certain types of physical evidence which they are not trained to look for.[7] This set of realities illuminates very clearly why profilers are best conceptualized as a single member of a larger investigative team, who depend on other team members to do their job competently. This set of realities also illuminates the reason why a good profiler should first conduct an equivocal forensic analysis before delving into the psychological aspects of a crime; they must be certain that the behavior they are profiling, and ascribing meaning to, is in fact the behavior that occurred.

The profiling process itself, which can begin after a thorough equivocal analysis has been performed, should not be based on inductive generalizations from statistical databases, such as with syndrome evidence, or be used to provide counsel with tailored expert testimony which serves one side of the courtroom in favor of the other, placing the profiler in the role of advocate. Rather, the profiling process at its best maximizes the potential of any existing physical evidence in seemingly motiveless cases involving criminal behavior of a violent, aberrant, sexual, and/or predatory nature. It further serves to illuminate physical evidence, and offender behavior, in a way that allows counsel to competently prepare for trial.

References

1. A. Burgess, R. D'Agostino, J. Douglas, C. Hartman, and R. Ressler, "Sexual Killers and Their Victims: Identifying Patterns through Crime Scene Analysis," *Journal of Interpersonal Violence* 1 (3): 288-308 (September 1986).

2. A. Burgess, J. Douglas, and R. Ressler, ed., *Sexual Homicide: Patterns and Motives* (New York: Lexington Books, 1988).

3. A. Burgess and R. Hazelwood, ed., *Practical Aspects of Rape Investigation: A Multidisciplinary Approach,* 2nd ed. (New York: CRC Press, 1995).

4. A. Burgess, J. Douglas, and R. Ressler, ed., *Crime Classification Manual* (San Francisco: Jossey-Bass Publishers, 1997).

5. D. DiMaio and V. DiMaio, *Forensic Pathology* (Boca Raton: CRC Press, 1993).

6. Vernon Geberth, *Practical Homicide Investigation,* 2nd ed. (New York: CRC Press, 1996).

7. F. Horvath and R. Meesig, "The Criminal Investigation Process and the Role of Forensic Evidence: A Review of Empirical Findings," *Journal of Forensic Sciences* 41 (6): 963-9 (November 1996).

8. Brent Turvey, *Criminal Profiling: An Introduction to Behavior Evidence Analysis* (London: Academic Press, 1999).

—by Brent E. Turvey, M.S.

Chapter 29

Computer-Aided Victim Identification

Introduction

Facial identification by visual means is routinely carried out throughout the world on fresh bodies by relatives and other acquaintances of the deceased as a legal requirement. In cases where there is mutilation of the facial features, advanced decomposition or skeletalisation of the head, however, visual identification is unreliable, undesirable or impossible. In such circumstances identification is usually achieved by other means, dental identification being the most practical and reliable method when antemortem dental records are available.[1] When it is difficult or impossible to obtain such dental records or other confirmatory evidence, such as fingerprinting, however, the forensic investigator may consider facial reconstruction if no comparative photographic material is available, or some form of superimposition of available photographs onto the skull. It should be appreciated that such methods are used in conjunction with other corroborative methods, such as the finding of personal belongings, and skeletal findings that may be present due to previous trauma, hospital therapy, congenital or acquired skeletal anomalies.

Excerpted from "Techniques in Facial Identification: Computer-Aided Facial Reconstruction Using a Laser Scanner and Video Superimposition," by A. W. Shahrom, R. C. Chapman, C. Blenkinsop, M. L. Rossi, P. Vanezis, and A. Gonzalez, in *International Journal of Legal Medicine,* Vol. 108, 1996, pp. 194-200. © 1996 by Springer-Verlag. Reprinted with permission.

283

Materials and Methods

Computer-Aided Facial Reconstruction Techniques

Facial reconstruction may either be three dimensional (3-D) from a skull or skull model or two dimensional (2-D) from radiographs and photographs of skulls. [2] The 3-D facial image may be reconstructed by either building muscle and other soft tissues onto a skull or plaster cast using clay or plasticine and then adding facial features, or by means of a computer-aided facial reconstruction technique.

We used a 3-D computer graphics system for reconstructing a face on the skull. The system used is based on acquiring the image using an optical laser 3-D scanning system (Facia Optical Surface Scanner by 3-D Scanners).[3-5] The skull of interest is placed on a skull holder, which can be slowly rotated through 360° in a horizontal plane under computer control. A thin beam of red laser light strikes a small cylindrical lens and fans out into a vertical line 0.7 mm wide. This line runs vertically down the skull, appearing as a thin red stripe. The form of the stripe running over the skull is viewed by a video camera with the room in partial darkness and a red filter in front of the lens. The output from the camera is digitised and passed through a digital comparator and further analysed by the computer to produce a 3-D skull image. The facial thickness tissue type which is to be given to the 3-D skull image is then selected. The software programme allows three selections: normal, thin, and fat. This is followed by entering 44 landmarks (peg markers) as described by Farkas[6] on the skull image. The software programme indicates the peg markers as a series of numbers 1-24, 31-44, and 53-58. The 'average face' thought to be representative of the deceased's skull (e.g., male, Caucasian, fat) can be selected from a database of scanned faces. Similar 44-peg markers are then entered on the average face. The skull and the facial images are then aligned with respect to orientation, position, and scale. The peg markers on both images are rechecked because the process of alignment may sometimes cause a slight change in their position. The 3-D skull image is then superimposed on the average image using the 'face change programme'. The peg markers on the skull are matched manually with those on the average face. On selection of the command 'face shift', the computer will proceed with reconstruction of the average face on the 3-D skull image automatically. The reconstructed facial image can he photographed directly from the monitor or printed out through a printer or videotaped. It can also be stored in a database for future reference.

Superimposition Method

The equipment consists of two video cameras, a television monitor, and a video mixing unit. The equipment used is of broadcasting quality. The preferred characteristics making a photograph likely to be chosen for the superimposition are:

1. It is recent.

2. It shows a smiling or laughing face with good dental landmarks to reduce the problem of getting a 1:1 ratio between the skull and facial photograph, and to provide better dental landmarks for superimposition.

3. It is full face (i.e., looking straight ahead) to minimise any problem of angulation.

4. It shows a large facial image to minimise any optical distortion that might occur during the enlargement process by the video camera.

The facial photograph is viewed through one of the video cameras. The focal length and focusing are adjusted in such a way that the facial image seen on the screen fills about four-fifths of the vertical length of the television monitor. The skull is placed on a skull holder that can be turned in all three planes and is viewed through the other camera. Since there is some difficulty in fine positioning of the skull, the facial photograph is rotated in the coronal plane to match the skull angulation along that plane. Manipulation of the skull position or angulation using the skull holder is done only in two planes, i.e., the sagittal and the horizontal planes. The two video images (images of face and skull) are mixed into one composite image. The video mixing unit provides convenient fade-in and fade-out of either image and also composite slicing (vertical and lateral wiping) of each image. A good match of the video superimposition is determined by analysing the corresponding landmarks on the skull and the face. One of the authors (AWS) used a cheaper video-transparency superimposition method for case 2. In this method the facial photograph is enlarged approximately to life-size and photostatted onto a transparency.

The skull is placed on a skull holder and adjusted to the same position as that of the facial photograph. It is viewed through a video camera and the image can be seen on a television monitor. The transparency is then superimposed on the skull image on the television monitor. The size of the skull image is increased or reduced by adjusting the focal length and the focusing of the video camera in such a way that the skull image fits the facial image. The landmarks used are the ectocanthions to correspond with the lateral aspect of the orbits; the anterior nasal spine (subnasal point) is expected to coincide with the uppermost part of the philtrum and the bite line of the teeth to coincide with the lip line of a closed mouth. If any teeth are present on the facial photograph, the skull image is adjusted in such a way that the size and position of the teeth on the photograph coincide with those on the skull. A lateral and vertical wiping effect can be achieved by positioning a piece of white cardboard in front of the skull and moving it sideways or up and down respectively. The superimposed image can be photographed directly from the television monitor or videotaped using a video recorder and a genlock as future evidence.

Case Reports

Case 1

Skeletalised remains were found in a wood. Anthropological examination of the remains suggested that the skeleton most probably belonged to a person aged between 20 and 30 years, male, and Caucasian in origin. The dead person was later positively identified through an antemortem dental record. The skull was sent to the Facial Identification Centre for a control study. The skull was scanned using the 3-D laser scanner, and the image was stored in the computer database. The skull image was then given a normal thickness of average Caucasian 'flesh' (from the database of Caucasian population) to reconstruct a facial image. The facial image was compared with a recent photograph of the dead person to study possible resemblance. There was some resemblance in the structure of the jaw, cheek bones, supra-orbital ridges, glabella, orbits, and the frontal bone. The nose showed no resemblance. The antemortem facial photograph of the missing person was superimposed onto the skull. There was a good match between the superimposed antemortem photograph and the skull image. Lateral and vertical wiping confirmed a good match between the various landmarks of the antemortem photograph and the skull image.

Case 2

Skeletal remains were found in a small bush. Examination of the scene showed some ashes and remnants of burnt clothing on the ground, suggesting the possibility that the body had been on fire at the time of death. Forensic anthropological examination suggested that the deceased was a Chinese man aged between 25 and 35 years with a height of between 152 cm and 170 cm. The time since death was estimated as 6 months to 1 year. The missing persons file was consulted, and the suspicion arose that the deceased person was a Chinese man who had been missing for about 10 months before the skeleton was found. A facial photograph was submitted by this person's family for the video-transparency superimposition process. There was a good match between the facial photograph and the deceased's skull. The deceased was tentatively identified as the person entered in the missing persons file, and the identification was later confirmed when the antemortem dental identification record of this person became available for comparison with the teeth of the skull.

A New Case

A further case was recently successfully concluded using our facial reconstruction technique together with confirmation obtained from DNA sequencing of DNA material taken from the skull and from living relatives of the person reported missing. This case will be the subject of a further comprehensive report.

Discussion

Facial identification of an unidentified body or skeletal remains can be divided into two stages: (1) the stage of reconstruction of the face and the publication of the reconstructed image through the mass media to get further information or the antemortem record of a suspected missing person, and (2) the stage of confirming or excluding the suspected identity of the body or remains with the missing person by superimposing the photograph provided by the relatives or friends on the skull of the dead person. The purpose of creating facial reconstruction images is to publicise the existence of an unidentified individual, in the hope that a relative or close friend of the deceased may come forward with extra information and antemortem records for the purpose of comparison and identification. A reconstructed facial image that is not an entirely life-like portrayal of the deceased during life may still be considered a success if it is sufficiently realistic to produce a good public response leading to identification.

In the past, the face has been reconstructed by sculpting clay or plasticine onto the skull or the skull model. This technique has been criticised by a number of authorities.[7-9] The difficulties associated with these techniques include lack of skin depth standards for various racial types, ages and body builds, and inability to predict soft tissue features of nose, ears, lips and eyes.[8] In addition, there is no scientific basis from which to extrapolate features such as hair colour and length, facial fatness, dimples and superficial scars.[10] Hair style interpretation is highly subjective and possibly misleading.

The computer-aided facial reconstruction method is more amenable to manipulation and can be improved with any drawing/paint programme in order to add any extra features or information that might be available at a later date. In addition, facial reconstruction can be completed rapidly. On average, a skull takes about one to two hours to be reconstructed.

A further advantage is that the "average face" thought to be representative of the deceased's skull can be selected from a database. With a bigger database and more experience in use of the technique, there is a better chance of getting the reconstructed face to resemble the true face of the decedent during life. To master a sculpting technique a forensic investigator needs to have years of experience before adequate skill and confidence can be developed. Computer-aided facial reconstruction can be mastered within weeks of learning the operation of the laser scanner and computer programme for the reconstruction of the face. However, the computer-aided facial reconstruction technique also faces similar problems to the sculpting method and does not escape similar criticisms. Further research needs to be done in relation to the skin depth standards for various races, ages and body builds, the prediction of the soft tissue features of nose, ears, lips, and eyes, and the prediction of the hair colour, style, and length to increase the chances of successful imaging. In case 1, there is some resemblance between the reconstructed image and the antemortem photograph. However, in our view, the resemblance is not very 'strong' and as far as the nose is concerned there is no resemblance at all. One of the reasons for the discrepancy is that the victim was of mixed ethnic origin, having Caucasian and Asian ancestry, which was only conveyed to us after the reconstruction. The average face used for the facial reconstruction was taken from a purely Caucasian population database. We believe this may be a major problem, since it is very difficult to predict mixed ethnic origin solely from the skull features. Mixed ethnic origin can have a strong influence on the shape of the nose, eyes, lips, and ears of a person, and these structures are important in determining the resemblance between the reconstructed facial image and the antemortem photograph. At the moment, we are accumulating data for the average face of both Asian and Negroid ethnic origin.

A further drawback is that the error of positioning the peg marks on the images may be as high as 2-3 mm in all directions from the 'true location'. This may affect the outcome of facial image reconstruction. Therefore, it is essential that the operator has sufficient experience to position the anatomical peg marks correctly on the skull and average facial images. Even though the anatomical peg marks have been defined, their exact locations may sometimes be difficult to position exactly on the images, because subjective judgement is required. Another problem is that the resolution of the image produced by the laser scanner may be as high as 2 mm, depending on the number of vertical planes scanned in the skull and face. Sometimes this inherent problem of the system does not allow the peg mark to be made on the exact location preferred by the operator. The operator cannot enter the peg mark within the 2 mm resolution area. To overcome this problem, the number of planes can be increased during the scanning process if this involves less than the entire circumference of skull or face. The database of average faces scanned from volunteers contains faces with closed eyes for the most part, because the volunteers prefer not to look into the laser light during the scanning procedure even though it is believed that the scanning procedure does not involve any risk to the eyes.[5] The reconstructed facial image may therefore also show a face with the eyes closed. To overcome this problem, it is preferable to select an average face with the eyes open. If this is not possible the closed-eye reconstruction can be improved with a drawing/ paint programme.

Photosuperimposition was widely recognised after the application of this method in 1935 by Glaister and Brash in their classic study of the Ruxton case.[11] This method is more rigid, since it requires a longer time to reproduce the life-size enlargement of the facial photograph and skull before they can be superimposed. In addition, it is difficult to obtain the correct angulation of the photograph of the skull without many attempts.

Our video superimposition method is more dynamic. The enlargement of the facial photograph does not require any laboratory photographic processing. A video camera is aimed at the facial photograph, and any enlargement is made by adjusting the focal length of the lens. Another video camera is aimed at the deceased's skull and adjusted to the appropriate size of the facial image. The adjustment is made after both video images are mixed using a video mixer unit. Even though the enlargement of the facial photograph is not life-size, the

1:1 ratio between the facial and the skull images can be determined using various landmarks on the face and the skull. McKenna, et al.,[12] stated that their most satisfactory method of enlargement was to use the dimensions of the anterior teeth in portraits. Bastiaan et al[13] suggested that establishing the correct enlargement using dentition measurements is the more quantitatively accurate superimposition technique when dentition is present. We agree with their opinion and we use the relative size of the teeth in a facial photograph to superimpose the relative size of the teeth on the skull after the enlargement using a video camera. Theoretically, if the skull and the facial photograph have originated from the same person, the enlargement of the teeth in the photograph and skull images to the same size (even if not life size) will cause the facial and the skull images to have 1:1 ratio. The problem with this method is that any error in determining the size of the teeth in the facial image may be magnified many times, depending on the ratio between the size of the face and the size of the teeth. For example, a 1-mm discrepancy between the enlargement size of the teeth in the facial to the skull images may magnify this error to 1 cm of the full face size if the size of the face is 10 times larger than that of the teeth. Dental landmarks are not only useful for obtaining a 1:1 ratio between the skull and the facial photograph, but also for comparison of any artefacts that can be found on the teeth such as broad dentition, malocclusion, rotated, tilted, or missing teeth. This may increase the probability of identification when there are matched dental artefacts in the facial photograph and the skull of the dead person. Sometimes the facial photograph may show no exposed dentition. In such a case, we subjectively enlarge both the facial and the skull images to the relative size of 1:1 ratio. Following that, we assess various landmarks, checking for example that: (1) both eyes are within the orbits, (2) the eyebrows coincide with the supraciliary arches, (3) the ectocanthions correspond to the lateral part of the orbits, (4) the uppermost part of the philtrum coincides with the anterior nasal spine (subnasal point), (5) the nasal cavity corresponds centrally with the nose as a whole, (6) the bite line coincides with the lip line of closed mouth, (7) the auditory meatuses on the skull coincide with those in the ears in the photograph, (8) the outline of the face encloses the outline of the skull with a reasonable thickness of facial soft tissue.

Chai, et al.,[14] have studied the selection of landmark points with the specification of 34 landmarks along eight reference lines (also called marking or determining lines) on the face and skull. The landmarks used here consist of the ectocanthion points at the left and right outer orbits along the ectocanthion determining line and the glabella, nasion, and subnasal landmarks along the front central determining line. These points and their determining lines were shown by them to have the highest probability of superimposition. Other researchers[11, 15, 16] have suggested that linear measurement of items within the antemortem photograph, such as fabric and other objects of known geometry, can be useful in establishing the correct enlargement factor. The establishment of the correct enlargement of the photograph of the skull and the photograph of the face is considered critical. Glaister and Brash[11] used the known dimensions of objects present in snapshots or photographic portraits, including a tiara headdress, the outline of the neckline of a dress, the heights of a door, a gate, and a wall. Gordon and Drennan,[15] Sekharan,[16] and Janssens, et al.,[17] used the linear pattern of a tie, the pattern on the border of a sari, and the diameter of a button on a sweater, respectively, to find the correct photographic enlargement and to yield successful superimpositions and probable identifications. Prinsloo[18] and Sivaram and Wadhera[19] used the combined anatomical landmarks and anthropometric measurements of the facial skeleton with the existing data for soft tissue thickness to estimate a magnification factor. Sekharan[16] suggested a standard interpupillary distance of 6 cm as the measurement from which life-size enlargements of antemortem photographs could be made in the absence of objects of known size in the antemortem photograph. This suggestion was proven unreliable by McKenna, et al.,[12] after measuring interpupillary distances in 75 Chinese subjects between the ages of 19 and 22 years. They concluded that there was too much variation for this to be used as an average figure for the basis of photographic enlargements. Bastiaan, et al.,[13] suggested that inherent in all superimposition procedures are assumptions and estimations that have to be made of the bony anatomical features on the antemortem photograph. The average thickness of tissue over bone has been recorded, and therefore, a calculation can be made of the soft tissue outlines on the skull. They also suggested that statistics drawn from flesh thickness data could be used to interpret a best-fit superimposition. We use a subjective estimate of facial thickness covering the outline of the skull from the superimposed facial outline in conjunction with other anatomical landmarks of the superimposed images.

Determination of the correct angulation of the skull to the photograph is another major problem in superimposition, irrespective of the method used. Therefore, selection of antemortem photographs with the face looking directly at the lens is desirable to overcome or at least minimize this problem. If the ideal (straight ahead) photograph is not available, the skull is oriented to the best possible position to match the facial angulation to that of the antemortem photograph. Even though our skull holder can be angulated in all 3-D planes, we prefer to adjust the skull holder in only two planes, i.e., along the median and horizontal planes. The matching of the images along the coronal plane is done by rotating the photograph on a round board, which can mark the angle of rotation. This allows easier manoeuvring of the skull holder than to when 3-D manipulation is practised. Sometimes, the photograph provided has shown some optical distortion of the face. An example of a facial photograph with optical distortion can be found on passports (in U.K.) when these have been taken with one of the instant cameras commonly available. Since we know the distance between the face and the camera lens is about 2 feet and the focal length of the lens is about 35 mm, we can simulate this when we image the skull to match the optical distortion for better and more accurate superimposition.

Video superimposition equipment used in our centre are of broadcasting quality and produce high-quality pictures. The only limitation is the quality of the original antemortem photograph. A substantial investment is required for this equipment. However, an alternative and cheaper video-transparency superimposition method is available for those who are interested in using this method as an extra tool to help in identification. One needs only a camcorder, a television monitor, and transparencies. The outcome is of reasonable quality but at an affordable price. The lateral and vertical wiping effect can be produced by moving a white card in front of the skull sideways and up and down directions respectively. However, there is an additional problem with this method. The television monitor has a slight curved surface. This causes some problems in matching the anatomical landmarks between the superimposed facial image on the transparency and the landmarks of the skull on the monitor as these landmarks move toward the periphery of the screen. Some courts have accepted the video superimposition method as an identification tool (Brown, personal communication).[12] Its value is highlighted when other methods of identification are not possible or are unreliable. However, we must stress that the degree of medical certainty of this method cannot be considered adequate for positive identification. It is used in combination with other corroborative evidence when confirmatory evidence such as fingerprinting, dental records, and DNA profiling are not available. The degree of medical certainty of this method increases when more anatomical landmarks on the antemortem photograph match those on the skull, especially when the dentition landmarks are also included. The value of superimposition has been challenged on the basis that the alignment and enlargement factors are too variable. De Vore[20] emphasised strongly that this method cannot be used for positive identification, since the magnification and angulation of the original picture are unknown. It has more value in exclusion than in positive identification. A misidentification by photographic superimposition of skull and antemortem photograph has been reported by Dorion.[21] The error was confirmed after positive identification using fingerprinting. This illustrates the danger of overestimating the capability of this method. In conclusion, despite some limitations in obtaining a positive identification, the computer-aided facial reconstruction and video superimposition methods are very useful in enhancing the process of identification especially in the case of severely decomposed or mutilated bodies and skeletal remains.

References

1. G. Gustafson, *Forensic Odontology* (London: Staples, 1966), 24-102.

2. W. D. Haglund and D. T. Reay, "Use of Facial Approximation Techniques in Identification of Green River Serial Murder Victims," *American Journal of Forensic Medicine and Pathology* 12: 132-42 (1991).

3. P. Vanezis, R. W. Blowes, A. D. Linney, A. C. Tan, R. Richard, and R. Neave, "Application of 3-D Computer Graphics for Facial Reconstruction and Comparison with Sculpting Techniques," *Forensic Science International* 42: 69-84 (1989).

4. A. D. Linney, A. C. Tan, R. Richards, J. Gardener, S. Grinrod, and J. P. Moss, "Three Dimensional Visualisation of Data on Human Anatomy: Diagnosis and Surgical Planning," *Journal of Audiovisual Media in Medicine* 16: 4-10 (1993).

5. J. P. Moss, A. D. Linney, S. R. Grinrod, and C. A. Mosse, "A Laser Scanning System for the Measurements of Facial Surface Morphology," *Optics Lasers Engineering* 10: 179-90 (1989).

6. L. G. Farkas, *Anthropometry of the Head and Face in Medicine* (New York: Elsevier, 1989).

7. C. C. Snow, B. P. Gatliff, and K. R. McWilliams, "Reconstruction of Facial Features from the Skull: An Evaluation of Its

Usefulness in Forensic Anthropology," *Journal of Physical Anthropology* 33: 221-28 (1970).

8. T. A. Rathbun, "Personal Identification: Facial Reproductions," in *Human Identification,* ed. T. A. Rathbun and J. E. Buikstra (Springfield: Thomas, 1984), 347-56.

9. J. S. Rhine, "Facial Reproduction in Court," in *Human Identification,* ed. T. A. Rathbun and J. E. Buikstra (Springfield: Thomas, 1984), 357-62.

10. M. Y. Iscan, "The Rise of Forensic Anthropology," *Yearbook of Physical Anthropology* 31: 203-30 (1988).

11. J. Glaister and J. C. Brash, *Medico-Legal Aspects of the Ruxton Case* (Edinburgh: Livingstone, 1937), 144-70, 245-59.

12. J. McKenna, N. G. Jablonski, and R. Feamhead, "A Method of Matching Skulls with Photographic Portraits Using Landmarks and Measurements of the Dentition," *Journal of Forensic Sciences* 29: 787-97 (1984).

13. R. Bastiaan, G. Dalitz, and C. Woodward, "Videosuperimposition of Skulls and Photographic Portraits— A New Aid to Identification," *Journal of Forensic Sciences* 3: 1373-9 (1986).

14. D. S. Chai, Y. W. Lan, C. Tao, R. J. Gui, Y. C. Mu, J. H. Feng, W. D. Wang, and J. Zhu, "A Study on the Standard for Forensic Anthropologic Identification of Skull-Image Superimposition," *Journal of Forensic Sciences* 34: 1343-56 (1989).

15. I. Gordon and M. Drennan, "Medico-Legal Aspects of the Wokersdofer Case," *Med J* 22: 543-9 (1948).

16. P. Sekharan, "A Revised Superimposition Technique for Identification of the Individual from the Skull and Photograph," *Journal of Criminal Law, Criminology, and Police Science* 62: 107-13 (1979).

17. P. Janssens, C. Hansch, and L. Boorhamme, "Identity Determination by Superimposition and Anthropological Cranium Adjustment," *Ossa* 5: 109-22 (1978).

18. I. Prinsloo, "The Identification of Skeletal Remains in Regina versus K and Others: The Howick Falls Murder Case," *Journal of Forensic Medicine* 1: 11-17 (1953).

19. S. Sivaram and C. Wadhera, "Identity of Skeleton—A Case Study," *International Criminal Police Review* 32: 158-160 (1977).

20. T. DeVore, "Radiology and Photography in Forensic Dentistry," *Dental Clinics of North America* 21: 81 (1977).

21. R. B. J. Dorion, "Photographic Superimposition," *Journal of Forensic Sciences* 28: 724-34 (1983).

— by A. W. Shahrom, R. C. Chapman,
C. Blenkinsop, and M. L. Rossi,
Department of Forensic Medicine and Toxicology,
Charing Cross and Westminster Medical School,
London, U.K.; and P. Vanezis and A. Gonzalez,
Department of Forensic Medicine and Science,
University of Glasgow, Glasgow, G12 8QQ, U.K.

Chapter 30

Computer-Aided Criminal Identification

A novel way of identifying suspects will soon be in the hands of law enforcement—a computer software program that lets investigators recreate the human head in three dimensions and then compare it to, or search through, one million faces in less than one second.

This software represents the latest and most sophisticated version of facial recognition technology, and Dr. Arsev H. Eraslan is the brain—or should we say the "face"—behind it. As the chief scientist at the National Institute of Justice's (NIJ) Office of Law Enforcement Technology Commercialization (OLETC) in Wheeling, West Virginia, Eraslan holds a doctorate in aerospace engineering. He has spent 20 years teaching and more than 30 years doing research for the National Aeronautics and Space Administration (NASA).

It was Eraslan's extensive experience that told him the two-dimensional mug shot/composite systems currently on the market could be improved. He knew there were newer and better technologies that would make the job infinitely easier and much more accurate. In November 1997, he began work to prove his theory by taking off-the-shelf technology originally created for the aerospace industry and combining it with 2,000 faces scanned in by the U.S. Air Force during a project to design new helmets and masks. The result was a program that can build a fully three-dimensional face.

"We have addressed the fundamental problem of all two-dimensional systems, which is that mug shots only have a front and a profile view.

From "I've Seen Your Face Before!" in NLECTC (National Law Enforcement and Corrections Technology Center) *Tech Beat,* Spring 1998, p. 8.

But most of the time people are captured on tape at an angled view," Eraslan says. "None of the existing methods can capture that to match it because the human head is three-dimensional."

Eraslan knew a three-dimensional problem required a three-dimensional solution. First, he divided the human face into 64 individual features. He then took the 2,000 three-dimensional scans done by the Air Force and sorted them into each of his 64 categories to create 256 possibilities for each feature. "We have 256 noses, 256 mouths, 256 foreheads, 256 chins. We can pretty much construct anybody's face using these parts," Eraslan explains.

The program also will be equipped with an automatic composite builder, which will allow the investigator to build a face while the victim describes the suspect. The investigator will be able to rotate the head to different angles and change the lighting to recreate the conditions that existed when the crime occurred. In addition, the software program will let investigators convert existing two-dimensional mug shots to three-dimensional. They will be able to match each facial feature with the three-dimensional features built into the program.

"I take a 3-D nose and turn it frontwise and see how it matches the front of your two-dimensional mug shot. Then I check it against your profile. If that doesn't work, I find another nose and compare it until I have a match. I do this with all the facial features until I construct a fully three-dimensional head. It's a new approach. It's tricky, but we're very excited about it," Eraslan says.

Each of the program's facial features is numbered. Comparisons are based on those numbers, which makes identification easier and faster. In fact, it is so fast that investigators will be able to search through one million mug shots in less than one second. "But the only thing we're comparing is 64 numbers to 64 numbers. This also means you need only limited storage. You can store 40 million mug shots in a PC [personal computer]," Eraslan says.

According to Eraslan, the facial identity program does not require expensive equipment. It will run on a PC equipped with a 200 MHZ Pentium processor. Agencies can keep the program entirely inhouse or set it up to network with other agencies.

Although the project is just six months old, Eraslan says he expects to have an alpha version and proof-of-concept demonstration ready by July 1998. If all goes as planned, NIJ will help commercialize the program through OLETC, which will work with a private vendor to make the program available to law enforcement agencies.

The National Institute of Justice is also developing other facial recognition technologies and applications. One application recently started with the ANSER Corporation will use various aspects of facial recognition technologies to enhance the operations of the National Center for Missing and Exploited Children.

For more information about the facial recognition software initiative at OLETC, contact Dr. Arsev Eraslan or Tom Burgoyne at OLETC by phone: (888) 306-5382.

Chapter 31

Bite Mark Evidence

Although bites and biting have been around as long as animals
with teeth have inhabited the earth, the science of bite mark identification is comparatively new and potentially valuable. Because of its
origin, biting is a primitive type of assault. It is often used as the
weapon of last resort. Consequently, bite injuries are frequently seen
in circumstances of forcible rape, skirmishes between young children,
and hand-to-hand mortal combat. Since biting may be part of fore-
play or other sexual activities, bite injuries are often seen in sex
crimes, particularly among male homosexuals.[1]

Identifying human remains by dental characteristics is a well-
established component of forensic science with a definite scientific basis. However, the whole arena of bite marks is a recent and still
controversial part of this discipline.

The history of the distinctive nature of tooth arrangement, and its
legal implications, is extensive. William the Conqueror reportedly validated royal documents by biting into a wax seal with his characteristic dentition. Debtors coming from Britain or Europe to America to
work as servants verified their agreements by biting the seal on the
pact in lieu of a signature and became known as *indentured servants.*

Excerpted from "Bite Marks in Forensic Dentistry: A Review of Legal, Sci-
entific Issues," by Bruce R. Rothwell, D.M.D., M.S.D., in *The Journal of the
American Dental Association,* Vol. 126, February 1995, pp. 223-32. © 1995 by
American Dental Association. Reprinted with permission of ADA Publishing
Co., Inc. For complete contact information for Dr. Rothwell, please refer to
Chapter 56, "Resources."

Although bite marks have only recently gained prominence, there have been cases and investigators for more than a hundred years. Various individuals have been recognized as being the first bite mark analyst. Several authors have mentioned Sorup as being the first such investigator; in 1924, he used transparent paper representations of a suspect's dentition to compare with life-size bite mark photographs.[2]

Possibly the earliest recorded bite mark case in the United States was *Ohio* vs. *Robinson* in 1870. Ansil Robinson was charged with the murder of his mistress, Mary Lunsford. In spite of evidence presented in court matching his teeth to bite marks on the victim's arm, Robinson was acquitted of the charge.[3] As precedent-setting convictions involving bite marks were relatively uncommon in the legal literature, it is difficult to establish the nature of early cases. Presumably, the first case involving a bite mark that led to a conviction sustained on appeal was a 1972 rape case, *Illinois* vs. *Johnson*.[3]

Most early forensic investigators analyzed marks left by dental casts in wax, clear overlays, and other mediums. Others attempted to simulate the consistency of human tissue by using articulated dental models to "bite" baker's dough and sponge rubber.[5] The problems of registering marks in the skin were studied,[6] and there were descriptions of photographic techniques to preserve evidence.[7]

With the advent of electron microscopy and computer enhancement, these new technologies were applied to bite mark analysis.[8] Methods to determine the ABO blood groups from the saliva on the skin were developed, and investigators tried to link bacteria and other organisms found in the bite marks to the oral milieu of the perpetrator. [9,10] In addition to the attempts to link marks left on human tissue to the dentition of the perpetrator, there were many instances of bites in food or other inanimate objects used as physical evidence to place the accused at the scene of the crime.[11,12] Although there were several attempts to systematically investigate bite marks and their application to forensic science, there was no general agreement about national or international standards of comparison.

Several famous cases, most notably Theodore "Ted" Bundy's serial murder trial, made bite marks a high-profile item with excessive media attention.[13] Because of the repellant nature of the biting of victims, bite mark evidence became highly sensationalized and prejudicial. Even popular fictional television series such as "L.A. Law" and "Quincy, M.E." depicted bite mark evidence used to convict wrongdoers.

More recently, there have been highly publicized trials involving bite mark evidence in which several dental experts on each side have argued convincingly that the marks did or did not implicate the accused. These wide divergences of opinion have led some to question the value and scientific objectivity of bite mark evidence.

Legal Status of Bite Mark Evidence

Admissibility. New scientific procedures are not automatically admitted into evidence in judicial proceedings; they must first satisfy rigorous scrutiny and analysis. The goal of such inquiry is protecting defendants from improper conviction based on methods and techniques that have not been established and accepted by the scientific community. Judges and juries usually do not have enough background to assess the scientific merit of new methods and procedures and must rely on experts within approved judicial guidelines. Bite mark evidence has been challenged on this basis both because of its perceived lack of scientific merit and its potentially prejudicial aspects.

The relevance and admissibility of new forms of scientific evidence depend on their general acceptance in the scientific community. Identification by fingerprint comparison was accepted first in U.S. courts in 1911 only on the basis of its general and common use and acceptance.[14] In 1923, the justification for admitting scientific evidence was established as a standard that would become known as the "Frye test."[15] This requirement for admissibility has three components:

- the principle must be demonstrable;
- it must have been sufficiently established;
- it must have gained the general acceptance of experts working in the particular scientific field(s) to which the evidence belongs.

Of course, the criticism of such a test is that the judicial admissibility of new techniques is often delayed. But because of the importance and relative weight placed on scientific evidence in trials, most legal scholars conclude that the Frye test is an important restraint on dubious methods.

The first case involving the admissibility of bite mark evidence was a 1954 Texas case, *Doyle* vs. *State*. In this instance, a piece of cheese found at the crime scene had tooth marks. The defendant, Doyle, was asked to bite into another piece of cheese, and a firearms examiner, not a dentist, compared the marks. At the trial, this examiner and a dentist testified that the marks were made by the same teeth. Although the dentist likely had no previous experience in evaluating bite marks, and the firearms expert presumably had no dental knowledge, the evidence was admitted. The court allowed the evidence because it appeared similar to fingerprint cases.

Most other cases involving bite mark evidence sidestepped the issue of scientific reliability even though there was often testimony to indicate a lack of plausibility in analysis. In a landmark 1975 case, *People* vs. *Marx,* the California Court of Appeals concluded that bite mark analysis was generally acceptable in the proper scientific community and thus admissible, in spite of the court's acknowledgment that "there is no established science of identifying a person from bite marks."[16] In a 1976 Illinois case (*People* vs. *Milone*), a major disagreement between authorities arose when the prosecution's experts asserted that the defendant's dentition was responsible for the marks in question, and four witnesses testifying for the defense maintained that the defendant's dentition was positively not responsible for the bite.[17] In this case, the court decided that the discrepancy in the opinions of the experts would not affect the admissibility of the evidence, but would rather influence the relative weight of the testimony.

After the *Milone* decision, the admissibility of bite mark evidence was explicitly established, and material of this nature has been routinely accepted in several legal venues. Although some legal scholars argue that bite mark techniques have never been critically examined and legitimately passed the Frye test, the admissibility of this type of evidence is generally no longer at issue.[18] There continue to be substantial questions about the validity of bite mark evidence and its scientific principles, but those questions must be considered by judges and juries listening to opposing witnesses, rather than by prior exclusion of evidence.

Impartiality. In legal circles, particularly in criminal defense, some have questioned the impartial, objective attitude of bite mark investigators. Most members of the forensic dental community are associated with law enforcement agencies. As representatives of police, coroners, or medical examiners, they could tend to identify with the prosecution in a trial.[19] Of course, that partiality does not necessarily exist, and many investigators go to great lengths to avoid any partisanship.

The process of bite mark evaluation, even without considering the techniques and methods, can reinforce prejudice. In most cases, forensic dentists rely on police agencies to provide them with suspects for evaluation and comparison with the bite marks, and this process produces a limited number of models. There is seldom an equivalent to an identification "lineup." Rarely, if ever, are investigating dentists offered models from individuals undoubtedly not involved in the crime.

Summary of legal considerations. Although there continue to be objections as to the relevance and appropriateness of bite mark evidence and its ability to pass the Frye test, the admissibility of such evidence is rarely questioned. It is up to the judge or jury to weigh the evidence presented by both sides and assess its relative value. The steps necessary to obtain bite mark evidence are reasonably well-established, and an investigator would be criticized for not following the appropriate steps. Presumably, an expert becomes defined by his or her knowledge of the correct manner in which a bite mark is processed.

Using Bite Marks: Methodology

Obtaining evidence from the victim. For bites on human skin, a potential bite injury must be recognized early, as the clarity and shape of the mark may change in a relatively short time in both living and dead victims. Bite marks appear most often as elliptical or round areas of contusion or abrasion, occasionally with associated indentations. There may be avulsion of tissue, or even pieces of tissue bitten off. There may be considerable bruising and wounds that have penetrated the skin.

Once the mark is initially evaluated, it should be examined by a forensic odontologist to determine if the dimensions and configuration are within human ranges. Since a large proportion of individuals (80 to 90 percent) secrete the ABO blood groups in their saliva, swabbing the area and a control area elsewhere on the body should be completed before the body is washed. The swabs, moistened with sterile distilled water, should be allowed to air-dry before their submission to a serological laboratory.[20]

Although there have been descriptions of using fingerprint "dusting" methods, photography is the primary means of recording and preserving the bite mark and is critically important in documenting the evidence.[21] Since the skin marks are apt to change over time, photographs provide the most reliable means of preserving the information. However great their value, photographs have considerable inherent limitations, and there are stringent requirements regarding the accuracy of reproduction. The basic difficulties involve replicating a three-dimensional object in a two-dimensional film and producing an image with true colors and spatial relations. Attention to procedure can help minimize these restrictions and create a reasonably reliable, consistent image for comparison.

Photographs should be made by experienced photographers using both color transparency and black-and-white film with a negative size of 35 mm or larger. Lighting, camera orientation, close-up capability, and stability are extremely critical. A camera support such as a tripod should position the camera perpendicularly to the long axis of the region. Photographs should be produced with and without a scale, and possibly other circular reference devices such as small metal washers.[7] There has been substantial discussion of the nature of the scale for bite mark photographs, including the inherent inaccuracy of small plastic rulers, the value of curved vs. rigid scales, and the need for placing other objects in the picture.[22] Many bite mark photographs are taken with substantial references. A scale developed by members of the American Board of Forensic Odontology has evolved as a standard, designated as the ABFO scale no. 2.[23]

In addition to the customary color and black-and-white films, some authors have recommended ultraviolet photography at the initial encounter and for a few days after.[24] The technique involves irradiating the bite mark with a UV light source and exposing black-and-white film through a UNA filter.[25, 26] With increased contrast printing, an image with additional details can be produced. In one article on the subject, two authors subjected themselves to being bitten under intravenous sedation for extended periods. The resulting marks were then photographed at various intervals with conventional films and UV techniques to demonstrate that images could be produced several days after the injury.[27]

When there are indentations in the skin, or to preserve the three-dimensional nature of the bitten area, impressions should be taken to fabricate stone models.[28, 29] This is done by fabricating custom impression trays and taking an impression of the mark and surrounding skin with a standard dental impression material. These impressions are then poured in dental stone to produce models. After the initial analysis is complete, there may be a need to preserve the actual skin bearing the mark. A ring of custom tray material can be made to fit like a hoop, closely approximating the skin, which can then be attached to the skin with cyanoacrylate adhesive and stabilized with sutures.[30] When the pathologist completes the autopsy, the bite mark can be excised with the supporting framework in place.

Obtaining information from the suspect(s). When suspects are identified, impressions and other dental data can be obtained by a qualified dental practitioner. There has been extensive debate in legal circles about the risk of potential self-incrimination by defendants in the process of furnishing dental information. Most jurisdictions, however, have allowed the procedures as similar to procuring fingerprints or facial photographs. Some police agencies obtain a search warrant from the court to permit dental impressions.

In addition to impressions for dental models, intraoral photographs and bite impressions can be secured from any potential suspects or from the victim in the situations where the perpetrator was bitten. In some special situations, dental radiographs, microbiologic cultures or salivary samples are indicated. These data should be procured as soon as possible to prevent alterations.

Analysis and evaluation. The standards for the collection of evidence from the victim and suspects have generally evolved into reasonably well-accepted protocols. There is still continuing controversy about the appraisal of bite mark evidence and the efforts to link it with a high degree of certainty to particular individuals. Even if all of the bite information is collected meticulously, the dental examiner's objectivity and methods are critical to the ultimate outcome. There are several cases in which forensic dental experts have arrived at opposite conclusions regarding the perpetrator of a particular mark. These extreme divergences of judgment can make the reliability of bite mark investigation questionable.

An effort to standardize the analysis of bite marks has resulted in guidelines by the American Board of Forensic Odontology.[31] As mentioned, the fundamental validity of bite mark inquiry has been challenged in court, generally because of the lack of standards and the widely differing results from separate investigators.[32] Although there has been some negative commentary on the principles proposed in the publication, they are a commendable endeavor in the pursuit of scientific order.[33]

The scoring system for evaluating bite mark evidence uses a relatively simple weighted compilation of points based on points of concordance between the mark and the dentition in question. The authors do not specify the confidence levels for making an indisputable match, but rather seek to "improve communication and impart meaning to the loosely used term, matching point. There was no attempt to indicate levels of confidence where certain scores indicated relative degrees of certainty. Although we can, with some diminished degree of bias, evolve a score for a particular bite mark and dentition, it has no established relevance to the degree of scientific certainty.

Problems in Bite Mark Analysis

Accuracy of the bite imprint. Although the accuracy of various dental impression materials is definitely established, there is considerable variability in the precision of the representation of marks on human skin or other objects. Not only is skin a poor medium for accurate impressions, but human tissues often contain curves and other irregularities that produce intrinsic distortion. Additionally, any stretching of the skin produces large amounts of distortion in the shape of the tooth marks and the size of the dental arches.[34] Some degree of distortion is found in all bite marks, and inattention to detail or photographic standards can increase this analytical deformation.[35] Some inanimate objects may initially produce reasonably good representations of tooth marks, but gross distortion can occur relatively rapidly in changing temperature or humidity.

The accuracy of tooth marks in skin can depend on the amplitude and direction of the biting forces, sucking action, whether the skin was penetrated and any movements by the assailant or victim during the biting episode. In addition, pre- and postmortem changes such as edema, hemorrhage, and lividity can result in radical modifications.[36] Complicating the issue further is the lack of suggestion to the investigator as to the extent and nature of the distortion. Thus bite mark registrations are often assumed accurate, although it is clear that it is rarely, if ever, true. Because of the inherent distortions of bite marks in skin, some investigators have even used human skin as a template to analyze and compare bite marks.[37]

Permanence. Unlike fingerprints, which are reasonably stable over the course of an individual's life, the dentition is capable of major changes in configuration, with and without professional intervention. Teeth can be lost by extraction, trauma, or exfoliation. The size and relationship of the arches can be altered by growth or orthodontic or surgical procedures. Various restorative materials can change the character of the biting surfaces or actual position of the individual teeth. Disease processes such as caries or periodontal disease can change the configuration or position of the teeth.

Uniqueness. The singular nature of an individual dentition is often assumed, but it has not been definitely established. We can argue that because of the endless variations in tooth position, size, shape, and other characteristics, each dentition is unique.[38, 39] But there is no study of large populations to establish this argument firmly. There is no conclusive demonstration of the distinctive nature of a single bite pattern.[40] Most forensic odontologists assume that bite patterns are characteristic and original, but this is not scientifically documented.

Many bite marks are incomplete registrations of the involved dentition. The theoretical studies promoting the concept of uniqueness generally include multiple teeth in both arches, which may have little relevance to actual cases in which only small portions of the dentition or only parts of the incisal edges are recorded. Possibly the most notable area of controversy in bite mark analysis is the minimum constitution and composition of a bite mark required for effective evaluation. Studies involving correspondence between 100 bite registrations made in ideal conditions and plastic overlays of the dentitions showed that several bite marks could be superimposed exactly with regard to one or more teeth, but none of the samples could be superimposed precisely unless all of the teeth were represented in the arch. It was concluded that no positive identification could be made unless there were at least four or five teeth marks present.[41]

Each bite mark circumstance has been generally treated as an individual entity. Although there have been published inquiries involving more than one bite mark, and descriptions of the distributions of bite marks in certain populations,[42] there is no central repository or inventory of bite marks and patterns, unlike fingerprints and ballistic information.

Analysis and comparison. In spite of a reasonably well-established approach to the acquisition of bite mark evidence, there is continuing dispute about the methods and emphasis of analytical procedures. Although the ABFO recommends a scoring system, it clearly states that "it is not the intent of these guidelines to mandate specific methods of analysis." As a result, many methods of comparing bite marks in skin with dental models have been proposed.

Most commonly, the forensic investigator compares life-size (1:1) representations (photographs or tracings) of the bite mark on skin and models of a suspect's dentition. This has been accomplished by a variety of means, from plastic overlays to imprints in wax or Styrofoam to templates of human skin. One author recommends using a photocopy machine to produce 1:1 paper reproductions of dental models to facilitate the tracing of tooth edges onto clear overlays.[43] In even the most careful process, each stage introduces errors. There is considerable interpolation and extrapolation required to take these inherent errors into account.

309

The few controlled studies of the accuracy of comparisons by bite mark examiners reported a fairly high rate of inaccuracy. In one 1975 study, experienced examiners could match bites in wax to the corresponding dentitions with a high degree of accuracy (99 percent), but 24 percent of the time, they were unable to correctly match bite marks in skin (porcine) with the appropriate dentitions.[44] It was further suggested that the accuracy rate could fall to as low as 9 to 20 percent if impressions were not taken or photographs were substandard.

There has been considerable interest in scanning electron microscopy, computerized image enhancement, and other similar "high-tech" procedures to analyze bite marks.[45, 46] Some advocate transillumination of the excised skin with a radiographic "hot light" to illustrate subcutaneous hemorrhages not otherwise visible.[47] Although these techniques enhance the apparent detail and visualization of marks in skin, we do not understand whether these augmentations represent artifacts or improvements.

Bite mark analysis is generally limited to comparisons of one or two sets of dental models with representations of the mark. There is rarely, if ever, any attempt to try to match the bite mark with a large number of dental models. As a result, it is impossible to determine if anyone else could likely have made the bite. In spite of the general lack of comparisons in a broader population, there are instances of bites in which two sets of teeth have matched identically with bite marks. In 1976, Sopher indicated that in one case, two suspects were "quite consistent" with the bite mark found on the deceased.[48] In the 1976 Milone murder trial, the defendant was convicted of a murder, largely on the basis of bite mark testimony. Later, another was found to have a dentition that exactly matched the bite mark. He subsequently confessed to the murder.[49] Although bite mark evidence usually connects perpetrators with victims, there are instances where such data have been instrumental in the acquittal of defendants. In one case, a man was acquitted, primarily on the basis of bite mark testimony, of a murder charge for which he had already served seven years in prison.[50]

A rational approach to bite mark evidence. These problems and limitations associated with bite marks do not necessarily relegate the whole field to question and subjectivity. But if bite marks, particularly those involving human skin, are approached in a rational, systematic way with full understanding of the innate limitations, they can be worthwhile forensic evidence.

Any mark suggesting a bite injury should have a preliminary evaluation and data collection including standardized photographs, drawings, qualitative description, and salivary swabbing. This should be part of the regular protocol of the medical examiner or pathologist when preparing for a postmortem examination. At this time, the pathologist and forensic odontologist can decide whether to proceed with a more complete workup. Certain elements, if present, make a particular bite mark case more amenable to extensive investigation and deduction. The preliminary analysis should allow a staged appraisal, ending when it is clear that the evidence does not warrant further investigation. There is considerable jeopardy in pursuing inadequate bite marks too far.

The bite mark's location is of prime importance because of the distortions and deformations that can occur on curved surfaces.[51] The nature and volume of distortion have not been quantified, so that the analyst cannot accurately interpolate the dimensions. The preliminary inquiry should indicate an estimated degree of distortion in a particular bite mark. Suspected extreme deformation precludes more extensive analysis.

Photographs and other recordings of the bite mark should be produced in accordance with the ABFO guidelines and special techniques considered. The goal should be producing accurate illustrations that faithfully represent the bite mark. Life-size enlargements should be produced precisely and reliably.

Records from suspects should be taken by a qualified dentist familiar with the techniques of bite mark analysis. These should minimally include dental models and intraoral photographs. The dentist may choose to include models from other individuals with similar demographic variables as controls. It is best to perform this analysis in a blind fashion, with the investigator unaware of the identities.

There is no consensus on the appropriate technical methods for evaluating the bite mark and potentially associated dental composition. Clear plastic overlays produced from the skin mark can be superimposed on the dental models for a preparatory appraisal. It is prudent to produce some sort of bite mark in wax or Styrofoam with the dental models either hand-held or in an articulated setup. These can then be compared with the photographs and drawings. The ABFO scoring system is a credible method of staged evaluation to produce a numerical tally. Although there is no information on the relative value of such a tally, it provides a logical format for moving from general to specific and produces objective estimations of the potential for agreement.

Often techniques such as electron microscopy and various image enhancers are used when there is minimal or clearly distorted information present in the bite mark—situations that may not warrant extraordinary means to produce matches. Unadorned methods can avoid extensive investigation of bite marks with minimal information.

Above all, the investigator should recognize the innate problems in bite mark examination and avoid expanding the analysis beyond rational boundaries. While it is important to extend and improve the methods used, it should be done scientifically and realistically. The forensic odontologist should make the difficulties and imprecision clear to police and other law enforcement agencies and encourage meticulous gathering of evidence. In addition, courtroom testimony should honestly depict the restrictions involved in bite mark analysis and candidly admit the areas where deficiencies exist.

Conclusion

Although there are questions about the scientific merit of some aspects of the evaluation process of bite mark evidence, numerous legal precedents allow for the admissibility of such evidence. The conflicts will now occur in the courtroom, with prosecution and defense witnesses arguing the relative merit and reliability of this material.

Likewise, the methods and techniques for gathering evidence in bite mark situations are becoming more established. The ABFO guidelines have gone a long way toward instituting standards for procedures such as photography, impressions, and swabbing. There appears to be little question as to the rational precision involved in impression procedures and the production of dental models from suspects.

Forensic dentists need to approach bite marks with a certain degree of skepticism and continually acknowledge their limitations. Bite marks with only minimal information should not be pursued beyond initial evaluation and evidence gathering. Bite marks with definite details should be evaluated along conventional lines, with allowances made for distortions and errors. When reporting on bite mark evidence, dentists should freely admit the inherent obstacles to accurate analysis and apply the bite mark evidence in a manner consistent with scientific principles. With the slow but rational enhancement of techniques along scientific lines, bite mark evidence can reinforce and expand its sound and logical basis.

Notes

1. R. A. Walther, "An Examination of the Psychological Aspects of Bite Marks," *American Journal of Forensic Medicine and Pathology* 5: 25-9 (1984).

2. F. Strom, "Investigations of Bite Marks," *Journal of Dental Restoration* 42: 312 (1963).

3. U. Pierce, D. J. Strickland, and E. S. Smith, "The Case of *Ohio* vs. *Robinson:* An 1870 Bite Mark Case," *American Journal of Forensic Medicine and Pathology* 11: 171-7 (1990).

4. *People* vs. *Johnson,* 8 Ill. App. 3d 457, 289 NE 2d 722.

5. G. Gustafson, ed., *Forensic Odontology* (New York: American Elsevier; 1966).

6. F. A. Keyes, "Teeth Marks on the Skin as Evidence in Establishing Identity," *Dental Cosmos* 67: 1165-7 (1925).

7. T. C. Krauss, "Photographic Techniques of Concern in Metric Bite Mark Analysis," *Journal of Forensic Sciences* 29 (2): 633-8 (1954).

8. R. Ouguid and G. S. McKay, "Bite Length Measurements and Tooth-To-Arch Relationships Obtained from Dental Casts Using an X,Y-Digitiser and Computer," *Journal of Forensic Science Society* 21: 211-23 (1981).

9. K. A. Brown, et al., "The Survival of Oral Streptococci on Human Skin and Its Implication in Bite-Mark Investigation," *Forensic Science International* 26 (3): 193-7 (1984).

10. T. R. Elliot, A. H. Rogers, J. R. Haverkamp, and D. Groothuis, "Analytical Pyrolysis of Streptococcus Salivarius as an Aid to Identification in Bite Mark Investigation," *Forensic Science International* 26 (2): 131-7 (1984).

11. J. J. Layton, "Identification from a Bite Mark in Cheese," *Journal of Forensic Sciences* 6: 76 (1966).

12. J. M. Cameron and B. G. Sims, *Forensic Dentistry* (London: Churchill Livingstone, 1974).

13. *Bundy* vs. *Florida,* So. 2d Aug 1979.

14. *People* vs. *Jennings,* 252 Ill. 534, 96 N.E. 1077 (1911).

15. *Frye* vs. *United States,* 293 F. 1013 (D.C. Cir 1923).

16. *People* vs. *Marx,* 54 Cal. App. 3d 100, 126 Cal Rptr. 350 (1975).

17. *People* vs. *Milone,* 43 Ill. App 3d 385, 356 N.E. 2d 1350 (1976).

18. A. P. Wilkinson and R. M. Gerughty, "Bite Mark Evidence: Its Admissibility Is Hard to Swallow," *Western State University Law Review* 12: 519-61 (1955).

19. "Qualifications and Requirements: Certification in Forensic Odontology," *ASFO Newsletter*: 2-3 (Spring 1990).

20. L. T. Johnson and D. Cadle, "Bite Mark Evidence. Recognition, Preservation, Analysis and Courtoom Presentation," *New York State Dental Journal* 55: 38-41 (1959).

21. J. R. Valerie and R. R. Souviron, "Dusting and Lifting the Bite Print. A New Technique, 1984," *Journal of Forensic Sciences* 19 (1): 326-30 (1984).

22. M. L. Bernstein, "Two Bite Mark Cases with Inadequate Scale Reference," *Journal of Forensic Sciences* 30: 955-64 (1985).

23. J. I. Ebert, "Discussion of the Bite Mark Standard Reference Scale—ABFO No. 2," *Journal of Forensic Sciences* 33: 301-4 (1955).

24. T. C. Krauss and S. C. Warlen, "The Forensic Science Use of Reflective Ultraviolet Photography," *Journal of Forensic Sciences* 30: 262-8 (1985).

25. T. C. Krauss, "Forensic Evidence Documentation Using Reflective Ultraviolet Photography," *Photo Electronic Imaging* 12 (2): 18-23 (1993).

26. R. E. Barsley, M. H. West, and J. A. Fair, "Forensic Photography. Ultraviolet Imaging of Wounds on Skin," *American Journal of Forensic Medicine and Pathology* 11 (4): 300-8 (1990).

27. M. H. West, J. D. Billings, and J. Fair, "Ultraviolet Photography: Bite Marks on Human Skin and Suggested Technique for the Exposure and Development of Reflective Ultraviolet Photography," *Journal of Forensic Sciences* 32: 1204-13 (1987).

28. B. W. Benson, J. A. Cottone, T. J. Bomberg, and N. D. Sperber, "Bite Mark Impressions: A Review of Techniques and Materials," *Journal of Forensic Sciences* 33 (5):1238-43 (1988).

29. J. C. Dailey, A. F. Shernoff, and J. H. Gelles, "An Improved Technique for Bite Mark Impressions," *Journal of Prosthetic Dentistry* 61 (2): 153-5 (1989).

30. R. B. J. Dorion, "Preservation and Fixation of Skin for Ulterior Scientific Evaluation and Courtroom Presentation," *CDAJ* 50 (2): 129-30 (1984).

31. American Board of Forensic Odontology, Inc., "Guidelines for Bite Mark Analysis," *Journal of the American Dental Association* 112: 383-6 (1986).

32. A. Hale, "The Admissibility of Bite Mark Evidence," *South California Law Review* 51: 309-34 1978.

33. R. D. Rawson, G. L. Vale, E. E. Herschaft, and A. Yjantis, "Reliability of the Scoring System of the American Board of Forensic Odontology for Human Bite Marks," *Journal of Forensic Sciences* 31 (1): 1235-60 (1986).

34. T. Furuhata and K.Yamamoto, *Forensic Odontology* (Springfield: Thomas, 1967), 98.

35. R. D. Rawson, G. L. Vale, E. E. Herschaft, N. D. Sperber, and S. Dowell, "Analysis of Photographic Distortion in Bite Marks: A Report of the Bite Mark Guidelines Committee," *Journal of Forensic Sciences* 31 (4): 1261-8 (1986).

36. J. C. Barbanel and J. H. Evans, "Bite Marks in Skin—Mechanical Factors," *Journal of Forensic Sciences* 14: 235-8 (1974).

37. M. H. West, R. E. Barsley, J. Fair, and M. D. Seal, "The Use of Human Skin in the Fabrication of a Bite Mark Template: Two Case Reports,"*Journal of Forensic Sciences* 35: 1477-85 (1990).

38. J. W. Beckstead, R. D. Rawson, and W. S. Giles, "Review of Bite Mark Evidence," *Journal of the American Dental Association* 99: 69-74 (1979).

39. R. F. Sognnaes, R. D. Rawson, B. M. Gratt, and B. N. Nauyen, "Computer Comparison of Bite Mark Patterns in Identical Twins," *Journal of the American Dental Association* 195: 449-52 (1982).

40. R. D. Rawson, et al., "Statistical Evidence for the Individuality of the Human Dentition," *Journal of Forensic Sciences* 29: 245-53 (1984).

41. F. Strom, "Investigation of Bite-Marks," *Journal of Dental Restoration* 42: 312-6 (1963).

42. R. D. Rawson, A. Richardson, and T. Bender, "Incidence of Bite Marks in a Selected Juvenile Population: A Preliminary Report," *Journal of Forensic Sciences* 29: 254-9 (1984).

43. J. C. Dailey, "Transparent Bite Mark Overlays," in D. C. Averill, ed. *Manual of Forensic Odontology* (ASFS, 1991).

44. D. K. Whittaker, "Some Laboratory Studies on the Accuracy of Bite Mark Comparison," *International Dental Journal* 25: 166-71 (1975).

45. W. L. Farrell, et al., "Computerized Axial Tomography as an Aid in Bite Mark Analysis: A Case Report," *Journal of Forensic Sciences* 32: 266-72 (1987).

46. T. J. David, "Adjunctive Use of Scanning Electron Microscopy in Bite Mark Analysis: A Three-Dimensional Study," *Journal of Forensic Sciences* 31: 1126-34 (1986).

47. R. B. J. Dorion, "Transillumination in Bite Mark Evidence," *Journal of Forensic Sciences* 32 (3): 690-7 (1987).

48. I. M. Sopher, *Forensic Dentistry* (Springfield, Ill.: Thomas, 1976).

49. L. Levine, "Forensic Dentistry: Our Most Controversial Case," *Legal Medicine Annals* 73: 77 (1978).

50. C. P. Karazulas, "The Presentation of Bite Mark Evidence Resulting in the Acquittal of a Man after Serving Seven Years in Prison for Murder," *Journal of Forensic Sciences* 29 (1): 355-8 (1984).

51. R. D. Rawson and S. Brooks, "Classification of Human Breast Morphology Important to Bite Mark Investigation," *American Journal of Forensic Medicine and Pathology* 5: 19-24 (1984).

—by Bruce R. Rothwell, D.M.D., M.S.D.

Dr. Rothwell is chairman of the Department of Restorative Dentistry, and director of Hospital Dentistry, School of Dentistry, University of Washington. He is also a consultant forensic odontologist to the King County Medical Examiner, Seattle, Washington.

Chapter 32

Latent Fingerprint Technology

Visualizing Latent Prints on Skin

Whether to stop them from fleeing, immobilize them, or dispose of them, murderers often grab their victims. What homicide detective has not wished for the ability to develop identifiable fingerprints of a suspect from the skin of a dead body? Crucial fingerprint evidence linking the perpetrator to the victim must be right there, but, until recently, attempts to retrieve those prints rarely met with success.

Skin possesses a number of unique qualities that distinguish it from other specimens examined for latent prints. Skin tissue grows and constantly renews itself, shedding old cells that might contain the imprint of an assailant's grip. Its pliability allows movement and, hence, possible distortion of fingerprints. As the skin regulates the body's temperature and excretes waste matter through perspiration, latent prints can be washed away.

In addition to these natural changes, the skin of homicide victims often is subjected to many harsh conditions, such as mutilation, bodily fluids, the weather, and decomposition after death. Further, during crime scene processing, many people might handle a body while removing it from the scene, which also can destroy existing fingerprints or possibly add new ones to the corpse's skin.

From "Hidden Evidence: Latent Prints on Human Skin," by Ivan Ross Futrell, in *FBI Law Enforcement Bulletin,* April 1996; and "New Reagents for Development of Latent Fingerprints," in *National Institute of Justice Update,* September 1995.

In spite of these hurdles, research conducted by the FBI Laboratory's Latent Fingerprint Section—in conjunction with police and medical authorities in Knoxville, Tennessee—proves that latent fingerprints can be lifted from skin if only investigators are willing to try. This article outlines the history and research that led to development of a workable method for developing identifiable latent prints on human skin.

History

The FBI has been involved in research on methods to develop identifiable latent prints on human skin for many years. In the early 1970s, FBI scientists reexamined existing methods using cadavers at a major university and the Virginia State Medical Examiner's Office in Richmond, Virginia. Most of these cadavers had been embalmed.

To create prints, these researchers applied a coating of baby oil and petroleum jelly to their hands and then touched areas of skin on the cadavers. At timed intervals, they then attempted to develop these latent prints, using primarily the iodine/silver transfer method. This method has five steps: heating iodine in an iodine fuming gun, directing the fumes onto the skin, laying a thin sheet of silver on the skin, removing the silver plate and, finally, exposing the plate to a strong light, which causes the prints to become visible.

The researchers developed identifiable prints in this fashion within a time frame that ranged from several hours up to several days after the prints were applied. It should be noted, however, that the researchers achieved these results under ideal laboratory conditions. It was not surprising that they developed latent prints composed of artificially introduced oily substances on embalmed cadavers. Yet, those early efforts provided important background data for subsequent research conducted in Tennessee.

In 1991, a police specialist from the Knoxville, Tennessee, Police Department contacted the FBI Latent Fingerprint Section to inquire about the FBI's experience and previous research on developing latent prints on skin. His own examination of numerous homicide victims had not produced prints with identifiable ridge detail, even though some cadavers exhibited observable outlines of fingers and palms. Out of these discussions arose a joint research project involving the Knoxville Police Department, the University of Tennessee Hospital, the Department of Anthropology at the University of Tennessee, and the FBI.

To develop a consistent and reliable technique for developing latent prints on skin, the researchers established a protocol significantly different from previous efforts. They decided to use only unembalmed cadavers and to place latent prints composed of only natural perspiration and sebaceous (oily) material. They felt that such conditions more accurately replicated field conditions faced by police investigators.

Research

The researchers first examined the body of a 62-year-old white female who had been dead for 9 days. Areas of skin were sectioned into numbered squares drawn on the body. One researcher placed latent prints on the skin by wiping his hand across his brow or through his hair and then touching the cadaver. The researchers then tried to develop the latent prints at timed intervals by employing several methods, including the use of lasers, alternate light sources, iodine/silver transfer, cyanoacrylate fuming (commonly referred to as "glue fuming"), regular and fluorescent powders, specially formulated powders, regular and fluorescent magnetic powders, liquid iodine, RAM, ardrox, and thenoyl europium chelate.

Most of these methods developed the latent prints up to approximately 1 hour after the prints had been deposited. For additional documentation, during the next several days, researchers tested the techniques on other cadavers, but most methods failed to provide consistent results.

The one technique that developed identifiable latent prints most often was glue fuming in conjunction with regular magnetic fingerprint powder. Similar to iodine/silver transfer, this method involves heating glue and directing the fumes onto the skin, then applying fingerprint powder to reveal the latent prints.

To test this technique further, researchers glue fumed several areas of skin containing sebaceous latent prints 2 hours after depositing the prints. Sixteen hours later, they applied various fingerprint powders to those areas. Using a fluorescent powder specially formulated for this testing, they developed a latent print of value for identification purposes. Initially, the researchers believed that the special fluorescent powder provided the key to obtaining usable prints, but additional tests proved that the type of powder did not matter as much as the amount of time allowed for glue fuming.

Glue Fuming Device

As they continued their research, the scientists realized that they needed an improved method for spreading glue fumes over the skin.

The earlier method used—forming an airtight plastic tent over a small area of skin or over an entire body—did not always work. It was impossible to distribute glue fumes evenly over the skin and extremely difficult to confine all of the fumes to the tent. In addition, when they removed the plastic tent at the end of the fuming process, the fumes often forced the researchers out of the work area. To alleviate these problems, one of the researchers, the police specialist from the Knoxville Department, developed a portable glue fuming chamber.

The glue fuming chamber contains a built-in heat source and a small electric fan. Glue is poured into a small disposable preheated aluminum pan and placed in the chamber. After approximately 5 minutes, the fan is turned on and the glue fumes flow out through a plastic hose attached to the top of the chamber. When set at maximum, the amount of fumes forced through the hose approximates the exhaust from an automobile on a cold day. This device enables the user to control the amount and time of the glue fuming much more easily than the tent method.

Using the new device, the scientists tested squares of skin to determine the optimal fuming time. They tried fuming in increments from 5 seconds up to 2 minutes. They obtained identifiable latent prints most often when glue fumes had been applied to the skin for 10 to 15 seconds.

Powders

In the early testing, it seemed that particular types and brands of fingerprint powders provided the best results. As the research progressed, however, it became apparent that this was not the case. More than 30 brands and several types of powders and applicators were tested. In the end, researchers determined that powder selection is less critical than ensuring that the glue fuming process is performed correctly.

Both fluorescent powders and regular magnetic powders produce identifiable prints. With nonmagnetic fluorescent powders, the best results are obtained by applying the powder with a feather duster rather than a conventional brush, which generally holds more powder. Too much fluorescent powder tends to overwhelm the latent print and the background. While fluorescent powders work, they do have some drawbacks. They generally cost more than regular magnetic powders, are more difficult to see, and require special light sources, filters, and additional photographic knowledge.

In comparison, regular black magnetic powders produce useful prints and cost much less. They also do not require special photographic skills. Indeed, technology does not need to be complex or costly in order to be effective.

Field Conditions

Developing latent prints under ideal laboratory conditions proved that prints could be obtained from human skin, but the researchers wanted to make sure that practitioners in the field could obtain similar results. In real life, homicide victims might not be found immediately, bodies might be exposed to the elements or other harsh conditions, or they might be taken to the morgue and refrigerated before they can be examined for prints.

To ensure that the process would work, the researchers simulated field conditions by testing cadavers that had been exposed to the elements for several days, as well as refrigerated corpses. They replicated potential time delays that could occur in the field by waiting for approximately 12 hours between the glue fuming (which could be done at the crime scene) and the application of fingerprint powders (perhaps conducted later at the morgue). The results showed that by following proper procedures, investigators could develop identifiable latent prints even under harsh conditions.

Recommendations

This research indicates that homicide victims should be examined for latent prints whenever investigators believe that the perpetrator touched the victim. If possible, bodies should be examined at the crime scene immediately after the coroner or medical examiner has completed an initial examination and granted permission. At a minimum, the body should be glue fumed at the scene to preserve the prints and help prevent contamination or obliteration of prints when the body is moved.

Ideally, bodies should not be refrigerated prior to examination for latent prints. The condensation that builds up on refrigerated bodies can have adverse effects by washing away the prints, reacting with the glue to distort the prints, or causing the powder to cake, thus losing the prints. Bodies that have been refrigerated should not be processed until the moisture evaporates, roughly several minutes, depending on ambient temperature. A control area of skin least likely to have prints can be tested to ensure that the moisture has dissipated.

Skin that is warm or near normal body temperature should be glue fumed for only 5 to 10 seconds. Colder skin should be glue fumed for a maximum of 15 seconds. Regular magnetic powders can then be applied. Any identifiable latent prints should be photographed first and then lifted using transparent lifting tape.

Visualizing Latent Prints on Other Porous Surfaces

Use of Ninhydrin

Technically, fingerprinting is a biochemical method for determining the structure of a protein in which the protein is split into peptides by digestion with protease, and the fragments are separated in one direction by electrophoresis and at right angles by chromatography. After staining with a reagent, the peptide fragments are seen to be in characteristic locations. Improving the processes for obtaining usable prints as evidence has led to a search for superior development reagents to aid in identifying latent fingerprints. National Institute of Justice (NIJ)-sponsored research found ways to enhance the properties (e.g., line resolution, fluorescence) of one of the most commonly used reagents, ninhydrin, via structural modifications. In addition, ninhydrin analogs were altered to expand their solubility to a wider range of organic solvents.

Previous Work on Ninhydrin

Ninhydrin was first prepared in 1910 by the English chemist, Siegfried Ruhemann, who also investigated the formation of the violet compound (Ruhemann's Purple, or RP) produced by ninhydrin's reaction with amino acids.[1] The significance of this discovery to forensic science went unnoticed until 1954, when Oden and von Hoffsten reported the use of ninhydrin as a fingerprint developing reagent that reacts with amino acids secreted from sweat glands.[2] Although the content of amino acids in a fingerprint residue is low (compared to the content of salts and fatty acids), the RP produced from the reaction of these amino acids with ninhydrin is deeply colored, and the developed fingerprints are usually highly visible. Thus, ninhydrin has long been known as one of the most affordable and useful reagents for visualization of latent fingerprints on porous surfaces (such as paper, wood, and walls).

In cases where the developed fingerprints are weak, secondary treatment with an aqueous zinc chloride solution can improve the print's line resolution quality. Zinc chloride-treated prints can be observed as "glowing" (fluorescent) when illuminated with light of a certain wavelength. In 1990, C. A. Pounds and coworkers introduced the reagent 1, 8-diazafluorenone (DFO), which is commercially available and used in the United Kingdom.[3] Unlike ninhydrin, DFO gives a weakly colored initial print; the main feature of this reagent is its ability to give a fluorescent print without secondary treatment. However, some investigators currently report difficulties with uniform print development using DFO.

Synthesis of New Ninhydrin Analogs

The NIJ-sponsored research group had previously prepared a compound, thieno[f]ninhydrin, that provided an initial print as deeply colored as one produced with ninhydrin as the reagent.[4] Thieno[f] ninhydrin also displayed excellent fluorescent properties without requiring the use of a metal enzo[f]ninhydrin, 5-methoxy-ninhydrin, 5-(methylthio)ninhydrin, thieno[f]ninhydrin, as well as to the extended series of 5-phenyl- and 5-thienylninhydrin derivatives, starting from the inexpensive bromoxylene in a short high-yielding synthetic sequence. When tested, 5-(2-thienyl)ninhydrin and 5-(3-thienyl)ninhydrin (2-THIN and 3-THIN) displayed properties (i.e., brighter fluorescence, better line resolution) superior to ninhydrin's as fingerprint developing reagents.[5]

Chemical Modifications Facilitating the Choice of Solvent

Ninhydrin is commonly used for fingerprint development on porous surfaces, which are dipped in the reagent solution or sprayed with it. The choice of solvent is important—different kinds of inks on documents can be affected by the solvent employed; the fingerprint itself can be smeared by an inappropriate solvent. Solvents used in forensic science must pose no more than a minimal safety risk, in terms of properties such as flammability or toxicity, and they must also be environmentally safe. Chlorofluorocarbons, such as trichlorofifluoroethane, had been the solvents of choice in ninhydrin formulations. When banned recently by the Environmental Protection Agency, a search was begun for acceptable substitute solvents, In the ninhydrin study, researchers found that some derivatives of the reagent, resulting from its reaction with higher molecular weight or "long chain" alcohols (i.e., hemiacetals), undergo the same color-forming reactions as ninhydrin, but they are substantially more soluble in organic solvents (e.g., ethyl acetate, methylene chloride, or toluene). Hemiacetals can be quantitatively obtained from any ninhydrin analog in a one-step procedure.

Practical Implications

Several synthetic approaches were developed and evaluated to provide a total of 21 new ninhydrin analogs. These reagents were evaluated for fingerprint visualization by forensic experts at the U.S. Secret Service and other law enforcement agencies, both in this country and in England, Switzerland, Australia, and Israel. The new methodology afforded two complementary reagents (2-THIN and 3-THIN), which displayed superior fingerprint developing properties. Large-scale production of 2-THIN has been initiated by Vinfer Ltd., a Northern Ireland manufacturer, to investigate its potential for commercialization.

This research has provided a viable solution to problems encountered by criminalists as a result of the prohibited use of chlorofluorocarbons.

Notes

1. S. Ruhemann, *Transactions of the Chemical Society,* 97: 2025 (1910).

2. S. Oden, and B. von Hofsten, *Nature,* 173: 449 (1954).

3. C. A. Pounds, R. Grigg, and T. Mongkolaussavaratana, *Journal of Forensic Sciences,* 35: 169-75 (1990).

4. A. Cantu, D. A. Leben, M. M. Joullie, and R. R. Hark, *Journal of Forensic Identification,* 43: 44-66 (1993).

5. R. R. Hark, D. B. Hauze, O. Petrovskaia, M. M. Joullie, R. Jaouhari, and P. McComiskey, *Tetrahedron Letters,* 35: 7719-22 (1994).

Chapter 33

Language-Based Author Identification

From Eyewitness to Questioned Document Examiner

Legal proceedings have long required some kind of authentication of documentary evidence. Until the 19th century, a document was typically authenticated by an eyewitness to its creation or signing (much as notaries do)—or by someone, such as a spouse, other close relative, or banker, who knew and recognized the writing. This kind of document authentication is still admissible testimony under the Federal Rules of Evidence (specifically Rule 901, "Requirement of Authentication or Identification").

But what if no such person is available or willing to testify in that regard?

In the early 19th century, another kind of document authentication came on the scene: comparison by an expert of the questioned document with known writing samples. Through the 1800s and into the early 1900s, most state courts allowed such expert testimony on the basis of court decision or state statute. In 1913, the United States Code permitted the admissibility of handwriting identification by expert testimony.

Despite the U.S. Supreme Court's 1923 ruling in *Frye* v. *United States* that scientific testimony should be limited by its "general acceptance" within the scientific community, questioned document examination (QDE) was, in a sense, immune from such scrutiny since

From "Who Wrote It?" by Carole E. Chaski, Ph.D., in *National Institute of Justice Journal,* September 1997, pp. 16-22.

any lawyer seeking to introduce it in court could argue that it was directly admissible by statute. When the Federal Rules of Evidence (FRE) were enacted by Congress in 1975, testimony based on "comparison by trier or expert witness"—that is, handwriting identification by a questioned document examiner—continued to be admissible through Rule 901.

In 1993, 70 years after *Frye*, the U.S. Supreme Court heard *Daubert* v. *Merrell Dow Pharmaceuticals, Inc.* (113 5. Ct. 2786), which resulted in major changes in the way that expert testimony is admitted as scientific evidence. The Court ruled that testimony, if it is to be considered "scientific," must be demonstrated to have characteristics shared by established sciences, like biology or chemistry.The Court listed some of those characteristics: empirical testing, known or potential rate of error, standard procedures for performing a technique, peer review and publication, as well as general acceptance in the scientific community.

Key criteria distinguishing scientific endeavors from others are stepwise procedures, identifiable (or discrete) units, measurement, replication, and predictability. The laboratory experiments conducted in high school embody those characteristics. So does cooking:

- A recipe is a procedure with steps that must be performed in a stated order.

- The ingredients in a recipe are separate, distinguishable items.

- The ingredients or units are measured using standard measuring devices.

- Anyone can repeat these procedures using the standard measures and standard tools.

- Anyone repeating the recipe in the same way with the same units, measures, and tools will get the same result.

In a *Daubert* hearing—one held to determine whether evidence can be admitted as scientific—Professor Barry Scheck attacked questioned document examination on the basis of its scientific foundation *(United States* v. *Starzecpyzel, 1995)*. District Judge McKenna agreed: "The *Daubert* hearing established that forensic document examination, which clothes itself with the trappings of science, does not rest on carefully articulated postulates, does not employ rigorous methodology, and has not convincingly documented the accuracy of its determinations."

Judge McKenna ruled that handwriting identification testimony could not be considered scientific and so would not fall under *Daubert* criteria for admitting scientific evidence. This ruling, however, would still admit handwriting identification testimony as long as it was perceived as "technical or other specialized knowledge" (as specified admissible by FRE Rule 702, "Testimony by Experts") rather than as science.

Judge McKenna's ruling initiated a series of judicial decisions from federal, state, and military courts challenging the admissibility of handwriting identification by expert comparison in various ways. For example, at the trial of Timothy McVeigh for the Oklahoma City bombing, after the defense requested a *Daubert* hearing on the proffered questioned document testimony, prosecutors withdrew such testimony and relied on other means of authenticating motel receipts, identification cards, and other documentary evidence.

The choices available appear to be not presenting handwriting identification testimony at all, presenting QDE as "technical" rather than scientific knowledge, or building a foundation for handwriting identification that meets *Daubert* criteria for scientific testimony.

Thus, questioned document examination is facing a steep legal and intellectual challenge to create an authentic science of document authentication via handwriting.

Toward a Science of Authorship: Handwriting Identification

In July 1996, the National Institute of Justice sponsored a workshop on developing a research agenda for questioned document examination. The workshop included questioned document examiners working in local, state, and federal law enforcement agencies; forensic linguists; attorneys; and experts in voice identification, computer engineering, neural networks, neuroscience, and statistics.

Workshop participants discussed this question: What would be needed to argue successfully in a *Daubert* hearing that QDE testimony is accurate, reliable, and based on sound, empirically tested principles? The fundamental requirement, workshop participants agreed, is empirical evidence to support the two central principles underlying handwriting identification:

- Each person's handwriting differs from any other's. Because this requires a comparison between documents from different people, the difference between individuals' writing is called interwriter variation.

- Each person's handwriting contains some variation. Because this requires a comparison between different documents from the same person, the differences within one person's handwriting samples are called intrawriter variation.

The workshop reached a consensus that proof of the foregoing principles is the highest priority for research.

For handwriting identification to be within the realm of the possible, a distinct difference must be detectable between interwriter variation and intrawriter variation so that, even if one's handwriting changes from document to document, it is still identifiably different from another's. Writing samples from one individual may differ, but an individual writing pattern exists in all of them.

If these principles are not proved true, the current approach of QDE should stop because testimony could be based on a false belief about the human behavior of writing and have very serious legal consequences. Thus, a prime scientific challenge to QDE is to demonstrate that its principles and methods meet or exceed the *Daubert* criteria for scientific evidence, such as by taking the following steps:

- Create a database by collecting samples from writers.

- Determine how to measure the samples. What characteristics should be measured (slant, height, etc.)? Which units of measure should be counted? What procedures should be established for measuring characteristics?

- Analyze statistically the results of quantifying handwriting samples.

Replication would test the hypothesis that handwriting is individually identifiable and validate the predictive ability of QDE to identify and differentiate handwriting samples.

The next step would be to determine how to apply these principles of interwriter and intrawriter variation—if proved true—to actual cases. Applying scientific criteria (stepwise procedures, identifiable units, measurement, replication, and predictability) would create a standard protocol for performing QDE, much like existing protocols for conducting DNA analyses.

But it would not be sufficient just to have a standard protocol that everyone agrees on (which itself may be difficult to obtain). The standard protocol must be tested to determine if it actually works and the rate at which it works correctly. The development and testing of a standard protocol is essential to demonstrating that handwriting identification is reliable. Reliability means that using the protocol on the same set of documents at different times under different circumstances—even by different people—will yield the same results.

Once a standard protocol for performing handwriting identification is tested and shown reliable, it can be taught as part of training for QDE.

At this point, yet another scientific challenge to QDE arises: the question of proficiency among examiners trained to use the standard protocol. Until a standard protocol is developed and practiced by questioned document examiners, proficiency tests may measure luck, visual acuity, persistence, or an odd talent, but not the ability to apply a scientific method to solve a problem in handwriting identification. (See "Recent Developments in Handwriting Identification" at the end of the article.)

From Pen and Pencil to Electronic Texts

Meanwhile, what kind of authentication is available if a document is not handwritten? Society is rapidly moving beyond pen and pencil and producing more and more electronic documents. Documents composed on the computer, printed over networks, faxed over telephone lines, or simply stored in electronic memory defy traditional handwriting identification techniques.

When authorship of an electronically produced document is disputed, analysis of handwriting and typing does not apply. In the case of networked printers—to which thousands of potential users have access—even ink, paper, and printer identification cannot narrow the range of suspects or produce a solitary identification. The language of a document, however, is independent of whether a document is handwritten or printed or faxed or stored electronically.

In the past 20 years, techniques of language-based authorship identification have been developing within university departments— classics, English, and applied linguistics—in Great Britain, Germany, Australia, and the United States. But if these methods of language-based document authentication were offered as scientific evidence in a criminal trial, one would expect a *Daubert* hearing to conclude in much the same way Judge McKenna ruled with regard to handwriting identification.[1] Even without such a ruling, language-based author identification needs to develop a sound scientific method if it is to serve justice and truth.

329

Foundation for Scientific Linguistic Identification

A good starting point for developing a scientific method of linguistic identification is to ask whether a theoretical foundation for language-based author identification exists within linguistic science.

Theoretical foundations for language-based author identification derive from various branches of linguistics. The following concepts are well founded and uncontroversial among linguists: dialect and idiolect, language processing, and metalinguistic awareness.

Dialect and idiolect. Dialect is a variation within a language, while an idiolect is an individual variation within a dialect. For instance, a speaker of the Southern American English dialect may say "John *might should* check his parking meter," while a speaker of Northern American English dialect would say *"Maybe* John *should* check his parking meter."

Because dialect is a group phenomenon, one might predict that Southerners who use "might should" are a fairly homogeneous group. But this is not necessarily so. One Southerner may use "might should" in statements only, while another may produce "might should" in statements as well as in questions such as "Should you might check the meter?" Even though Southerners can be identified by their Southern American English dialect, they can be individuated by their idiosyncratic uses of the dialect, that is, by idiolect.

The theoretical notions of language, dialect, and idiolect suggest that individual identity in language is feasible. But can we control and manipulate idiolectal features, or is language use unconscious enough to be reliably indicative of a specific person? To answer, from a theoretical perspective, one must consider language processing.

Language processing. In normal language processing, we communicate so quickly that we can finish each other's sentences. Typically we do not even remember the exact words we used but do remember the gist of a conversation long after it has concluded. The form (or syntax) is disposable, while the message (or semantics) is durable. In normal language processing, the construction of the form is automatic or unconscious. Automatic or unconscious control of language enables us to do all we are doing while we are speaking (selecting and retrieving words, combining words into phrases and larger units, attaching phrases to other phrases and larger units) while we as communicators focus consciously only on the meaning of our message.

From the perspective of automatized processing, linguistic production (especially syntactic structures) would appear to be very difficult to control. The more automatic a behavior, the more reliably it indicates a personal identity. Fingerprints are reliable indicators of individuality because, normally, we do not control them. Likewise, syntactic structures may be so automatic as to be reliable indicators of individuality.

Metalinguistic awareness. Although unconscious control of language is normal behavior, we can distance ourselves from language and make conscious commentary about it. This ability to think consciously and talk about language itself (rather than the message language conveys) is called metalinguistic awareness.

The possibility of metalinguistic awareness raises the question of linguistic disguise. Suppose someone is so sensitive to language, so metalinguistically aware, that such a person can overcome the automatization of language processing and actually change natural patterns to such a degree as to imitate the idiolectal patterns of another speaker and suppress one's own idiolectal patterns. Research has already shown that adults vary in their metalinguistic abilities.[2] Therefore, until more is known about metalinguistic awareness in adults, the theoretical position should be taken that linguistic disguise is possible depending on the author's particular level of metalinguistic awareness.

So, because the notion of individual identity in language is credible, language-based author identification is theoretically feasible. Because some kinds of linguistic production, especially syntactic processing, are unconscious, detection of authorship through reliable linguistic patterns is also feasible. Because individual awareness of and sensitivity to language varies, an individual may be able to manipulate linguistic patterns; thus, disguising authorship is also theoretically possible.

Basic Steps toward a Science of Linguistic Identification

Since language-based author identification seems theoretically feasible, a scientific method that results in an identification would require analytical approaches and technologies—some taken directly from linguistic theory, others to be developed for this application of the theory—enabling repetitions of a stepwise procedure to yield consistent results that could be tested statistically.

Standard procedures for analyzing a document into syntactic structures—noted above as difficult to manipulate or disguise—are already available from theoretical linguistics. Having the analytical method at the ready leads to the question, What sort of documents should be assembled on which to apply the standard analytical procedure?

A database of documents should be assembled with the principles of linguistic performance in mind. If we compare two different document types, say a business letter and a diary entry, some differences in the linguistic patterns will be at least in part due to the differing social context and communicative goals of business letters and diary entries. A person's idiolect will vary depending on the document type being produced. Further, since this database is being constructed for forensic application, the document types should be similar to the document types found in actual cases—similar, rather than same, because one would not request, for example, actual suicide notes or actual threatening letters or actual ransom notes from human subjects. So the database should contain several writing samples from each writer, and these writing samples should be similar to document types found in actual forensic cases.

Once the document database is assembled and each document is analyzed into its syntactic structures, the next step is to examine writing samples for idiolectal markers—those fragments of syntactic structures that serve to identify idiolects, or individual language patterns. DNA typing provides an interesting analogy. We share an enormous amount of DNA; only a minute fraction distinguishes us as individuals. So, analogous to DNA, the bulk of linguistic patterns are shared, and the minor quantitative variation is where we need to look for idiolectal markers.

There is no list of idiolectal markers available from linguistic theory. Thus, we need standard operating procedures for how to determine idiolectal markers in documents of varying size, type, and authorship.

As with QDE, when evidence of the idiolect and standard operating procedures are developed for performing language-based author identification, proficiency testing of forensic linguists can be designed and conducted on a regular basis.

Progress in Scientific Linguistic Identification

An NIJ Visiting Fellowship provided the opportunity for developing a computer system—Automated Linguistic Authentication System (ALAS), which has two main components. The first is a database of documents (see "The Writing Sample Database" at the end of the article). The second embodies natural language parsing programs that "process" documents in the writing sample database by assigning syntactic labels to the words, phrases, and larger units of each text, which can then be quantified and used statistically to categorize texts into authorship clusters.

Currently, ALAS is being used to analyze writing samples from a small subset of subjects to search for idiolectal markers—that is, syntactic structures or combinations of syntactic features that can both discriminate between documents authored by different writers and group together documents written by the same person. Texts of varying lengths were examined to determine which markers are feasible to use depending on the amount of text available, taking into account the special problem of very short texts typical of forensic cases.

In a pilot study, ALAS parsed and computed the syntactic distribution in writing samples from two subjects. These subjects, known as 016 and 080, are both women, white, in their 40s, with 2 to 3 years of college education and similar dialectal backgrounds. Since these sociological features may affect linguistic performance, one would expect that the two women might be similar—perhaps indistinguishable—linguistically. Indeed, in response to the first writing task, both discussed their fear of dying and leaving their children motherless. ALAS analyzed three samples of 343, 557, and 405 words from subject 016, and one sample of 240 words from subject 080.

The first task was to discover whether any linguistic features were constant through different samples of one subject's writing so that such features could be used to identify the subject's writing. One linguistic feature exemplifying an "identifying ability" is the number of combinations per sentence. The combinations tested here were both clauses per sentence and phrases per sentence. On average, writer 016 produced 5.4 clauses per sentence in text 1, 5.13 clauses per sentence in text 2, and 3.75 clauses per sentence in text 5—and 23.5 phrases per sentence in text 1, 24.85 phrases per sentence in text 2, and 22.33 phrases per sentence in text 5. When the measures of these combinations for the three writing samples are examined statistically, one may conclude that the three texts were written by the same person.

The second task was to find out whether any linguistic features could discriminate between different writers. For this purpose, three writing samples were compared from 016 with the 240-word sample from subject 080. One linguistic feature exemplifying a "differentiating ability" is the variant structures of prepositional phrases. The most frequent form of the prepositional phrase is a preposition followed by a noun phrase. Variant forms of the prepositional phrase include a "stranded" preposition, as in "what are you up to?," or prepositions followed by verb phrases, as in "tired of living a lie."

When computing the ratio between the most frequent form of the prepositional phrase and the variant forms, one finds that writer 016's ratios are 18:1, 38:7, and 38:3 for her three samples. Writer 080's ratio is 11:5 for her one sample. Statistically, the chance of these documents coming from the same source is 2 percent; put another way, the chance that these documents were written by different authors is 98 percent, which, of course, is the case.

But an idiolectal marker must serve both to identify and to differentiate. So a third task is to test whether any linguistic features had both "identifying" and "differentiating" ability and so could serve as idiolectal markers.

For this purpose, measures of the feature differentiating subject 080 from subject 016—ratio of types of prepositional phrases—were compared with the measures of this same feature within the writing samples of subject 016. The feature differentiated between 016 and 080. Would it also have an identifying ability for 016? Statistical testing of the three samples of subject 016 did not detect statistically significant differences among the three samples' ratios of prepositional phrase types. This suggests that the samples were written by the same person. Thus, the ratio of prepositional phrase types serves both to discriminate between the writing samples of 080 and 016, and to cluster together the writing samples of 016.

An exciting finding of this pilot study is that idiolectal markers were found in writing samples that are well under 1,000 words in length. Because such small writing samples can be used for syntactic analysis, the method is forensically applicable—in contrast to other techniques, which require much longer texts. The pilot study indicates that language-based author identification may be possible with samples in sizes actually found in kidnaping, homicide, and libel cases. Much more work, however, is needed.

At this point, the essential conclusion this and other pilot studies demonstrate is that a syntactic method of analysis, which is grounded in linguistic theory and implemented within a computer program, may be the route to an authentic science of language-based author identification.

Investigative Uses of Language-Based Author Identification

Even though language-based author identification has a long way to go before achieving status as scientific testimony, it certainly can be used effectively now as an investigative tool.

On April 29, 1992, Michael Hunter died of a lethal injection of lidocaine, Benadryl, and Vistaril. One of his two roommates, Joseph Mannino, reported the death. The other roommate, Gary Walston, was out of town.

A fourth-year medical student, Mannino was only weeks away from his medical degree. He admitted giving antihistamine to Hunter for a migraine headache. After an autopsy report showed the presence of lidocaine, Mannino denied injecting Hunter with the drug, which can induce central nervous system collapse. He declared that Hunter must have injected the drug himself.

Mannino produced computer disks containing suicide notes from Hunter. Detective W. Allison Blackman of the Raleigh, North Carolina, Police Department contacted Dr. Carole E. Chaski about the posssibility of determining the authorship of the suicide notes on the basis of the language used.

Detective Blackman gathered almost 10,000 running words of documents spontaneously written by Hunter, Mannino, and Walston. Dr. Chaski's analysis of the syntax, vocabulary, and punctuation patterns of the documents, with statistical testing, showed that the suicide notes were most likely not written by Hunter or by Walston but by Mannino. Soon after, Mannino was charged with first-degree homicide.

Through his attorney, Mannino admitted to writing the phony suicide notes. Due to ambiguous test results concerning the level of lidocaine in Hunter's blood, Mannino was convicted of the lesser charge of involuntary manslaughter. In the sentencing phase of the trial, Judge Stephens said, "It's terrible that Michael Hunter died. It's terrible that the defendant unlawfully caused his death. But to give the impression that Michael Hunter took his own life, I find that extremely aggravating in this case" (*Raleigh News and Observer,* July 28, 1994).

Mannino was sentenced to seven years in prison.

Recent Developments in Handwriting Identification

Electronic approaches to verifying interwriter variation are under way. The Secret Service used the German-based FISH computer program, which measures the pixel positions of handwriting scanned into digital format. Funded by the Federal Bureau of Investigation (FBI), Professor Kam of Drexel University and his students are developing another automated system for measuring pixels in digitized samples of handwriting from 400 bank robbery notes.

The FBI has formed the Technical Working Group on Documents (TWGDOC). A TWGDOC subcommittee has already begun work on documenting standard procedures for questioned document examination.

Proficiency testing of document examiners has been undertaken by Professor Kam. The most recent test revealed that trained document examiners and untrained laypersons with comparable educational backgrounds match handwriting samples correctly at approximately the same level, with each group making correct matches 87 percent of the time. However, trained document examiners made false positive matches 7 percent of the time, compared to 38 percent for untrained laypersons.

The Writing Sample Database

The Writing Sample Database—a major component of the Automated Linguistic Authentication System—is designed to take into account general statistical sampling issues and linguistic performance. Decisions about selecting the types of subjects for inclusion were based on a variety of factors, such as a subject's availability, the prominence of writing in the subject's normal lifestyle, dialect similarity or dialect grouping, generally equivalent education level, and representation of both genders and several ethnicities. Factors considered in selecting topics for writing samples from the subjects included document type and similarity to actual types of questioned documents. Writing tasks assigned to subjects included narrative essays describing traumatic events and personal influences, business letters, personal letters, and threatening letters.

Data were collected from two groups: criminal justice majors at a community college and business and nursing majors at a private 4-year college. Subjects wrote, at their leisure, on 10 topics.

At present, the Writing Sample Database includes samples from 98 persons, almost evenly divided between males and females, ranging in age from 18 to 49. Almost three-quarters of the subjects are white; the rest are black or multiracial. Because the writing samples were collected in a community college environment, writing is part of the subjects' lifestyles, and the subjects generally share equivalent educational levels and dialect backgrounds. The texts produced by the subjects contain approximately 100,000 words. Some subjects contributed as few as 50 words while others produced several thousand.

Notes

1. In technical report 95-IJ-CX-0012-01, *A Daubert-Inspired Assessment of Currently Available Language-Based Methods of*

Authorship Identification, I show that previous methods of language-based identification either violate well-established principles of linguistic theory or do not flow from linguistics but from literary studies and thus lack a scientific method. In their reviews, Crystal and Goutsos found similar problems with McMenamin's work (see David Crystal,"Review of *Forensic Stylistics* by Gerald R. McMenamin," *Language* 71: 2, 381-5 (1995); and Dionysis Goutsos, "Review Article: *Forensic Stylistics,*" *Forensic Linguistics* 2: 1, 99-113 (1995)). On the issue of replicability, Tiersma and Finegan report problems in previous methods, including lack of publication, lack of peer review, and nonreplicated results (see Peter M. Tiersma, "Linguistic Issues in the Law," *Language* 69: 1, 113-37 (1993); and Edward Finegan, "Variation in Linguists' Analyses of Author Identification," *American Speech*: 334-40 (Winter 1990)). Hardcastle was unable to replicate results using Morton's CUSUM method (see R. A. Hardcastle, "Forensic Linguistics: An Assessment of the CUSUM Method for the Determination of Authorship," *Journal of the Forensic Science Society* 33: 2, 95-106 (1993)). At this point, language-based authorship identification would fail a *Daubert* hearing.

2. Metalinguistic ability in adults is related to literacy level (Carole E. Chaski and Randall Engle, *Cognitive and Metalinguistic Characteristics of Adult Illiterates,* Technical Report (State of South Carolina Commission on Higher Education, 1990); C. E. Chaski, "Segmental Manipulation and Metalinguistic Ability in Adult Literates and Pre-literates," Linguistic Society of America Annual Winter Meeting, Philadelphia, Pennsylvania: 1991); and also to training in disciplines related to language (Hayley Davis, "Ordinary People's Philosophy: Comparing Lay and Professional Metalinguistic Knowledge," *Language Sciences* 19: 1, 33-46 (1997)).

— by Carole E. Chaski, Ph.D.

Carole E. Chaski is an NIJ Visiting Fellow. After earning her doctorate in linguistics at Brown University, she taught syntax and computational linguistics at the University of South Carolina and North Carolina State University. She has consulted for law enforcement agencies since 1992.

Chapter 34

Diatom Test for Drowning Victims

Introduction

The diatom test for drowning has proved to be a useful, reliable, and valid test for the postmortem diagnosis of drowning in hundreds of cases of drowning in Canada. In this brief overview, the rationale, validity, and applications of the test will be described. The diatom test for drowning remains an important adjunct to the medicolegal investigation of bodies found in water. A greater role for the test is becoming apparent in unusual deaths and homicidal drownings.

What Are Diatoms

Diatoms are aquatic unicellular plants that represent the most abundant single source of oxygen producers in the biosphere. The most distinctive feature of this unicellular organism is its extracellular coat or frustule, which is composed of silica. The vast structural diversity of the frustule leads to a remarkable number of morphologically distinctive varieties of diatoms. Recent estimates indicate that there are in excess of 100,000 different species of diatoms. Diatoms are most often encountered in naturally occurring bodies of water such as lakes,

From "The Forensic Value of the Diatom Test for Drowning," [Online] undated. Available: http://www.erin.utoronto.ca/academic/FSC/FSC239Y_ DROWNING.htm. Produced by Michael S. Pollanen, Ph.D., Forensic Pathology Unit, Office of the Chief Coroner, 26 Grenville St., Toronto, ON M7A 2G9 Canada. For complete contact information, please refer to Chapter 56, "Resources." Reprinted with permission.

rivers, oceans, seas, ditches, and puddles. Some diatom species have preference for water of specific salinity thus allowing general distinction between freshwater and marine diatom types. In addition, some diatom species are more frequently associated with soil and puddles than lakes. Fossilized diatoms are another major source of frustules in the biosphere, although, these frustules are derived from long dead diatoms. Such diatoms are mined for commercial use and are as forensically important as live freshwater contemporary diatoms. Mined fossilized diatoms are used in several commercial products including abrasive cleaning agents and polishes.

Some important features of diatoms are their population dynamics and ecology. Diatom populations are constantly in flux and these fluxes are the result of complex and poorly understood nutrient and aquatic cycles. The net result is a monthly periodicity in the abundance of live aquatic diatoms with blooms of diatom populations in the spring and autumn (i.e., seasonal maxima). In addition, there are temporal and spatial variations in diatom concentration in any body of water in response to local factors including mineral content of water, temperature, water stratification, and acidity. A poorly understood aspect of diatom ecology is the variation in the species and genus distribution over seasons. These ecological characteristics of diatom populations have great, and under utilized, forensic significance. Among the most important forensically relevant feature of diatom populations is the monthly variation in water concentration of diatom frustules that should, a priori, affect the outcome of the diatom test for drowning during various times of the year.

Rationale for the Diatom Test for Drowning

In the drowning process, water is inhaled, and enters the systemic circulation via the lungs. If diatoms are present in the drowning medium, the diatoms "embolize" to organs and tissues such as the bone marrow. Therefore, the presence of diatoms in the femoral bone marrow is an indication of antemortem inhalation of water. If diatoms are detected in the bone marrow (a positive test) this implies that: (i) drowning caused death or was a contributing factor to death, and (ii) the individual was breathing upon entry into the water.

The silica-based frustule of the diatom allows for the easy extraction of diatoms from human tissues by digestion of tissues in concentrated acid. Although other methods for diatom extraction have been advocated, the acid digestion method and centrifugation has been the most consistently applied and gives highly reproducible results. Various tissues have been used as starting material for the extraction of diatom frustules. Bone marrow removed from a femur is the preferred tissue of choice in our experience. The advantage of the bone marrow extracted from an intact femur is that contamination can be minimized or eliminated since the marrow is extracted from a "closed" organ that can not be soiled by diatoms from some external source.

The Validity of the Diatom Test for Drowning

The Diatom Controversy

The forensic pathology community has been polarized in its general acceptance of the diatom test as a definitive diagnostic test for drowning.[1-12] The practical result of this polarization is that the medicolegal communities in the United Kingdom, Europe, and Asia apply the test with greater frequency than in North America and elsewhere in the world. This is in part due to the origin of the test in Europe and because much of the research on the test is derived from laboratories in Europe. Some investigators believe diatoms may be present in the tissues of non-drowned people thus limiting the medicolegal utility of the test. The experimental support of this proposal in limited and contradictory, however, further research is warranted.[2, 5, 7, 8, 10, 11] In recent studies, new evidence for the reliability of the test has emerged.

Incidence of Positive Diatom Tests Correlate with Diatom Blooms

The utility and validity of the diatom test for drowning was recently studied using a retrospective analysis of 771 cases of drowning mostly from Ontario, Canada, over the period 1977 to 1993.[13] Freshwater drownings accounted for 738 of the cases and 33 cases were drownings in bathtubs, pools, or toilets. Diatoms were recovered from the femoral bone marrow of 205 cases (28%) of freshwater drowning and four cases (12%) of domestic water drowning. There was a monthly variation in the frequency of positive test outcomes. The monthly variation was strongly correlated with the periodic cycle of diatom blooms that occurs in freshwater. Positive diatom tests were characterized by a limited number of distinctive diatom species per case, and a restricted quantity and size range of diatom frustules. These results indicated that the diatom test for drowning will identify approximately 1 in 3 victims of freshwater drowning and may be useful in the assessment of deaths occurring in bathtubs. The correlation of the outcome of the diatom test for drowning with diatom blooms provided powerful evidence for the reliability of the test.

Concordance of Diatom Type in Bone Marrow and Drowning Medium

The most commonly applied method for demonstrating diatoms in human tissues is digestion of the organic component of the sample with nitric acid and isolation of the insoluble diatom frustules. [10, 11] The microscopic analysis of the frustule allows direct comparison with diatoms that are present in samples of the putative drowning medium. Thus, the microscopic comparison of diatoms from tissue and water allows an opinion to be rendered regarding possible common origin of the diatoms (i.e., if the diatoms in the tissue could have originated in the water from which the body was recovered).[14] In a recent study, 52 cases of freshwater drowning with diatoms in the femoral bone marrow in which a sample of the putative drowning medium was also collected, were analysed.[15] The same types of diatoms were found in the bone marrow and putative drowning medium in 47 cases (90%) indicating that the water samples were representative of the site of drowning in at least 90% of freshwater drownings. In the remaining 5 cases (10%), the diatoms in the water samples did not match those in the bone marrow indicating that the site of body and water sample recovery were likely geographically remote from the site of drowning. In an additional 34 cases of putative drowning in water that lacked detectable diatoms, 29 cases (85%) lacked diatoms in the bone marrow. These data indicated that the true positive rate of the diatom test for drowning is at least 90%.

Use of the Diatom Test for Drowning

Accidental and Suicidal Drowning

The diatom test is routinely applied to open-water and domestic drownings in three main circumstances: (i) accidental drowning, usually in the summer months; and (ii) suicidal drowning usually in psychiatric or elderly individuals; and (iii) drownings in bathtubs complicating natural disease (e.g. epilepsy, coronary artery disease).

In cases of accidental or suicidal drowning, the diatom test can be an important corroborating adjunct to death investigation. In some cases, the diatom test can be extremely helpful in establishing a cause of death in the absence of the classical findings of drowning. This is best illustrated in cases of drowning with extensive aquatic putrefaction in which postmortem findings may not indicate drowning as a cause of death due to decompositional changes. In addition, isolated body parts may be recovered from lakes after being dismembered by turbines or ship propellers. In the cases, the diatom test may be the only evidence of death by drowning.

Homicidal Drowning

The diatom test has successfully applied to homicidal drownings in two main circumstances: (i) confirmation of a diagnosis of drowning made at postmortem examination; and (ii) detection of drowning in cases of homicidal deaths with extensively decomposition or postmortem burning of the body. Homicidal drowning is an infrequent method of homicide and, since it may be difficult to detect at autopsy, may go undetected. In Ontario, some cases of homicidal drowning have been detected using the diatom test as the primary investigative tool since scene investigation and postmortem findings, in these cases, were not immediately indicative of drowning as a cause of death. This is particularly the case if the body is transported from the site of drowning to a "dry" site on land. The diatom test for drowning as been admitted as evidence in courts in Ontario, British Columbia, and some states in the Unites States of America. In Ontario, the diatom test has been an integral component of the prosecution of several cases of murder.

In the Ontario experience, most cases of homicidal drownings occur as a complication of other injuries such as strangulation or blunt force head injury. The injured individuals may be drowned after the initial assault or the assailant may "dispose" of the victim in a watery environment. In the latter circumstance, the assailant may believe the victim to be dead at the time of immersion into the water. However, the presence of diatoms in the bone marrow is an indication that the victim was breathing at the time of submersion and the cause of death was, at least in part, drowning. In selected circumstances, specific types of diatoms recovered from the marrow can be matched with putative sites of drowning. Such an analysis may implicate a particular site of submersion and help identify the scene of death.

A Final Word

The postmortem diagnosis of drowning remains one of the most enigmatic issues in forensic pathology. Application of the diatom test in the context of a complete death investigation remains one of the most significant and sensitive methods for the diagnosis of drowning. The widespread availability of the diatom test can facilitate the medicolegal investigation of a variety of cases including decomposed bodies found in water, and obscure homicidal drownings.

References

1. D. A. Neidhart and R. M. Greendyke, "The Significance of the Diatom Demonstration in the Diagnosis of Death by Drowning," *American Journal of Clinical Pathology* 18 (4): 377-82 (1967).

2. N. Foged, "Diatoms and Drowning—Once More," *Forensic Science International* 21: 153-9 (1983).

3. N. I. Hendey, "The Diagnostic Value of Diatoms in Cases of Drowning," *Medicine, Science, and the Law* 13 (1): 23-34 (1973).

4. J. V. Pachar, and J. M. Cameron, "The Diagnosis of Drowning by the Quantitative and Qualitative Analysis of Diatoms," *Medicine, Science, and the Law* 33 (4): 291-9 (1993).

5. A. J. Peabody, "Diatoms and Drowning—A Review," *Medicine, Science, and the Law* 20 (4): 254-61 (1980).

6. ———, "Diatoms in Forensic Science," *Journal of the Forensic Science Society* 17: 81-7 (1977).

7. W. U. Spitz and V. Schneider, "The Significance of Diatoms in the Diagnosis of Death by Drowning," *Journal of Forensic Science* 9 (1): 11-18 (1964).

8. W. U. Spitz, *Drowning, in Medicolegal Investigation of Death, Guidelines for the Application of Pathology to Crime Investigation,* ed. W. U. Spitz and R. S. Fisher (Springfield, Ill.: C. C. Thomas, 1973).

9. J. Timperman, "The Detection of Diatoms in the Marrow of the Sternum," *Journal of Forensic Medicine* 9 (4): 134-6 (1962).

10. ———, "Medico-Legal Problems in Death by Drowning: Its Diagnosis by the Diatom Method," *Journal of Forensic Medicine* 16 (2): 45-75 (1969).

11. F. Thomas, W. Van Hecke, and J. Timperman, "The Detection of Diatoms in the Bone Marrow as Evidence of Death by Drowning," *Journal of Forensic Medicine* 8 (3): 142-4 (1961).

12. — — —, "The Medicolegal Diagnosis of Death by Drowning," *Journal of Forensic Science* 7 (1): 1-14 (1962).

13. M. S. Pollanen, L. Cheung, and D. A. Chaisson, "The Diagnostic Value of the Diatom Test for Drowning. I. Utility: A Retrospective Analysis of 771 Cases of Drowning in Ontario, Canada," *Journal of Forensic Science* (March 1997).

14. N. I. Hendey, "Letter to the Editor, Diatoms and Drowning—A Review," *Medicine, Science, and the Law* 20 (4): 289 (1980).

15. M. S. Pollanen, "The Diagnostic Value of the Diatom Test for Drowning. II. Validity: Analysis of Diatoms in Bone Marrow and Drowning Medium," *Journal of Forensic Sciences* (March 1997).

—Michael S. Pollanen, Ph.D., Forensic Pathology Unit, Office of the Chief Coroner of Ontario, Canada

Chapter 35

Drugs and Explosives Detection

This [chapter] looks at three aspects of the search for ways to detect illicit substances such as illegal drugs and explosives. The first part examines how specialists are trying to improve the already striking ability of dogs to zero in on specific "odor signatures." The second part explores the wishes and wants of law enforcement and aviation security officials with regard to technology for detecting explosives. The third part describes a novel way of capturing the boundary layer of air that surrounds every human as a means of sampling for residues of illegal substances.

Unlocking the Secrets of Supersniffing Dogs

In Sydney, Australia, Jamie begins a busy day with grooming, exercise, and a health check. He then travels to the airport for the day's first task, inspecting cargo from a number of jumbo jets parked on the tarmac. From the airport, he moves to the location where mail is imported to check half a million or so articles. Next, he goes to the waterfront to search a ship—and the day isn't over yet.

Jamie, an athletic, black Labrador retriever trained by the Australian Customs Service to search for narcotics, epitomizes the unrivaled ability of dogs to locate objects through their sense of smell. Yet, it is not fully understood how dogs do what they do and why they are

Reprinted with permission from *Chemical & Engineering News,* Vol. 75, No. 39, September 29, 1997, pp. 24-7, "Detecting Illegal Substances," by A. Maureen Rouhi. © 1997 by the American Chemical Society.

so good at it. Basic studies of canine olfaction and breeding are help-ing researchers figure out the secrets of the dog's exquisite detection capabilities. They are also generating knowledge that may be used to enhance the technology of canine detection and to design detectors based on canine olfaction.

In the U.S., the rising frequency of criminal bombing incidents has increased the visibility of dogs as explosives detectors. Last June, for example, bomb-sniffing dogs were called in several times to assess a bomb threat at an office building just a few blocks from the White House. And as a result of the recommendations of the White House Commission on Aviation Safety and Security, chaired by Vice Presi-dent Al Gore, the Federal Aviation Administration (FAA) has estab-lished a program that makes detector dogs available to all major U.S. airports in case of a security alert.

Those who have seen dogs in action swear they work. Dogs can find people, bombs, land mines, illicit drugs, illegal agricultural produce—anything that has a discrete odor that they have been trained to find. But skeptics question the wisdom of relying on a tool for which a sci-entific basis has not been fully established.

"The greatest disadvantage now to the use of dogs as detectors of illicit substances—terrorist bombs, illegal narcotics, and chemical and biological warfare agents—is that we don't know how they work," says James A. Petrousky, a chemical engineer and a program manager at the Department of Defense's Office of Special Technology, Fort Wash-ington, Md. "Would you want your safety to depend on something not well understood?" he asks.

Petrousky also coordinates the Multiagency Canine Substance Detection Working Group, formed by federal agencies that use dogs—such as FAA, the Secret Service, the Customs Service, and the Fed-eral Bureau of Investigation—to pursue the mutual goals of understanding and enhancing canine detection technology. The wide interest in this group's work is evident from its funding, which, Petrousky says, comes not only from member agencies but also from others such as DOD, the Technical Support Working Group of the National Security Council, and the Office of National Drug Control Policy, as well as several foreign governments.

Unlike machines, dogs do not come with precise specifications, notes Susan F. Hallowell, a research chemist and acting program manager of airport security technology integration at FAA. She ex-plains: "If a vendor comes to me with an explosives detection sys-tem, the first thing I'll ask for is the data package: How does the device work? What does it detect? What is the detection limit? What is the probability of detection? What is the mean time between failure?"

The heightened interest in canine detection is keeping scientists very busy finding answers to such questions about dogs. Among them is James M. Johnston, a professor of psychology and director of behavioral research at the Institute of Biological Detection Systems, Auburn University, in Alabama. His federally funded research is coming up with very interesting results.

One of the nagging questions concerns the limit of detection: How small an amount of a material can dogs detect?

When tested with methyl benzoate, a degradation product of cocaine, the limits of detection of dogs range from 5 to 27 ppb, Johnston's studies indicate. Data for other compounds are being compiled, and similar levels of sensitivity are expected for most compounds.

This level of sensitivity is comparable with those of most analytical instruments and is not extraordinary, comments Petrousky. "The dog's supersensitivity is a myth," he says. "Rather it's the dog's accurate and discriminating detection ability that makes it invaluable."

Another question: What is it really that dogs respond to when they're being trained to recognize various substances through smell?

Using nitroglycerine-based smokeless powder, Johnston finds that what humans expect the dog to be smelling—nitroglycerine, in this case—is not in fact what the dog is responding to. Indeed, when a type of nitroglycerine-based smokeless powder is presented to a dog, the odor the dog associates with the material, the odor signature, is composed of acetone, toluene, and limonene.

The finding that explosives have odor signatures unrelated to the energetic component has serious implications in training. "In the dog world, some people think the dogs should be alerting to the explosive component," says Johnston. "If you force the dog to recognize the component of your choice, you may be making the dog's job much harder." That's because most explosives have very low vapor pressures.

Even though nitroglycerine comprises the bulk of the smokeless powder tested, because of its very low vapor pressure (0.00026 mm at 20° C), very few molecules are in the air at any time. Components with higher vapor pressures will have more molecules in the air even if they are present only in minute amounts in the material. If the canine nose has the appropriate receptors, these components would be far easier for the dog to smell.

Knowing the odor signature of target materials will help in the design of training aids. FAA, for example, is supporting an effort to study whether dogs can reliably find explosives after training on reconstituted odors. Such aids would not have the safety problems associated with using actual explosives to train dogs nor the security problems of illegal drugs.

Odor signatures will also help explain false-positive responses. People have reported bomb-sniffing dogs alerting—that is, signaling they have found something—on materials unrelated to explosives, says FAA's Hallowell. In such a situation, more dogs are brought in to sniff the material. "If all the other dogs also [alert], we conclude that it might be something that, to the dogs, smells like explosives," she explains.

"It doesn't mean the dog is wrong," explains Johnston. The dog may have detected the odor it was trained to smell, but the scent may be coming from some other material that has the same odor signature as the target substance. For example, a dog trained to look for explosives based on ammonium nitrate may alert at the scent of ammonium nitrate in garden fertilizer.

Johnston's group is identifying the odor signatures of other substances such as illicit cocaine and additional explosives. "As we build a library of signatures, we will understand [false alarms] better and even predict the kinds of false-positive responses we can expect," he says.

Johnston is now beginning to explore other issues that need to be addressed. One is the dog's real-time sampling capability, a major advantage of dogs over machines.

The real advantage of dogs is that they "go to source." That is, dogs find things, whereas machines now can only verify. As Petrousky puts it, "Machines are very good in answering the question, Is this particular sample cocaine? But only a dog can answer in a timely manner the question, Is there cocaine in this room?"

As a sampling device, the dog is remarkable, says Johnston. It takes little sniffs while it moves briskly back and forth, using the tiniest whiffs of an odor to decide whether to keep sniffing at a particular area or move on. If it senses an odor of interest, it will follow that odor and quickly locate the point of highest concentration. And then it alerts, as trained.

"The dog is obviously very good in localizing a source," which current state-of-the-art systems cannot do, says Johnston. "If we understand how the dog does that, it might tell us how to program or develop instruments that can."

Another issue that needs to be addressed is calibration. Many factors, internal and external, can affect canine olfaction, including heat stress, toxins, injury, and even disease at presymptomatic stages.

Right now, with dogs, there's no "press-to-test" button to check if the system is working effectively—a major disadvantage, says Petrousky.

What's needed is some means of checking the dog's nose before the dog is deployed, "just like highway troopers test their radar guns before they go on patrol," says Johnston. "If you're the handler of a dog that searches for land mines, you definitely want to know if your dog's nose is working as well as it usually does," he adds, "because sniffing is just a behavior, and dogs will keep sniffing when they can't smell anything."

But it's not all about the nose. Although most dogs have a keen sense of smell, only a few can be trained to be detector dogs like Jamie, the Australian Labrador retriever. Even at an early age, Jamie exhibited a trait that Australian researchers now have found to be a key determinant of good detector dogs.

That trait is called independent possession. It relates to how well a dog remains motivated to play a game that's used in training, explains Kathryn A. Champness, breeding manager at the Royal Guide Dogs Associations of Australia (RGDAA), Kew, Victoria. In collaboration with RGDAA and the Australian Customs Service, Champness completed a Ph.D. degree at the University of Melbourne on the development of a breeding and rearing program for drug detector dogs.

Training of Australian drug detector dogs is based on hunting for a toy that is scented with a narcotic odor. When a dog finds the toy, the handler rewards it with lots of praise and a game: The handler plays tug-of-war with the dog, and when she gets the toy off the dog, she throws the toy, and the dog chases it and brings it back.

By observing techniques used by the Australian Customs Service, Champness arrived at several traits that are important for work as detector dogs; for example, high chase/retrieve drive, possessiveness of toy, strong hunt drive, good stamina, stable temperament, and positive response to praise.

These traits are moderately heritable, Champness found. Therefore, a program that breeds selectively for these traits should be successful. But because other factors such as the environment or gene interactions also play a significant role in the expression of these traits, "progress by selective breeding will not be as rapid as it would be if the traits were highly heritable," explains Champness.

The most highly heritable character is related to the dog's possessiveness of its toy. Champness says the trait was assessed in three ways. One is mental possession, or how well the dog stays focused on watching its toy all the time. Another is physical possession, or how strongly the dog holds on to its toy when it has retrieved it. But the

351

most highly heritable is independent possession, which is how well the dog remains focused on playing regardless of input from its handler.

This finding "ultimately was very nice for us," says Champness. "Because we're really after dogs that are totally focused on playing this game and don't get distracted by other things."

Champness also studied the effect of environment and found that dogs need to be exposed to the training games as juveniles in order for the characteristic to be expressed in adulthood.

Guided by these findings, the Australian Customs Service now has a very successful breeding program for detector dogs. Before the breeding program was in place, the service recruited dogs from pounds, shelters, and private breeders, says John Vandeloo, manager of the service's National Breeding and Development Centre. Not only was the supply insufficient, the quality of the dogs was unreliable. Less than 50% graduated as detector dogs, and there was no guarantee of the dog's working life. The cost was about $17,000 per detector dog per eight-year cycle (eight years being the average working life of a Labrador retriever).

Now the service has a steady supply of dogs suitable for training as detector dogs. "Each generation is getting better and better," says Vandeloo. As a result of better selection of dogs for training, the cost per detector dog per eight-year cycle has dropped to only $3,600.

The Australian Custom Service's use of detector dogs, such as Jamie, must contend with a point widely regarded as a disadvantage of dogs as detectors: They can't be used for routine screening because their duty cycles are short.

"Australian customs has to use the dog as a broad screening tool because of the millions of people and articles moving across borders," says Vandeloo. "We like to put them out front so they're constantly working."

There's a lot of diversity in what they do on any given day, as Jamie's average schedule shows. Such diversity is good, because canines, like humans, need variety. "If you just keep throwing them bag after bag on a conveyor belt—humans lose interest and so would dogs," says Vandeloo.

Optimizing rest time is also very important. For example, the travel time from one job to another should be a rest period. "Some dogs never shut down," says Vandeloo. "In between jobs, they may go stir crazy in the back of the van, barking, carrying on. By the time they reach the next job, they're tired."

Thus, part of the training is teaching the dogs to respond to a "trigger," for example a harness. "Once we put the harness on, it's like turning on the power, and the dogs are very enthusiastic," Vandeloo explains. "Once we take the harness off, the dogs know to cool off, relax, and conserve energy."

By late afternoon on Jamie's average day, the local police may have called, needing the assistance of a dog. And Jamie finishes the day by searching two or three premises.

Champness first tested Jamie when he was about six months old, during the very early stages of her research. "I had the gut feeling right then that he was very special," she recalls. He's been working in the field very successfully and also works as a stud. His offspring are also performing very well. "Jamie's success is living confirmation that I was doing the right thing," she says.

Dog Talk: Extracting Unambiguous Answers to Questions

There's a story in the dog research community about a dog being tested for its limits of detection. Seemingly confirming the myth of supersensitive odor-detecting abilities of canines, this dog appeared to be able to detect the target even at infinite dilution of samples. It turns out this dog was responding to a change in air pressure whenever it was presented with a sample—and not to the target.

Stories such as this reflect the difficulty of quantifying canine olfaction. Dogs respond to stimuli other than what researchers think they are presenting. Dogs are unable to speak and answer questions directly, and some methods that have been used to detect a dog's response to stimuli are subjective, relying on the experimenter's interpretation of sometimes subtle behavior.

Researchers at the Institute for Biological Detection Systems, Auburn University, in Alabama, have developed psychophysical methods that allow objective and unambiguous communication with dogs during testing. They eliminate competing stimuli when testing the ability of a dog to detect an odor and they teach the dog to use levers to signal clearly their response to a stimulus.

"We do it by testing the dog in a semi-sound-proof chamber," says James M. Johnston, the institute's director of behavioral research. The chamber takes away visual and auditory distractions, leaving the dog to respond only to odor.

The wooden chamber is big enough to comfortably accommodate fairly large dogs. The walls are insulated to muffle sounds, and the inside is painted gray. When a dog steps in, all it sees is an aluminum panel with a hole in the middle and levers on either side. Attached to the bottom of the panel is a pan where food appears whenever the dog performs a task correctly.

At the back of the panel is a glass chamber through which air is constantly flowing. During testing, vapor from odorous substances is inserted into the air stream, which the dog samples through the hole in the panel. Generating and delivering the samples requires especially designed vapor generators and close collaboration with the institute's chemistry laboratory, supervised by Cindy C. Edge.

The dogs are trained to stick their noses in the hole for at least one second, to ensure uniform access to the odor. They are also taught to communicate what they are smelling by pressing either lever: the right if it's the target odor, and the left if it's clean air. If they respond correctly, the dogs are rewarded with food on an intermittent schedule.

The limit of detection—or odor threshold—is found by providing the dog with a range of concentrations of the target and determining the point at which the dog's accuracy is no better than what it can achieve by randomly choosing either lever.

Identifying the detection odor signature is more complicated. The dogs work with three levers: the right for the target odor and the left for clean air. And they press a middle lever when they're smelling neither clean air nor the target odor—that is, anything else.

Using this setup, Johnston has acquired some basic facts of canine olfaction. For example, odor thresholds do not vary greatly from dog to dog, at least for those dogs they have tested, which came from dog pounds. Also, to dogs, 99% nitroglycerine doesn't smell like nitroglycerine-based smokeless powder.

Johnston says there are a lot of issues that need to be examined, such as the effects of age, sex, neutering, diseases, and veterinary drugs on odor thresholds or the relationship between detection odor signatures and the biochemistry of the dog's nose. "The dog is an impressive detection instrument," he says. "We just need to generate the science to understand it."

Better Detectors Needed for Varied Threats

As a result of the crash last year of TWA flight 800 off the coast of Long Island, New York, the Federal Aviation Administration (FAA) has embarked on a major upgrading of U.S. aviation security. At the same time, the agency continues to support research for even better, cheaper, and faster bomb detectors. Other groups here and abroad hope advances in explosives detection will benefit not only aviation security but also local law enforcement and counterterrorism.

Upon the recommendation last year of the White House Commission on Aviation Safety and Security and with funds provided by Congress,

FAA is buying and deploying 54 units of the CTX 5000. This commercial detection system, made by InVision Technologies, Foster City, Calif., is the only one that has passed the agency's strict performance criteria. The move reflects "a change in national philosophy as to who is responsible for purchasing bomb-detecting equipment," says Lyle O. Malotky, FAA's scientific adviser for civil aviation security.

In the U.S., this responsibility used to rest squarely with the airlines. In response to the loss of TWA flight 800, which initially was suspected to have been caused by a bomb, "Congress and the Administration basically said [bomb detectors in airports are] important enough that perhaps the federal government should have a role in at least priming the pump to get the technology out there," Malotky says.

The CTX 5000, which is based on computer tomography and costs about $900,000 per unit, is doing "an adequate job" in screening checked-in luggage for explosives, says Malotky. More important, he says, it's giving FAA and U.S. policymakers a "baseline of equipment performance" under operational conditions.

"We would like to have equipment that is faster, has lower nuisance alarm rates, and is less expensive" than the CTX 5000, says Malotky. So far, a better system does not exist. "It may well be that we have looked at all the ways to detect the presence of explosives," he notes. "If indeed there are technologies left to exploit, we could use them to make the next revolutionary jump in capabilities."

An airline crash is sure to capture headlines whatever the cause, but especially if it's due to a bomb explosion. Yet more bomb-related incidents occur outside of aviation, and technology to deal with everyday threats—whether in U.S. towns and cities or in troubled areas of the world—is practically unavailable.

The latest statistics from the Federal Bureau of Investigation show numbers of criminal bombing incidents in the U.S. rising from 1990 to 1995. Except for the bombings of New York City's World Trade Center in 1993 and of the Alfred P. Murrah Federal Building in Oklahoma City in 1995, most are relatively small events that involve small homemade devices and don't do serious damage. However, the number of significant incidents is increasing, and the devices are becoming more sophisticated, according to David G. Boyd, director of the Office of Science and Technology of the National Institute of Justice, Washington, D.C.

"It's important to remember that [in the U.S.] bombings of big targets such as in Oklahoma City are very rare," says Boyd. "But at the local level, bombings are not infrequent and bomb squads are called out regularly."

In case of a bomb threat, the first response usually has to come from local authorities, such as the local police department, explains Boyd. However, these local units are the least trained, least funded, and least equipped of all law enforcement forces when it comes to dealing with bombs, he says.

The general rule is that local law enforcement doesn't "have anything at all in terms of bomb detection equipment," says Boyd. Although bomb detectors are available commercially, they are not practical for local bomb squads. "Most are expensive," he says, explaining that most police departments cannot afford any equipment that exceeds the cost of a laptop computer. In addition, most commercial equipment requires trained operators. "Police departments have a tough time sending people for training," says Boyd, because staff sizes are very small.

The ideal equipment for local bomb squads and first responders should cost no more than $10 and be so small it can be worn like a badge or on a belt or stuffed in a pocket, says Boyd. "It should be so reliable that it never misses the real thing and only false alarms once or twice a year."

That's a tall order, especially for Boyd, whose office engages in R&D of technologies to meet the needs of local law enforcement. And he acknowledges: "We're not close to where we would like to be."

Although criminal bombings are a tough problem, what U.S. local law enforcers have to deal with is probably a fraction of what their counterparts in Israel have to face day by day.

Jonathan Shoham, head of Israel's Branch for Counterterrorism and Detection of Explosives, explains the magnitude of the job: "We have to identify explosives on a person getting into a bus or a cinema or an airport check-in hall. We have to find it in a journalist's camera pointing at the president, in a bag or carry-on luggage of someone getting on an aircraft, in a cargo container, in an envelope sent to your house, or in a car traveling toward a government building. And all that as quickly, as precisely, and as cheaply as possible."

Shoham admits it would be very difficult to use technology to find a suicide bomber or to stop an attack in a crowded open market. "It's a complicated area," he says, and he hopes the explosives detection research community will share knowledge "to create new ideas to help deal with a threat that influences the lives of all of us."

Bomb detection technology would be very useful at strategic sites — at border crossings, for example. Shoham says it would help to have technology that could alert border agents to people carrying explosives as the individuals pass through without anyone stopping them.

Another place where technology may be applied is in shopping malls. Something like a handheld metal detector to check people for explosives can diminish the threat at such targets, he says.

In the end though, says Shoham, the citizens' perception of the threat is what really matters. He says Israelis know they live in a threatened area. And they're willing to pay for security, for example by arriving very early at airports to be questioned or by accepting the presence of security agents almost everywhere.

By contrast, in the U.S. for example, "TWA flight 800 was in the news for a while," Shoham notes. "But now," he wonders, "how many people are still thinking of security?"

Sampling Body Heat, Skin Flakes

The demand for tighter aviation security has accelerated the development of portals for explosives detection. These passageways are similar to the familiar metal detector portals in airports, but explosives detection portals signal an alert in the presence of traces of explosives that may be sticking on the skin and clothing of people who have been handling or may be concealing explosives.

How these portals take a sample and bring it to the detector—the so-called front end of an integrated detection system—is an important issue. Some portals use a barrier that comes in contact with a person's body and clothing. Others blow currents of air to dislodge explosive traces from the person.

These sampling methods are inefficient and may even be counterproductive. Sampling by contact is not only intrusive but useless unless the barrier touches the contaminated area. Blowing air currents to dislodge explosive traces further dilutes the sample and could lead to its loss.

So researchers are looking to natural processes for a better way.

In the comic strip "Peanuts," the character named Pig-Pen is stubbornly dirty, invariably followed by a trail of dust. It appears Pig-Pen's dusty envelope is not unique, just an exaggeration of an air boundary layer that naturally surrounds any human body. That phenomenon now is being applied to sampling of trace explosives by Huban A. Gowadia, a mechanical engineering graduate student, and Gary S. Settles, a professor of mechanical engineering and director of the Gas Dynamics Laboratory at Pennsylvania State University, University Park.

Skin is usually warmer than ambient air and heat flows from the body to the surroundings, creating a freely moving boundary layer, explains Gowadia. For a person standing still, the layer begins at the ankles and moves up the torso, becoming thicker and moving faster and with more turbulence as it travels upward. Finally, swirling at the ate of about 40 L per second, it takes off from the shoulders and the head in the form of a thermal plume.

At the same time, humans constantly shed their outer skin layer. So much is shed that up to 90% of environmental dust in homes and offices is composed of human skin flakes, says Gowadia. Because the flakes are very small, they move freely through clothing and into the motion of the boundary layer. Thus the moving layer is a particle-laden flow, transporting skin flakes at about a third of a milligram per second for an average body surface area of 1.8 sq meters. Carried along are any materials lodged in the flakes, such as body fluids or traces of cosmetics, perfume, or explosives.

Gowadia believes the sheer numbers of skin flakes in the human plume provide a large cross-section to which trace explosives will attach. "In fact," she says, "explosive traces on skin and clothing will likely be shed continuously along with skin flakes and textile fibers without the need for external agitation."

The skin-flake-laden human plume provides "a simple and elegant approach" to sampling for explosives detection portals, says Gowadia. In research supported by the Federal Aviation Administration (FAA), she is developing a sampling system that will collect a person's natural thermal plume and filter the airborne particulates, made up mostly of skin flakes. Her preliminary tests show that explosive traces from samples concealed under clothing can be found easily in the thermal plume.

Susan F. Hallowell, a research chemist and acting program manager of airport security technology integration at FAA, says the Penn State research is "really quite novel." And she is not surprised that imaginative approaches are coming from areas other than chemistry.

"Chemists have been so fixed on detector development, and that's exactly what we got: very well developed detectors that have no front ends," says Hallowell. " We're going to have to reach out to other disciplines to develop novel sampling systems."

—by A. Maureen Rouhi, C&EN *Washington*

Part Five

Advances in Crime Investigation

Chapter 36

Crime Laboratory Developments

It has been a long time since forensic science has had as much public attention as it has in recent months. Several high-profile criminal cases have featured hours of grueling testimony—witnessed by millions of viewers—during which defense attorneys attacked every aspect of evidence collection and analysis. The media spotlight illuminated for the public what police have always known—that forensic science is one of the more underfunded, understaffed and underequipped areas of law enforcement.

Indeed, crime labs have been treated almost as an afterthought for years—housed in cramped, inadequate quarters and limited in their ability to purchase the kind of sophisticated and expensive equipment needed to keep up with ever-changing technologies.

While recent media attention certainly highlighted crime lab deficiencies, it also shed new light on the vital role the lab plays in the criminal justice process. The result has been a renewed interest among crime lab directors and police administrators in lab accreditation, personnel certification, and standardization of equipment and analysis techniques, as well as in upgrading facilities and acquiring state-of-the-art equipment.

Accreditation

Of the 330 crime labs in the United States, only half are accredited by the American Society of Crime Lab Directors (ASCLD). Kevin

From "Spotlight on . . . Crime Laboratory Developments," by Lois Pilant, in *The Police Chief,* June 1997, pp. 31, 32, 34-7. Reprinted with permission.

Lothridge, ASCLD president and director of the Pinellas County Forensic Science Laboratory in Largo, Florida, notes that the number of accredited facilities also includes labs in Australia, Hong Kong, Singapore and New Zealand. Surprisingly, it does not yet include the FBI lab, which is planning to apply for accreditation later this year.

Many years ago, ignoring accreditation had few repercussions. It was an expensive, tedious and time-consuming process, and few labs had the money, time or personnel to devote to such an effort. Besides, courtroom attacks on the science, the evidence or the lab's procedures were rare. Forensic science was more about corroboration than identification.

But as new discoveries opened up the realms of physics, chemistry and biology, analytical techniques grew more sophisticated, and so did juries, defense attorneys and the public. Today, expectations are higher, and lab personnel are expected to be letter-perfect.

"Part of the [O. J.] Simpson case fallout was that we've seen much longer and stiffer cross-examinations in court," says Ron Urbanovsky, director of the Texas Department of Public Safety's statewide system of crime labs. "Testimony that used to take two to three hours now takes eight to 12 hours, and it's grueling. We are asked to be perfect in a non-perfect world."

Urbanovsky admits, though, that not all of the reverberations from the Simpson case have been negative. "It makes us all better," he said. "It ensures that we do things the right way, and that we have the right controls in place."

Those controls took center stage when Simpson's defense team failed to make headway in its attacks on the science of DNA profiling, and instead attempted to establish that the evidence had been somehow contaminated by collection methods, analysts and crime scene technicians, and/or chain-of-custody procedures.

The Simpson case was the first time anyone talked about accreditation and certification on the stand in front of millions of people," Lothridge says. "It was obvious that it doesn't matter how good we are in the lab; they can still attack the evidence before it gets to there. The result is that the jury can never get past the fact that the evidence may have been tainted before it got to us."

More labs are seeking accreditation as a way to ensure quality control. It is a check of the lab system—of its policies, procedures, physical space, security and housekeeping. The National Forensic Science Technology Center, a nonprofit spin-off of ASCLD, is available to assist unaccredited labs. The center's consultants do pre-accreditation inspections and help labs review and write policies and procedures.

Certification

Although the idea of certifying lab employees has been around for many years, it has only been through the efforts of the American Board of Criminalists (ABC) that testing and certification procedures have been put in place. Admittedly, the idea was not easy for some to accept, and there were those in the profession who were against it entirely. Despite objections, however, the ABC now has a program that certifies lab personnel with a Diplomate, Fellow, or Student certificate. It conducted its first round of testing at the 1993 annual meeting of the American Academy of Forensic Sciences.

A Diplomate certificate is awarded to those who successfully complete a general knowledge examination. A Fellow certificate goes to those who complete the general knowledge exam and at least one specialty exam, and meet proficiency testing standards. For example, a specialty examination in forensic biology would consist of a core set of questions on fundamental principles, with two separate tests on DNA and traditional serology. A similar approach is used for trace evidence, with a test based on core principles, as well as a module in paints and polymers hairs or fibers. Requirements are that the candidate have an earned bachelor's degree in a physical science, a certain number of years' experience before taking the general exam and additional experience in his chosen specialty.

By ensuring that lab personnel are all held to the same standard, certification helps analysts fend off courtroom salvos about their experience, background and training, says Jose Almirall, a criminalist in the Trace Evidence Section of the Metro-Dade Police Department's crime lab in Miami. "The product we provide is expert knowledge and expert opinion. As the material has gotten more difficult to understand, the nature of testimony has gotten harder. The burden is now on the expert to make that material understandable to a jury of non-scientists. Defense attorneys use this to their advantage; some consider it to be their job to create some sort of doubt about our procedures, our abilities, or our background. Fifteen years ago, an expert witness would give an opinion in court, and nobody would doubt it. That is not the case today," Almirall says. "Physical evidence can be complex, which means that we need to be scientists . . . . We used to take police officers and train them, but in areas like DNA analysis, it requires a sophisticated and in-depth knowledge of the field. We're now hiring Ph.D.s in molecular biology for these special areas."

Like accreditation, certification is voluntary. And while it is not required by any federal or state law, its importance is increasing as science becomes more sophisticated and lab personnel become more specialized. "A generalist will not survive very well anymore," Lothridge says. "The advanced technologies make it too hard to shift gears. The generalists are still in place in some labs, but in most other places, lab personnel are becoming highly specialized. Certification will only further professionalize what we do and who we are."

Standardization

In the medical field, laboratory samples are pure, pristine, precisely formulated. But in the crime lab, evidence might consist of a bit of glass, a speck of paint, a partial print, a single cell. It is never exact and rarely pristine. Because of this, a single set of standards for the various types of analysis has never been devised, except in the case of arson analysis and DNA profiling. And with no definitive set of standards, a lab's techniques, protocols or methods are easy prey for defense attorneys.

"The equipment can be different from one lab to the next, and the training I have had may be different from what another analyst has had," says Almirall. "If I'm analyzing gunshot residue, I might use a scanning electron microscope, where another criminalist might use atomic absorption. They both work. They both lead to the same answer. But I'll use a microscope because I happen to have one, and he may use atomic absorption because that's the equipment he has in his lab."

The lack of regulation is complicated by the fact that no two labs are alike. "We need a total solution," Lothridge says. "We need standard methods, training on those methods using various techniques; and databases for each specialty Then we need to make sure everyone has the same instrumentation available."

E30, the forensic science committee of the American Society for Materials and Testing, is attempting to set standards for the field. But the process is slow, Lothridge explains, because it is essentially consensus-driven. "We have no one-stop shopping place to get our standards. We have to develop a large consensus of people, and that can take years. We need to develop standards, but we also need funding to do it. The most likely source for that is the federal government."

Equipment and Supplies

When properly collected, physical evidence does not have memory lapses. It cannot lie, and it cannot be corrupted or impeached. Therefore, patrol officers, crime scene technicians and detectives must be exceedingly careful when collecting evidence. Not only will they be challenged in court, they will also find that the importance of physical evidence is increasing as the significance of confessions diminishes. Twenty years ago, confessions figured in about 75 percent of murder cases; today, they are instrumental in about 50 percent. Today, juries or courts want corroborating evidence and expert opinions.

Evidence should be marked when it is removed from its original position, and property labeled to ensure identification at a later date. Each item should be placed in a separate container, such as a test tube, jar, bottle, plastic bag, envelope or carton. The containers should be sealed so they cannot be opened without breaking the seal.

Chain of custody begins at the time of possession, and must be faultlessly maintained if the evidence is to be admissible in court. Departments should limit the number of people who handle evidence, keeping accurate records of the date, time and reason it moves from one place to another. These records can be kept by way of a receipt system, bar coding, labels that cannot be altered or a comprehensive computer tracking system. Companies that sell evidence collection supplies—including Fitzco, Kinderprint, Esty Specialty Products, Becton Dickinson, and ODV, Inc.—all agree that the money invested in something more sophisticated and tamper-proof than brown paper lunch sacks will pay off. "A defense attorney is smart enough to know that if he can break the evidence, he can break the case," one company representative says. "Police departments have a lot of cases lost because they refused to spend money on evidence collection supplies."

Companies offer all types of supplies, such as drying bags and drying racks for evidence intended for DNA analysis, evidence bags that have heat seals and tamper-proof labels, fingerprint powders and reagents, sexual assault kits, gunshot residue collection kits, vacuums for collecting evidence from crime scenes, protective syringe containers, evidence tape, specially designed mailing boxes that prevent breakage, chain-of-custody forms, and integrity seals. Also available are light sources to detect latent prints, devices that transfer prints to film from surfaces like human skin, fabric, concrete or carpets; protective gloves made of latex, or gloves that are water- and cut-resistant; and foams and lotions that protect officers from the penetration of body fluids, most bacteria, and caustic chemicals.

There are also a host of companies that offer software programs to track evidence, generate reports, assign case numbers and chart monthly statistics. One progam can do blood spatter analysis, another digitizes crime scene photos and stores them on a disk. Of course, as with all types of equipment, departments should always check with a neighboring agency or get referrals from the company to make sure the equipment or software program does what the salesperson promised.

Lab personnel need not only the best equipment and supplies, but the right training and the ability to connect with other forensic science professionals."We're heavy into training here," says Texas' Urbanovsky. "We think our people need to be properly trained, so we give them in-service training and outside training at workshops at scientific meetings. If necessary, we send them back to school to learn more about their specialty."

According to Commander Tom Lannon, director of the Phoenix Police Department's Crime Laboratory, continued proficiency testing also should be required. "We need a system for administrative review of reports, and the ability to do a technical review to make sure another person can follow the procedures and get the same results," he says. "This kind of quality control, which is all part of the accreditation process, is very serious. It can mean the difference between conviction and acquittal."

Training is doubly important in agencies where officers wear more than one hat. Says Lothridge, "There is a big margin between the well-trained, well-equipped metro agencies and the small agencies that don't have resources, where the guy who is the patrol officer is also the crime scene technician and the booking guy. If they are faced with a major crime, evidence collection is key. They need to have the training to handle it. You don't want them to miss something because they don't know the new techniques."

The Future

Much has changed in the past few years. DNA analysis has undoubtedly had the most profound impact on forensic science in the past 10 years. Where investigators once relied on fingerprints or blood typing, DNA profiling has scientists identifying and excluding suspects with population statistics that number in the millions. The costly and slow RFLP process has been shortened using PCR, and is expected to be further shortened, and made less expensive, as labs conduct PCR-based analysis using Short Tandem Repeats, or STRs. The science has been automated with the use of a thermocycler and computers that record, digitize, and electronically enter data into a computer for analysis. Not only has automation made the process faster, it has reduced the need for "hands-on" help and, therefore, the possibility of human error.

Forensic scientists are able to do more with fingerprints today than ever before. Using various chemicals and laser light they can detect latent prints that at one time would have been impossible to discern. In addition, crime labs are coming out of the basements and into facilities that have sterile environments for DNA analysis, and separate ventilation systems to avoid contaminating lab personnel or other department workers.

Computer programs such as Drugfire and the Integrated Ballistic Identification System (IBIS) work in much the same way an automated fingerprint identification system does. Instead of fingerprints, however, these programs catalog, store, and link cartridge casings and projectiles to crimes. Using a microscope connected to a computer workstation, the analyst collects the individual characteristics found on a fired casing or projectile, and enters the images into a computer. The computer translates these data into a mathematical algorithm, which is then stored in a database. The database can be searched for possible matches. A "hit" enables the lab to connect a single weapon to multiple crimes, or link weapons to unsolved shootings or repeat offenders. Although these programs can be used on cartridge casings and projectiles, there currently is no way to swap information between the two. The Department of Justice is currently doing an interoperability study to address the problem.

When Lothridge looks into the future of forensic science, he sees a continued focus on accreditation, standardization and certification, as well as a dazzling array of technologies that will better enable crime labs to corroborate evidence, and help to redirect investigations that may have veered off course:

- A remotely operated microscope that can be controlled via the Internet. Evidence would be sent to an appropriately equipped lab, mounted on the microscope and controlled by the original agency. Such a device is currently being studied by the Department of Energy's Oak Ridge lab.

- A miniature, belt-worn computer that lets the wearer take digital images of a crime scene. The technology has already been developed by the Pacific Northern National Laboratory in Hanford, Washington.

- Miniaturized DNA profiling equipment to make analysis field portable.

- Databases for paint, glass, and other types of trace evidence. The FBI already has a wealth of information on analyzing and identifying different types of duct tape, which is commonly used to bind victims.

Even significant scientific advances, however, cannot make up for the current inadequacies of the laboratory system, Lothridge says. "The criminal justice system is like an hourglass, with the lab at the neck of the glass. If we're going to put 100,000 more officers on the street, we're going to have more crimes to investigate and, therefore, more evidence. The crime lab at the neck of that glass has its limitations—only a certain amount of sand can get through. We need to increase our funding of crime labs if we want to widen the neck of the hourglass, and consistently provide the necessary, timely analysis that law enforcement agencies require. If we did that, we could save the entire criminal justice system many times more than it spent on us in the first place."

—*by Lois Pilant*

Chapter 37

The Potential of DNA Testing

Since before the turn of the century, at a time when Sir Arthur Conan Doyle was spinning his tales of Sherlock Holmes, objective scientific evidence has been routinely used to investigate crime. Today, although most crimes continue to be solved through confessions and eyewitness accounts, forensic evidence—most often drugs, fingerprints, firearms, blood, and semen—has come increasingly to be used to establish the truth. In the past few years alone, major technological advances have been made in fingerprinting, the development of computerized fingerprint databases, and, perhaps most familiar because of recent sensational criminal cases, DNA testing.

Advances in technology have helped DNA testing to become an established part of criminal justice procedure. Despite early controversies and challenges by defense attorneys, the admissibility of DNA test results in the courtroom has become routine. More than 200 published court opinions support this use, and DNA testing standards have been developed and promulgated. Last year there were more than 17,000 cases involving forensic DNA in this country alone. Questions about the validity and reliability of forensic DNA test methods have essentially been addressed.

DNA's promise of using evidence invisible to the naked eye to positively identify the perpetrator or exonerate the innocent suspect is being fulfilled. Thanks to DNA, biological evidence is now used in new

Excerpted from "The Unrealized Potential of DNA Testing," in the U.S. Department of Justice, Office of Justice Programs publication, *NIJ Research in Action,* June 1998, pp 1-8.

ways, and many more sources of evidence are available than in the past.Yet the potential of DNA may be greater than its accomplishments thus far. Realizing that potential means first overcoming a number of limitations—in procedures for testing DNA evidence and systems to collect and access DNA information.

An Enhanced Role for Biological Evidence

As a result of the development of DNA testing, biological evidence—evidence commonly recovered from crime scenes in the form of blood or other body fluid—has taken on new significance. Traditional blood and saliva testing have been rendered obsolete. DNA is found in these substances and in fact in all body tissues and fluids. Because DNA testing is more sensitive than traditional serologic methods and DNA is able to withstand far harsher environmental insults, DNA testing may be successful when traditional testing is not.

Because the DNA molecule is long lived, it is likely to be detectable for many years in bones or body fluid stains from older criminal cases in which questions of identity remain unresolved. The result is that DNA testing applies to a vastly wider array of specimens than conventional testing and is much more powerful in analyzing biological evidence than any previous technology.

Expanding the Range of Evidence

Virtually all biological evidence found at crime scenes can be subjected to DNA testing. At most crime scenes, there are many kinds of biological evidence: not only blood and hair but also botanical, zoological, and other types of substances. Blood evidence was revealed in one study to be found in 60 percent of murders and in a similar percentage of assaults and batteries. Hair was found at the scene of 10 percent of robberies and 6 percent of residential burglaries.

Multiple sources. In this country, DNA testing has been conducted primarily in cases of sexual assaults from vaginal swabs and semen stains. By contrast, In England the majority of DNA database matches involve burglaries, with the evidence tested consisting of blood found at sites of forced entry. Saliva, skin cells. bone, teeth, tissue, urine, feces, and a host of other biological specimens, all of which may be found at crime scenes, are also sources of DNA. Saliva may be found in chewing gum and on cigarette butts, envelopes, and possibly drinking cups. Fingernail scrapings from an assault victim or a broken fingernail left at the scene by the perpetrator may also be useful DNA evidentiary specimens. Even hatbands and other articles of clothing may yield DNA. DNA testing of urine is becoming common to establish whether a particular individual is truly the source of the specimen in which illegal drugs have been identified.

The array of evidence that can be found at crime scenes and subjected to DNA testing suggests its unrealized potential. For despite the abundance of evidence. and despite the advantages of DNA testing, little of this evidence is recovered from crime scenes, less is submitted to crime labs, and still less is analyzed. (See "Sexual Assault Cases: Need for More DNA Processing," at the end of the article.)

The potential for more sources. For certain kinds of DNA-laden biologic evidence, the potential has yet to be fully explored. Hair cells are an example. During a violent confrontation, hair may be transferred between the victim and the perpetrator. Traditionally, forensic scientists have been able to identify the source of this evidence on the basis of its general appearance and structural features, but rarely has it been possible to determine the source definitively. Because an individual's DNA may be detectable in his or her hair, DNA testing technology is likely to change substantially the significance and use of hair evidence.

The superficial skin cells that an individual sheds in the hundreds of thousands every hour may be prevalent at crime scenes. Their presence raises the possibility of subjecting such trace biological material to DNA testing.

Recently researchers have reported that DNA can be recovered from fingerprints, which are therefore another possible source of trace specimens that may be valuable as evidence.

Back to the Future

The longevity of the DNA molecule means its power extends not just to the present and future but also to the past. Specimens that in many cases are years or even decades old—dating to the time when DNA testing technology was not yet available—can be tested, resulting in overturned convictions and release of the innocent.

The exoneration of Kirk Bloodsworth is an example of how the past was revisited with DNA evidence. In this case, a Baltimore court, using an anonymous tip, identification from a police artist's sketch, eyewitness statements, and other evidence, found Mr. Bloodsworth guilty of sexually assaulting and murdering a young girl. Later he was retried and again found guilty. But in 1993, more than 8 years after his arrest, prosecutors compared DNA evidence from the victim's clothing to Mr. Bloodsworth's and found the two did not match. He was subsequently released and then pardoned.

As of this writing, dozens of other inmates have been released on the basis of similar evidence. A number of examples of cases in which DNA testing furnished new evidence that resulted in the release of people wrongly convicted have been published.

Limitations to Overcome

The fact that much forensic biologic evidence remains unrecovered and unanalyzed is only one obstacle to realizing the full potential of DNA testing. Other limitations stem from lack of sufficient laboratory funding, time-consuming testing methods, inability to test in the field, and the challenges of automating DNA evidence databases. These problems are serious, but new developments suggest they can be overcome.

Laboratory testing—funding low, processing slow. For the full potential of DNA evidence to be realized, forensic laboratories must have resources sufficient to test the evidence submitted to them. But laboratories are notoriously underfunded, and many already face heavy backlogs of work. Law enforcement agencies are often forced to distribute scarce resources among a range of pressing needs, and the labs vie for funding in this highly competitive environment.

Exacerbating this difficulty, and explaining why limited testing is done, are the slow, costly testing methods currently used. Because they are so time-consuming, crime laboratories must prioritize cases to be processed and specimens to test. It is not possible, given the deadlines imposed by the needs of the courts, to analyze all potential evidentiary specimens submitted. Thanks to the development of new methods of analysis, however, crime laboratories' ability to process DNA evidence within a reasonable time is expected to improve substantially within the next few years. (See "In the Pipeline: New and Improved Testing Technologies," at the end of the article.)

Field testing—being tested. Investigatory leads often grow cold within a very short time after a crime is committed. Suspects vanish, witnesses disperse, and potential physical evidence may persist for only a limited time or may be disturbed in some way, even by normal activities. Although faster processing in the laboratory is important, in many cases the ability to secure critical information by field testing at the crime scene might significantly enhance the likelihood of a successful resolution.

Field testing should not replace laboratory testing; instead it may powerfully augment investigations conducted at crime scenes. It could be used to screen potential DNA evidence specimens for those most likely to produce results and, through preliminary analysis conducted at the scene, to help develop investigative leads. Oral swabs could be used to collect DNA samples from those willing to submit to the procedure. Of course, more powerful, confirmatory testing in the controlled environment of the laboratory should continue to be conducted to ensure absolute confidence in the results. The role of preliminary analysis in the field would be to eliminate certain individuals as suspects, arguably always a more important role for DNA evidence than incrimination.

Steps are now under way to realize the potential of field testing DNA evidence. Recently, a truly portable microchip-based prototype field-testing instrument has been developed. The instrument, which produces findings within 30 minutes, is currently being upgraded and made available commercially. The National Institute of Justice is sponsoring the development of other types of portable field instruments.

DNA databases—in their infancy. Without computerized searching and without suspects, evidentiary testing, no matter how powerful, can do little more than link crimes together and is of little use in solving them. In the same way that fingerprint registries and then automated fingerprint identification systems each dramatically enhanced the utility of fingerprint evidence, the development of DNA databases and networks can substantially augment DNA profiling.

Information in the database, which consists of DNA test results from individuals convicted of certain categories of crime and DNA from the scenes of unsolved crimes, can be compared to results of evidence obtained at recent crime scenes to find associations. This creates DNA databasing's greatest advantage: its use as an investigative tool in cases where there are no suspects. However, jurisdictions must process suspectless cases to produce "cold hits" (matches lacking previous leads). Databanking in the United States is still limited, but as with testing technologies, it continues to evolve.

The Status of Databanking

In the United States. Today almost all states have legislation related to DNA databanking, most of it focusing on collecting and testing

373

DNA from individuals convicted of sexual assaults and often homicides. In some cases the legislation requires collection from all convicted felons. Although DNA databanking was proposed almost 10 years ago, and although databanking has been almost universally adopted at the state level, the concept of its development in this country is still rudimentary.

The limitations are partly due to the definition of offender categories in the legislation. For example, rapists who plead to a lesser offense not covered by a particular state databanking law are therefore not subject to it. Similarly, in some states DNA collection laws are inapplicable to juveniles involved in the criminal justice system. In other instances DNA is not collected until an offender is released, instead of at intake, making it impossible to match the offender's DNA to that in a case opened during incarceration. Other problems stem from lack of funding and the incompatibility of the states' genetic testing system. Of the 47 states that have passed legislation, the program is operational in only 36, and of that number most programs are severely backlogged.

In the United Kingdom. Compared to the United States, the United Kingdom has moved far more aggressively to establish a national DNA criminal database. Specimens are collected from a wider range of offense categories than the sexual assault category targeted by most State programs in the United States. The number of DNA profiles entered thus far in the United Kingdom is now nearly 200,000 with an expected increase to more than 5 million specimens in the next decade.

The United Kingdom has taken other steps to increase the utility of its database. Specimens are taken upon arrest rather than, as in virtually all the States in the United States, on conviction. Databank staff tell police investigators the chances are about 1 in 2 of finding the perpetrator through a DNA match.

In testing technology, the United Kingdom has switched completely to automated STR, which is able to discriminate among every man, woman, and child in the country. By contrast, most databanking in the United States uses RFLP results. (For an explanation of RFLP and related terms, see "A Primer of DNA Testing Technology.") Laboratory processes in the United Kingdom have been streamlined and automated and therefore are generally more efficient than those at the U.S. state level.

The most important distinction between the two countries is that the United Kingdom views databanking as a primary investigative tool. It is used, for example, for "mass screens" or "intelligence-led screens," in which targeted canvassing is conducted in a certain area or among a certain pool of suspects. The approach has been used with great success: Since 1995 at least 17 high-profile cases have been solved in this fashion.

Officials in the United Kingdom believe that their DNA testing program has actually reduced overall law enforcement costs by eliminating extensive traditional police investigations in some cases.

Toward a national system? Because the United Kingdom databanking system is based nationally, it is central and uniform, not an aggregate of many different, incompatible State systems. Our "patchwork" system is improving, however, because of systems developed by the FBI, Federal support for State DNA databanking, and the convergence of DNA typing methods.

The CODIS system (COmbined DNA Index System) is a national investigative support database. Developed by the FBI, it is used in the national (NDIS), State (SDIS), and local (LDIS) DNA Index System networks to link the typing results from unsolved crime cases in multiple jurisdictions or to those convicted of offenses specified in the DNA databanking laws passed in 47 States. By alerting investigators to similarities among unsolved crimes, CODIS can aid in apprehending perpetrators who commit a series of crimes and in this way prevent other offenses by the same person. The 77 laboratories in the 36 States participating in CODIS have produced 126 case-to-case "hits" and 76 case-to-offender "hits."

For CODIS to work efficiently, all forensic laboratories must use reliable and compatible DNA test systems so that data can be compared. To that end the Violent Crime Control and Law Enforcement Act of 1994 promotes uniform standards for forensic DNA testing and provides Federal support to State and local law enforcement agencies to improve their DNA testing capabilities so they can participate in CODIS. Also, to establish minimal compatibility among laboratories, the FBI has promulgated a core set of RFLP genetic loci (specific places in DNA) and will promulgate a core set of STR loci.

On the Horizon

Improved testing technologies are ensuring more efficient and effective DNA evidence processing; advances in technology and databanking promise to widen the use of DNA evidence as an investigational tool, and new sources of biologic evidence are being explored. Nevertheless, we are still far from full realization of the potential of DNA testing. As laboratories improve their ability to process DNA evidence quickly, and as the courts' expectations of the use of DNA test results increase, there will be greater emphasis on initial collection of evidence at the crime scene.

Initial collection of evidence is a key link in the chain of events leading to successful testing, but it is also a vulnerable link. Currently the groundwork is being prepared to strengthen specimen collection and preservation, with more structured crime-scene teams and more formalized evidence collection procedures being established in many jurisdictions. The aim of these teams is to ensure that all potential evidence is recovered and properly preserved for testing, and especially to minimize the possibility of contamination.

Today much evidence is not retrieved, submitted to the lab, or analyzed. Crime tabs are neither adequately funded nor fully supported. Database registries are not comprehensive and not fully utilized. People still get away with murder. But if the potential of DNA testing can be fully realized, their chances are likely to be greatly reduced.

Sexual Assault Cases: Need for More DNA Processing

Case processing of rapes could be improved if, in more instances, the DNA evidence were submitted to laboratories and tested. Currently, in only a relatively small proportion of all rape victimizations is DNA recovered and tested. For DNA databasing of people convicted of sexual assaults, the situation is similar: samples are not collected, and many of those that are collected are not tested.

A recent FBI survey revealed that of all rapes, less then half were solved by the police and less than 10 percent were sent to crime laboratories. And because crime laboratories are not able to work all cases submitted, in only 6 percent of the 250,000 rape cases was the recovered DNA tested, leaving a backlog of several thousand cases awaiting processing (see below).

Of all convictions for sexual assaults (whether felonies or misdemeanors) from which DNA collection is legislatively mandated for database matching purposes, DNA was obtained from less than half the individuals, and in less than one-third were the samples DNA typed (see below). This proportion is an improvement over the past; however, of the overall, cumulative number of DNA samples collected (452,000 in the 35 States participating in the COmbined DNA Index System [CODIS]), only 20 percent have been typed. Exacerbating this limited databasing is that the mismatch between DNA typing systems prevents comparison searches; for example, most casework is now performed using PCR (polymerase chain reaction) analysis, while RFLP (restriction fragment length polymorphism) typing is performed on the vast majority of collected DNA database samples.

Fortunately, the situation is improving for rape cases: these low DNA utilization rates represent a substantial increase in DNA testing over the previous year (19 percent for DNA typing casework and 30 percent for DNA databasing. However, for nonsexual assault crimes, DNA testing is limited or in some cases even nonexistent.

Table 37.1. Incidence of Rape vs. DNA Databasing

Rapes	No.	%	DNA Databasing (sexual assaults)	No.	%
Victimizations	250,000	(100)	Convictions	165,000	(100)
Investigated by police	100,000	40	DNA collected	80,000	48
DNA submitted to crime labs	22,000*	9	DNA typed	45,000	27
DNA processed by labs	16,000	6	DNA not typed	35,000	73
Backlog in labs	6,000	—			

*Of the remaining 78,000 rape cases in which DNA was not submitted, 48,000 remained unsolved. The rest (30,000) were solved without the use of DNA evidence.

Note

These data were presented by Stephen Niezgoda, CODIS Program Manager, FBI, at the American Society of Crime Laboratory Directors' 25th Annual Symposium on Crime Laboratory Development, San Antonio, Texas, September 18, 1997. Data on number of rapes are from the Bureau of Justice Statistics National Crime Victimization Survey; the other data are from the FBI's *1997 CODIS Survey of DNA Laboratories*. The survey used information from the States for the period January 1996 through June 1997, and projected data to the end of fiscal year 1998.

In the Pipeline: New and Improved Testing Technologies

More rapid processing of DNA evidence should be possible within the next few years as a result of improvements in testing technology now under way.

The first widespread use of DNA tests in the criminal justice community involved RFLP (restriction fragment length polymorphism) analysis, which was informationally rich but took a long time—about 6 weeks. Recent nonradioisotopic methods have considerably reduced the turnaround time of RFLP. Nonetheless, it is anticipated that RFLP testing will eventually be supplanted by PCR (polymerase chain reaction)-based technology.

It takes only days to perform PCR-based dot/blots and, more recently, STRs (short tandem repeats). Moreover, current STR marker sets produce as much information as RFLP tests and can be used with extremely small and degraded DNA specimens. STRs have recently become commercially available, but already they are anticipated to supercede less informative dot/blot systems.

Developments that will further automate DNA analysis are being developed as an outgrowth of the Human Genome Project. These include robots, microchip-based instrumentation, and mass spectrometry. The run time of such instruments may be only minutes or even seconds. Performance of 100 STR analyses within an hour using an automated mass spectrometer has been demonstrated in a research setting.

Support for development of microchip and mass spectrometric work in forensic DNA testing is being provided by the National Institute of Justice. Today the resulting systems are in operation in only a few research centers, but are likely to become available in the next few years.

Note

The Human Genome Project (HGP) is an international, 15-year effort, begun in 1990, to discover all the genes in the human body's DNA and determine the complete sequence of DNA. A major focus of HGP is development of automated technology for the sequencing process.

A Primer of DNA Testing Technology

DNA is the chemical deoxyribonucleic acid, which stores the genetic code of the human body—the hereditary blueprint imparted to us by our parents. DNA is useful in forensics because it is present in all cells, is the same throughout the body, and does not change in the course of a person's life. Perhaps most important, for each individual (except identical twins) the DNA sequence (the order of the DNA building blocks) is different, making each person's DNA unique.

RFLP

The first type of forensic DNA test to be widely used by crime laboratories was restriction fragment length polymorphism (RFLP), based on the variation among individuals in the length of the DNA fragments. In the RFLP method, DNA is extracted and cut by an enzyme into restriction fragments, which are suspended in a gel, divided up by size, and transferred from the gel by blotting onto a membrane. In order for the examiner to see the fragments, they are identified by radioactively labeled probes, and the membrane is placed over an x-ray film. The radiation from the probe exposes the film and produces a picture of the DNA fragments, called an "autoradiogram."

A match is made when the patterns produced by DNA from an evidence stain and those from a suspect's sample DNA are found to be the same. An estimate of the statistical probability that this evidence is from a suspect rather than someone selected at random is then calculated. RFLP is powerful but is relatively insensitive, cannot be applied to degraded specimens, and is tedious and time consuming, taking about 6 weeks. More recently, to avoid the precautions needed to handle radioactive samples and to speed processing time, other labeling systems have been adopted, including chemiluminescent and fluorescent methods.

PCR

If a forensic sample is too small for RFLP testing or if the DNA is degraded, polymerase chain reaction (PCR) testing may be used to obtain a DNA typing result. PCR is a method of preparing samples in which the targeted DNA is copied many times (amplified). Two DNA molecules are produced from the original molecule; the procedure is repeated many times with a doubling of DNA fragments every time. Eventually millions of copies of a DNA sequence are produced. Although PCR is very sensitive, permitting analysis of as little as a single copy of DNA, this sensitivity also makes the sample susceptible to contamination. NIJ has provided support for the development of PCR as well as RFLP testing standards.[1]

Reverse Dot/Blots

The original application of PCR to DNA testing involved what is called dot/blot analysis. In a given region of DNA, there is a finite number of possible sequences ("alleles") between individuals, and a probe can be developed to determine the alleles present. In reverse dot/blot analysis, used by some forensic laboratories. amplified DNA binds to probes attached to a membrane. Membrane strips produce a blue dot in the presence of the bound, amplified DNA. Although these tests may be useful in many circumstances, their discriminatory power is low compared to other DNA typing methods, and one specimen may be contaminated with DNA from another person.

STRs

It is possible to amplify regions of the DNA molecule that show variation in DNA fragment length between individuals rather than using the RFLP method of isolating and cutting out these regions. The forensic community has found that smaller sets of fragments, called short tandem repeats (STRs), are preferable for several technical reasons. The technique of using STRs is easier and faster than RFLP, and the analysis can be performed with a number of different automated and semiautomated methods, such as capillary electrophoresis, [2] which is particularly rapid and highly automated.

Notes

1. In cooperation with the Office of Law Enforcement Standards of the National Institute of Standards and Technology, NIJ has initiated development of standards for the RFLP and PCR testing methods.

2. NIJ provided support for applying capillary electrophoresis to forensics.

— by Victor Walter Weedn and John W. Hicks

Chapter 38

Product Tampering and the FDA

By the time the mouse and its Pepsi-can coffin reached FDA, Fred L. Fricke and his team of chemists and microbiologists didn't have much to work with.

The mouse, found dead in a can of Diet Pepsi in New York, had already been examined by Pepsi officials. From there it went to a veterinarian on the East Coast. Next stop was a pathologist in Utah. Finally, the dissected mouse was sent to Fricke at FDA's Forensic Chemistry Center in Cincinnati.

Fortunately, the mouse's teeth were still intact. "We measured the spacing between the teeth and the pattern of bite marks on the can," explains Karen A. Wolnik, director of the center's inorganic chemistry branch. "From those measurements it was determined that his lower teeth had left marks on the inside of the can and his upper teeth had gnawed the outside, right at the pull-tab opening."

Wolnik says that pattern demonstrated the mouse had been inside the can when it bit the lid. But because the can lid with the pull-tab opening is in one intact piece throughout manufacturing, the mouse couldn't have bitten the lid or gotten into the can until after it was opened. The evidence was used to convict a tamperer who had falsely claimed to have found the mouse inside the can when she opened it. (Under the Federal Anti-Tampering Act, it is a felony to tamper with foods, drugs, devices, cosmetics, and other consumer products.)

From "FDA's Forensic Center: Speedy, Sophisticated Sleuthing," by Isadora B. Stehlin, in *FDA Consumer* magazine, July-August 1995.

"Every week we get something that's suspected tampering," says Fricke, director of the forensic center. "It never slows down."

FDA established the center in 1989 to provide the agency with a team of forensic science experts who can respond immediately to all tampering incidents and provide expert advice and scientific evidence to FDA officials. The 30 chemists and three biologists unravel the scientific mysteries of tamperings and other criminal activities involving FDA-regulated products through careful observation and high-tech instruments.

The center has inorganic chemistry and organic chemistry branches. The organic branch uses organic analytical detection methods—such as infrared spectroscopy, gas and liquid chromatography, and mass spectrometry—to separate and identify the components of mixtures. The inorganic branch uses tools such as digital image analysis and scanning electron microscopy to detect physical evidence of tampering or counterfeiting, and ion chromatography, atomic absorption, and inductively coupled plasma spectrometry to measure inorganic components of mixtures.

Most cases require the expertise of both branches. "There's no division [of responsibilities] that's really sacred," says R. Duane Satzger, director of the organic branch. "When we get a case, both branches sit down and talk about it and decide how to address the situation."

For example, he explains, a syringe might first be examined by the inorganic group. Wolnik's staff would use light microscopy to examine the syringe. If, during this examination, they observed some kind of liquid in the needle of the syringe, Satzger's staff would use chromatographs or mass spectrographs to identify the liquid. Electron microscopy might be used to detect decomposition and other physical changes to the syringe that might have occurred if the syringe had been submerged in soda or come in contact with poison.

Tylenol, Grapes, and Cyanide

In 1980, Fricke, Satzger, and Wolnik worked at the forensic center's predecessor, FDA's Elemental Analysis Research Center in Cincinnati, where they conducted research and developed procedures for detecting toxic and nutritional trace elements in foods and drugs.

In 1982, when the first Tylenol tampering occurred, FDA chemists developed elemental "fingerprinting" techniques that allowed the authorities to trace the cyanide back to the manufacturer and the distributor. "The identity and relative amounts of various elemental constituents in a suspect sample form a distinct pattern that can be used for comparison with other samples, much like actual finger-prints," explains Wolnik.

The next few years saw more cases of cyanide in Tylenol and other pain relievers, as well as other types of tampering. "We applied the "fingerprinting" techniques to various poisons," says Fricke. They also developed "fingerprints" for inorganic substances such as metal and glass.

By the time cyanide was discovered in Chilean grapes in 1989, the center had developed expertise in detecting cyanide and other poisons in drugs and processed foods. But they had very little knowledge about what effect the cyanide would have on the fruit and vice versa. Would the poison become more or less toxic? Would it do something to the fruit that would be obvious to consumers?

"We didn't have a lot of answers at that time about what would happen," says Fricke. To keep FDA from being caught off-guard in the future, the agency redirected the focus of Fricke's lab from elemental to forensic research.

The lab's primary function shifted to research on what happens when poisons are added to foods and drugs. The "fingerprinting" tech-nique used for comparing items of evidence was expanded to include many chemicals. In addition, the lab began developing screening meth-ods for poisons so it could respond rapidly to any suspected tamperings. Since then, the lab has developed techniques to screen for more than 250 of the most toxic poisons commonly available to the public.

The forensic lab is also the only laboratory facility in FDA espe-cially equipped for, and experienced in, ultra-trace elemental analy-sis. Using a specialized type of mass spectrometry called inductively coupled plasma/mass spectrometry, the lab's chemists can find con-taminants in amounts as small as parts per trillion.

Tracking Down the Source

There are three points at which a foreign object or other contami-nant can get into a product:

- *During manufacturing.* "There are legitimate things that can go wrong during manufacturing," says Wolnik, "and there are rare occasions of employee sabotage."

- *While the product is in distribution.* These are cases in which someone tampers with a product and returns it to the store shelf looking as untouched as possible so the purchaser is un-likely to detect the tampering. Frequently the perpetrator has a single victim in mind but tries to make the crime look like random tampering. "It's a crime similar to blowing up an airplane to kill one person," says Wolnik.

- *After purchase.* Those are the false report cases, such as the false claims of Pepsi tamperings during the summer of 1993.

Many clues help the forensic lab's people zero in on the time and place of contamination, including the amount of physical deterioration of foreign objects, the breakdown of poisons into chemical components, and physical measurements of containers. But they won't tell the public what those clues are. "We don't want to hand out a blueprint to would-be tamperers," says Fricke.

The process for identifying poisons and other chemical contaminants is something the scientists will share. Separation of the different chemical components of a mixture is one of the most frequent techniques used and requires some type of chromatography.

Chromatography separates complex mixtures by measuring migration rates of component molecules through columns and through coatings on chromatography plates. "We'll compare those components with a control and we'll be looking for differences," explains Satzger. "We won't try to identify everything in the sample. So if there are 20 components that we can separate in the suspect sample and only 18 in a control, we'll zero in on those two extra components."

Identification usually requires infrared spectroscopy or some form of mass spectrometry. Gas chromatography/mass spectrometry is used for volatile components. Liquid chromatography/mass spectrometry is the usual choice for nonvolatile ones. Ion chromatography and atomic spectrometry are used for inorganic components.

Even after suspect components are identified, the sleuthing may not be over. Sometimes components that show up in lab tests are part of a bigger picture.

"We've done studies to show that when you put sodium hypochlorite (bleach) in soft drinks it breaks down into several different components," says Wolnik. "So we look for elevated breakdown products of the sodium hypochlorite. That's where the sophistication [of our lab] comes in. Any lab can run a test for bleach in soft drinks. But if they don't find any bleach it doesn't necessarily mean bleach wasn't in there. It just means that [the bleach] may have been changed by the material."

Even when the final lab results are in, FDA's work may not be done. "A lot of what we do isn't the be all and end all," says Wolnik. "It just really helps focus the investigation. We work closely with [FDA] agents and investigators so we know what kinds of questions they're interested in answering. As we learn things, we provide information to the investigators which may help direct their investigation."

Leftovers

One of the toughest obstacles the forensic lab faces is the condition of samples when they reach the lab. Like the mouse in the Pepsi can, samples have frequently been studied by other authorities first, leaving very little for the forensic lab to work with.

"It's infrequent that we get the sample first," says Wolnik. "That alone makes our analysis difficult. We have to spend some time thinking about what analyses we want to do, and what order we want to do them in. We can't afford to waste what little sample is left."

Another problem is damage or contamination of the samples. For example, Wolnik says during the 1982 Tylenol tampering incident, the medical examiner unintentionally contaminated the cyanide from some of the poisoned capsules with sodium during his analysis. He then sent the contaminated capsules to FDA.

"In forensics, you want the evidence as close to the condition in which it was originally found as possible, and you want to preserve that," says Wolnik.

That was not the case on March 19, 1993, when Bobby Joe Johnston of Oklahoma City, suffered burns to his lips and tongue after drinking from a can of Pepsi. The hospital where he was treated took a sample of Pepsi from the can and determined it was highly caustic. The hospital called the fire department, which retrieved the can and the rest of the six-pack Johnston had purchased. The fire department treated the cans as hazardous materials instead of forensic evidence, however.

"They put the five unopened cans in a glass container, set the open can on top of the others, and went home for the weekend," says Wolnik. "When they checked it on Monday, the corrosive material had eaten through the open can and dribbled onto and through another can, causing the second one to explode. When we finally got the sample, we had to reconstruct what came from the contaminated can and what came from the other previously unopened can. It ended up being fairly tricky."

However, the lab was eventually able to confirm that sodium hydroxide (lye) had been added to the can after it was opened and could not have been in any of the unopened cans. "We did studies to see how long it would take [for sodium hydroxide] to eat through a can," says Wolnik. The FDA chemists found that highly caustic solutions such as lye ate through the can in a matter of hours. "That proved that it couldn't have happened during manufacturing." Johnston was convicted of tampering on June 3, 1993.

Beyond Tampering

While tampering cases are the main focus of the forensic lab, there are other activities—such as illegal sale and use of unapproved drugs, counterfeit drugs, and economic fraud—that require the lab's expertise.

For example, the drug clenbuterol, which isn't approved in the United States for any use in either people or animals, is sometimes used illegally in show animals, including cattle, pigs, and sheep, to increase muscle. If those animals are subsequently slaughtered, anyone who eats the tainted meat might experience symptoms such as increased heart rate, muscle tremors, dizziness, nausea, fever, and chills. "We developed methods to analyze animal retinas for clenbuterol residues," says Fricke. This is significant, he explains, because while clenbuterol residues may show up in various tissues, almost any use will leave residues in the retina.

Counterfeit products require a combination of high-tech analysis to compare ingredients with the real product and careful study of the labels and packages.

The lab has uncovered evidence to support charges of economic fraud as well. Two such cases involved substandard stainless steel on imported surgical instruments and purported nutritional products that didn't contain any of the listed ingredients.

The procedures and techniques the forensic lab has developed better prepares the agency to meet these types of emergencies. Still, "every sample that comes in is like a separate research project," says Fricke. "We have to decide what procedures and methods to apply, and there still are many cases that require new procedures. And, always, we have to do this as quickly as we can."

—by Isadora B. Stehlin

Isadora Stehlin is a staff writer for *FDA Consumer.*

Chapter 39

The National Center for Forensic Science

In a move that will expand its ability to offer support and service to state and local law enforcement, the National Institute of Justice (NIJ) has opened the National Center for Forensic Science (NCFS) at the University of Central Florida (UCF) in Orlando. This new center, now part of the National Law Enforcement and Corrections Technology Center (NLECTC) system, will focus on research and training in the area of arson and explosives.

UCF has been known for many years for a prestigious forensic science program, a component of its Chemistry Department, which offers science-based baccalaureate degrees in two tracks: trace analysis and serology, according to department chair Glenn Cunningham, Ph.D. With program graduates currently employed by laboratories at all levels of local, state, and federal government, a perfect foundation exists for a partnership with NIJ and its NLECTC system.

"We survey our alumni every so often just to see what they think about our program here, what changes need to be made, and what kind of problems they need help with in the field," Dr. Cunningham says. "A couple of years ago they told us they wanted more training in handling situations where there might be arson or explosives involved. We felt there was a need we could fill. We talked to NIJ about forming this national center. We then prepared a proposal for the agency's review. A planning grant was then approved and funded," he says.

From "More Fire Power for Bomb and Arson Investigation," in the NLECTC (National Law Enforcement and Corrections Technology Center) newsletter, *Techbeat,* Spring 1998, p. 3.

To determine what scientists needed and to keep from duplicating work done by other labs, UCF hosted a national needs symposium in August 1997 that was attended by more than 50 experts. The experts were divided into two working groups—one on arson and one on explosives analysis—and asked to identify problem areas. Their responses were then turned into a specific set of tasks and goals for the center, as follows:

- Develop a restricted access electronic library for forensic and law enforcement professionals. This library will link to databases of other organizations and associations to provide a comprehensive source of expertise and research materials. It will be accessible to lab personnel and to crime scene technicians, who can tap into it from onsite laptop computers. This online access will include procedural guidelines, information on unfamiliar types of evidence, and contact names of individuals with in-depth experience in a particular area.

- Provide support for the development of standard protocols for the collection and analysis of fire and explosion debris.

- Offer supplemental training via the Internet and through distance education and professional seminars.

- Conduct fundamental research to scientifically validate evidence collection and analysis procedures.

The symposium also resulted in the selection of a 13-member advisory board that includes forensic scientists from local, state, and federal crime laboratories.

"We met extensively with representatives from the Federal laboratories, including the FBI (Federal Bureau of Investigation) and ATF (Bureau of Alcohol, Tobacco, and Firearms), to make sure there wouldn't be any project overlap," Dr. Cunningham says. "We now have some of their top people on our board. We'll use the working groups and our advisory board to direct our research and training initiatives . . . no point in us duplicating research that is being done by the ATF or the FBI. They already do superb research in these areas," he says.

Dr. Cunningham notes that a World Wide Web site is already in place, and work on the center's electronic library is under way. There is even a newsletter, appropriately titled *Debris*. Center staff also are developing new training courses for crime lab and law enforcement professionals. In the future, he says, the center will partner with the university's Institute of Simulation and Training, which currently focuses on using computer simulation to train in emergency preparedness. According to Dr. Cunningham, the institute's ability to do computer modeling can be extended into the area of molecular modeling to simulate explosions.

"We believe in strength in numbers and in a strong partnership between government, industry, and academe," says Marilyn Cobb Croach, UCF's director of federal relations. "We have an amazing research base here, with the Naval Air Warfare Center, the U.S. Army Simulation Training and Instrumentation Command, the U.S. Air Force's Simulation and Modeling Office, and the U.S. Marine Corps Program Office, all located in Orlando. We believe we can join with these partners to take the knowledge to the professions that need it," she states.

For more information about the National Center for Forensic Science, call (407) 823-6469, fax (407) 823-3162, or e-mail natlctr@pegasus. cc.ucf.edu. The center maintains a Web site at www.ucf.edu.ncfs. Or, you may access NCFS through the NLECTC Web site, JUSTNET, at http://www.nlectc.org.

Chapter 40

Child Fatality Review Teams

Conservative estimates place the yearly number of child abuse and neglect fatalities at 2,000 (Grayson, 1995). Additionally, there is general agreement that the actual incidence of child abuse deaths is poorly documented. In fact, no single health, social service, law enforcement, or judicial system exists to track and comprehensively assess the circumstances of child deaths (Durfee, Gellert, and Tilton-Durfee, 1989).

In response to his concern that child homicide victims were being missed, in 1978, physician Michael Durfee set up a system to retrieve cases from coroners' records. He was later joined in his efforts by a public health nurse with a background in child abuse cases. Together, they began to establish a protocol for review of potentially suspicious child deaths.

In many cities, multidisciplinary child fatality review teams exist. The American Academy of Pediatrics has developed guidelines and procedures for child death investigations. Two benefits of such a team review is to develop data about causes of child deaths to prevent such tragedies and to assist law enforcement in identifying suspect indicators to focus an investigation.

Law enforcement is critical in responding to a missing child report. Missing children reports are difficult case types to investigate because they are situations with minimal information, maximum pressure,

From "Missing Children Found Dead," by Rubin D. Rodreguez, Jr., et al., in *Journal of Psychosocial Nursing and Mental Health Services,* Vol. 36, No. 6, 1998. © 1998 by SLACK Inc. All rights reserved. Reprinted with permission.

and the need for an immediate solution. Law enforcement needs to know about available resources, especially in the area of child homicides.

These cases are special in their own right. The typology and motivations are believed to be different in the suspects and victimology from adults, thereby requiring the need for a specialized investigative approach to the case. However, the academic, clinical, and criminal justice literature are silent on the subject.

This article seeks to contribute to the quantitative and qualitative literature on child fatalities. The quantitative analysis is to provide suspect indicators or profile characteristics from analyzed cases to assist investigators of missing children in focusing their search to a suspect.

The qualitative analysis provides brief case vignettes to sensitize law enforcement and clinicians to the various motives and circumstances of child homicides. If similar circumstances appear in a case where the suspect is unknown, it is reasonable to hypothesize that some actions or circumstances may be common or identifiable in similar case types, based on knowledge obtained from prior case analysis.

National Center for Missing and Exploited Children

The National Center for Missing and Exploited Children (NCMEC) receives thousands of calls per year regarding missing children. One of the mandates of the NCMEC is to help law enforcement recover or locate the child; however, there is also a mandate to disseminate information to law enforcement. Every day, newspapers nationwide publish accounts of children being victimized: strangers who abduct and kill; the neighbor who seduces and kills; and the mother and father who kill their child. The NCMEC wanted to know the why, how, and where of deceased missing children.

Realizing that the Center's files contained a wealth of information that, when analyzed, could be extremely useful to the investigator, this project was initiated.

The Deceased Child Project

As part of an internal review of case files, the staff of the Case Enhancement and Informational Analysis Unit conducted a 10-year record review of cases where the children were deceased when recovered. This search yielded data on 210 usable cases reported as missing and recovered deceased between April 1982 and August 1992. Within the 210 cases, 143 cases were identified as homicides. The remaining cases were either death as the result of accident or suicide.

Methodology

Key variables were determined by the staff at NCMEC. The data were first checked as to total population and then as homicides only. Data were entered on a code sheet and a Pearson correlation was run on all variables. The initial correlation analysis indicated areas for further investigation or changes. Variables such as suspect's relationship to victim, and original caller, were reduced to six groupings: natural family; step family; foster family; extended family; close friends; and strangers. Cause of death was reduced to four groups: unknown; accidental; suicide; and homicide using NCMEC groupings. Prior convictions were reduced to five groups: crimes against minors; violent crimes; adult sex crimes; felonies; and misdemeanors.

Using the groupings of variables, the Pearson correlation was run a second time with some correlations dropping out of significance and others becoming significant. A two-dimensional cross tabulation (Chi square) was conducted to test for statistically significant differences with variables as a function of other variables (e.g., sex of victim versus cause of death).

Some statistically significant results emerged and confirmed prior knowledge developed through law enforcement investigative experience. It is important to note that the absence of statistical significance also shows what not to identify as important indicators of potential suspects (e.g., strangers and family members are equally likely to take the victim across state borders).

Findings

Total Population

The predominant cause of death with children who have been reported missing to the NCMEC is homicide (68%). This category is far ahead of accidental (16%), unknown (12%), and suicide (4%).

Differences were noted between sex of victim and cause of death. More girls, 124 or 59%, were found dead in the missing population than boys, 86 or 41%. The number of female victims increased when looking at homicide figures: 66.4% are girls and 33.6% are boys. Caucasian girls were the largest victim group, followed by Caucasian boys, African-American boys, and African-American girls.

Gender was significant in deaths by accident and suicide. Of the non-homicide cases, accidental deaths were predominantly boys (82%) and by drowning. Additionally, more males committed suicide than females. Of the eight suicides, five were boys and two were under age 12. No girls under 12 committed suicide.

Girls were victimized more often by members of the opposite sex; boys were victimized more often by the same sex. Children between the ages of 6 and 17 comprised the largest victim group, with the majority of missing children in this study abducted by people they knew.

Homicide

Girls were more likely to be murdered by males than by females, with strangulation (manual or by ligature) being a frequent cause of death. Of the cases where molestation occurred, girls were the largest victim group by a wide margin. In those cases where a parent killed the child, when the father was the perpetrator, the average distance from the site of reported abduction to site of disposal or recovery was 350 miles. In those cases where the mother was the perpetrator, the average distance was 5.6 miles.

Children younger than 4 were equally likely to have suspects of either sex. Although boys ages 5 to 12 had some female suspects, the majority were male; however, all male victims older than 12 had male suspects. Girls younger than 5 and ages 5 to 12 had either females or males as suspects, but for girls older than 12, the majority of suspects were males.

Weapons and Homicide

For all ages, more girls than boys are murdered without weapons. Older boys are more likely to be murdered using a weapon than by physical means. Children of both sexes younger than 5 are more likely murdered through physical means than by weapons. As children increase in age, boys ages 5 to 12 are murdered with weapons, although the majority of girls are physically murdered. The majority of boys older than 12 are killed with weapons, although the majority of girls are killed by other means.

Female suspects in this sample did not use a gun or knife to kill and did not kill children older than 12. Of the 13 male victims older than 12, 11 or 85% were killed with a gun or knife. Of the 30 girls older than 12, 13 or 43% were killed with a gun or knife. Of the 24 victims younger than 5, only boys were killed by male suspects using a gun or a knife. Of the 24 victims younger than 5, 15 had male suspects (six male and nine female victims) and nine had female suspects (five male victims and four female victims).

Suspect Relationship to Victim

When the victim is a girl, the offender is more likely to be a close friend or stranger. The leading suspect category for boys is close friends, followed by family members, then strangers. Younger than 5, the predominant suspects are family members. Between the ages of 5 and 12, the close friend and stranger category are tied at 23 victims each (46 out of 66). Older than 12, the leading suspect category becomes close friends (22), followed by strangers (14).

Gender and Molestation

A higher percentage of homicide victims are molested than in the total sample. More girls are molested than boys; however, the percentage of boys molested in the homicide population is higher than the percentage of boys molested in the total population.

The majority of molested girls are killed by physical means (32 of the 43). The remaining 11 die by gun or knife. More girls killed by weapon are molested than not (11 yes, four probable versus two not). More boys killed with weapons are listed as not molested than being molested.

The largest age group for molested children is between 5 and 12. No victim younger than 5 was reported molested. The majority of molested children between the ages of 5 and 12 were killed by physical means (46 out of 66), and 24 of these were molested. This compared with seven molested and three probable molestations out of 20 victims killed with a weapon.

Suspect Relationship, Victim Age, and Gender

The largest category of victims (19) are girls between the ages of 5 and 12 who are killed by strangers. The second largest number of girls killed (15) are also aged 5 to 12 and are killed by close friends. These two groups are more than twice the size as the comparable boy group (four and eight, respectively). The largest boy group are those younger than 5 who are killed by family members (10). The second largest group of boy victims (those ages 5 to 12) are those killed by suspects in the close friend category (eight). The 5-to-12 age group is also killed by strangers and family members (four and three, respectively).

Case Examples and Suspect Indicators

Case 1

Case 1 was called in to NCMEC by the mother, who reported that she had car trouble while driving along the highway with her sons. The mother reported that while she was looking under the hood of the car to see what was wrong, a van pulled up, and someone came up from behind and put a cloth over her head. She claimed that she did not get a good look at the van and did not hear it pull up. After she managed to free herself from the cloth placed on her head, she returned to the car to find that her children were gone.

The NCMEC hotline operator who took the initial report commented that "the mother seemed too calm" while she was describing the events that had occurred that day. When the case manager called the mother the following day to gather further information, he made a notation in his report that "mom seems too calm." That same evening, the mother confessed to authorities that she had killed her two sons.

The mother took the police to the location where she had placed the bodies, which was about 10 miles from her home. They were found behind a hill, located in a ditch, hidden from view. The mother indicated she killed the children by smashing their skulls with a sledge hammer. Her reason: she didn't have enough food to feed them. According to the authorities, this mother had a history of violent criminal behavior (she had tried to kill someone by burning down a house).

Case 2

Case 2 involved a grievance over a custody dispute. When the father realized he had lost custody of his two sons, ages 4 and 6, he quickly tricked his ex-wife into letting him take the children for a visit. He then took the children 1,200 miles away to hide with some of his relatives in another state. The father finally killed both boys by shooting them in the head with a 12-gauge shotgun. During his confession, he told authorities that his "ex-wife was a horrible person, and [his] sons asked [him] to kill them rather than go back to their mother."

The bodies of the two brothers were located more than 1,200 miles from the site of the abduction. The father was described as having an explosive personality with a previous criminal history that included family violence charges and attempted assault on his ex-wife (the mother of the two victims).

Case 3

Case 3 involved an 11-year-old girl who was reported missing on Halloween night. Within several days, the police received a handwritten map from the abductor showing them where they could find the child's body, as well as a statement to "please give the girl a decent burial." It took the police several days to find the body because many of the landmarks on the map were not accurately placed. Every detailed item on the map, however, was found by the police. The body was eventually found in the root system of a large overturned tree.

After the body was located, the police began receiving anonymous letters through the mail, in the form of riddles to be answered. The riddles were based on ancient Egyptian and Greek mythological figures and had to be answered within a set period of time "or another victim would be taken by Christmas." The answers to the riddles had to be placed on the front page of the local newspaper.

After conferring with a friend about the difficult riddles, the police officer realized that the riddles were coming from "Sesame Street." The television show was running a week-long special on mythology. At that point, the police realized they were dealing with "an organized killer operating at the level of a child."

The letters were traced to a post office box and finally led the police to Fred, a 16-year-old adolescent who knew the victim from seeing her in the neighborhood and was preparing to kill her younger sister. The police described Fred as "having an abnormal childhood and being a 'Ted-Bundy type,' ready to explode." He had no previous criminal history, but did have some behavioral problems in school.

Case 4

Case 4 involved Fran, a 15-year-old girl, who was the third in a series of four victims by the same abductor, a white male in his late 20s. He claimed that he "has kidnapped and sexually abused other children in the past."

The victim was abducted from her home. She was found shot to death in an area 20 to 30 miles northwest of the abduction site and had been sexually molested.

This abductor's method of operation (MO) consisted of answering furniture advertisements in the local trade papers to search for people with children in the home. When he found his victim, he would stop by the home again after he knew the parents had gone out and abduct the child. The abductions took place whenever his wife went away on business, because he liked to take his victims to his home and "play with them" before returning them to the location of their abductions.

Fran was kept hidden in a closet in the abductor's house for his sexual gratification. The abductor claimed that they "were in love," but when he caught her trying to escape, he shot her in the back. According to the authorities, the truth was that his wife was returning home sooner than he had anticipated and he had to get rid of his victim as quickly as possible.

His last victim, Susan, was the individual who finally led the police to the abductor. She too was abducted and kept in his closet; authorities believe that she also would have been killed if she had not escaped. The victim asked her abductor if she could "go outside to play for awhile." He agreed, and Susan escaped by running to the nearby interstate and flagging down a motorist. Susan's story linked the abductor with the abduction and rape of two other female victims, and with the abduction and murder of Fran.

Case 5

Case 5 is of Michael, age 13. Witnesses claimed they had seen a driver "stop his car, get out, and follow the victim," who was on a bicycle. The man was then seen "dragging the child back to his car, kicking and screaming." By the time the witnesses doubled back to the area, the car and victim were gone.

Michael's decomposed body was located 7 miles from town on a rural road in a hunting campground. The abductor had continued on the same highway on which the abduction took place; it was a direct route to a hunting cabin.

The information on the abductor highlights the escalation of his criminal activity from childhood to adulthood. The abductor, Brian, was 26 years old. As an adolescent, he was diagnosed as having a behavioral disorder, unsocialized aggressive reaction with schizoid tendencies, and a predisposition to sexual deviation. At 13, Brian kidnapped a 15-year-old male at knife-point. He let the boy go after tying his hands and molesting him. Brian was placed in a treatment center; the case never went to trial.

At 16, Brian forced a 12-year-old male onto his bicycle. He took the boy to a field and forced him to ingest pills, fondled and choked him, leaving him for dead. For this crime, he was tried as an adult and placed in a county youth home.

At 23, after finishing his time in the youth home, he was working and arrested again. He pled guilty to "contributing to the delinquency of minors," by offering 13- and 15-year-old boys money to pose nude for photographs. At 25, a man believed to be Brian picked up a 13-year-old boy, got him drunk, and fondled him before driving the boy home. When Brian's roommate was questioned about the incident, he said that "Brian was scared because he had been fooling around with boys again."

At 26, Brian was back in his home state, driving a gold station wagon. At about this time, a 14-year-old boy was forced into a brown station wagon while riding his bicycle, in an area about 2 miles from Brian's residence. His body was found and Brian is currently a suspect in this homicide.

Later the same year, Michael, age 13, was taken from his bicycle and forced into a light-colored Jeep, which Brian had bought after trading in his station wagon. It is believed that he then took the victim up to the hunting camp, where he molested and killed the victim. The body was found 2 weeks later, naked and bound with rope, so badly decomposed that the cause of death could not be determined, although strangulation is suspected.

Law enforcement officers noted that when Brian, as an adolescent, would be questioned about a crime, he would vehemently deny all accusations. Later, he would pedal his bike back to the police station, sit down, and "lay it all out." Police officers said he did not brag about the crimes or appear embarrassed, rather, just stated the facts about what happened. When police began questioning local citizens living near the hunting lodge where Michael was found, one woman claimed that a man matching Brian's description "knocked on the door and asked to use [their] .22 to 'shoot some bats he found in his cabin.'" The neighbors refused to give him the gun.

Police began a manhunt for Brian when he fled the state. An FBI agent followed him to a trailer park where he was staying with friends. As soon as police were able to have a warrant issued for him, they returned to find an empty trailer. Upon entering the trailer they found several short-wave radios, all of which were tuned to the various police bands in the area. Brian knew they were coming and was one step ahead of them. He remains at large.

Discussion

The analysis of the 210 missing children found deceased has forensic, motive, and educational implications.

Forensics

Many cases lacked forensic testing and resulted in a high number of "probably molested" cases. Forensic testing for sexual abuse and molestation is indicated in all cases. If the victim is a girl, she will have even a higher chance of being molested. Additional suggested forensic tests are: DNA tracing; HIV, pregnancy for female victims; and use of drugs or alcohol.

Motive

Knowing the motive of a homicide assists in classifying the crime (Douglas, Burgess, Burgess, and Ressler, 1992). When molestation is a motive, law enforcement can review suspect files for sex offenders of children. Whatever method caused the child's death, molestation was probably the main reason for the child's abduction. Motive in other than molested cases needs to be studied, such as argument, conflict, anger, and domestic violence.

Suspect Indicators or Profile Characteristics

When there is an unsolved homicide and only victim data, the following suspect indicators or profile characteristics may assist in focusing an investigation toward possible suspects.

For children missing and found deceased younger than 5, check family members. As the child enters the 5-to-12-age group, the stranger and acquaintance becomes the leading suspect category. When the child is older than 12, the leading suspect comes from the group called close friends, which is closely followed by strangers.

Parent and Community Education

For parent education, the fact that more boys die by accident suggests either that boys probably take more chances in the water (boating, swimming) than do girls, or caretakers are less vigilant and instructive about safety with boys. The number of child suicides also has implications for parents and mental health professionals to be aware of early signs of depression in children, especially boys.

Education is important in instances of child exploitation and abuse. Establish a community hotline (through the police department) for persons noted to be following or watching children. Educate people to look for strangers as well as people in the close friend category around areas where kids congregate, such as paper routes, playgrounds, and shopping malls. Law enforcement needs to pay careful attention to children who report that they think they have been watched or followed.

References

Douglas, J. E., A. W. Burgess, A. G. Burgess, and R. K. Ressler. *Crime Classification Manual.* New York: Free Press, 1992.

Durfee, M. J., G. A. Gellert, and D. Tilton-Durfee. "Origins and Clinical Relevance of Child Death Review Teams." *Journal of the American Medical Association* 267: 3172-5 (1992).

Grayson, J. "Child Fatality Review Teams." *Virginia Child Protection Newsletter* 46: 1-4 (Fall 1995).

— by Rubin D. Rodreguez, Jr.; Cathy Nahirny; Ann W. Burgess, R.N., D.N.Sc.; and Allen G. Burgess, D.B.A.

Rubin D. Rodreguez, Jr., is Senior Analyst, Child Abduction and Serial Killer Unit, FBI Academy, Quantico, VA; Cathy Nahirny is Case Analyst, National Center for Missing and Exploited Children, Arlington, VA; Ann W. Burgess, D.N.Sc., is van Ameringen Professor of Psychiatric Mental Health Nursing, University of Pennsylvania School of Nursing, Philadelphia, PA; and Allen G. Burgess, D.B.A, is President, Data Integrity Inc., Waltham, MA. Address correspondence to Ann Wolbert Burgess, D.N.Sc., University of Pennsylvania, School of Nursing, 420 Guardian Drive, Philadelphia, PA 19104.

Chapter 41

Hair Assays and Urinalysis in Drug Detection

Estimates of the incidence and prevalence of drug use among juveniles have been derived, historically, from self reports obtained during interviews. However, comparison of survey responses with urinalysis results has shown that self-reported drug behavior does not accurately reflect the extent of drug use. Urine-based testing consistently detects more drug use than is revealed by self reports, suggesting that estimates based on surveys alone underreport drug use. But for several major drugs of abuse, urinalysis affords too narrow a detection 'Window.' For example, the maximum retrospective period allowed by urinalysis for detecting cocaine or most opiates at currently accepted cutoff values is approximately 48 to 72 hours, as determined by the rate at which these drugs clear the body. This limited detection capability, as well as problems associated with implementing a urine monitoring program (i.e., the need to refrigerate samples and to observe the voiding of specimens), makes validation of new drug testing methodologies a priority.

Hair analysis is one such methodology. Hair entraps drugs or their metabolites for much longer periods than urine and represents an alternative medium for estimating the use of rapidly excreted drugs. In 1993, the National Institute of Justice (NIJ) funded a project designed to replicate the findings of an earlier study[1] that had examined drug use among juvenile offenders using self reports, urinalysis,

From "Hair Assays and Urinalysis Results for Juvenile Drug Offenders," by Tom Mieczkowski, Ph.D., in the U.S. Department of Justice, Office of Justice Programs publication, *NIJ Research Preview,* April 1997.

and hair assays. The original study showed that hair analysis revealed seven times as much cocaine use as was detected by urinalysis. The findings from the replicated study confirmed those made earlier, although only a fourfold difference was found between hair and urine assay results for cocaine. In addition, the drug assessment instrument used in the study, COMPASS,[2] was able to identify sample members at risk for substance abuse independently from the bioassay or self report.

Study Methodology

The target population consisted of 426 juvenile detainees, between 14 and 18 years old at two sites: Cleveland (Cuyahoga County), Ohio (185 male detainees, of whom nearly 72 percent were black), and St. Petersburg (Pinellas County), Florida (241 male and female detainees, of whom approximately 6 percent were black). Participation in the study was voluntary. At the Cleveland site, a juvenile detention facility, eligibility was restricted to youths arrested or apprehended less than 48 hours prior to interviewing; the Florida site, also a juvenile detention facility, included referrals from schools, parents, and similar sources. All juveniles were approached, recruited, and interviewed according to NIJ's Drug Use Forecast (DUF) system protocol. Following the interview and collection of a urine specimen, hair specimens were gathered, and the COMPASS assessment was administered to all subjects.

Urinalysis was performed using EMIT™ (enzyme multiplied immune test), an objective, machine-readable method. Specimens were analyzed for the 10 drugs standard to DUF: cannabinoids, cocaine, opiates, PCP, methadone, amphetamine, diazepines, methaqualone, barbiturates, and phenylpropanolamine. Hair specimens were analyzed for evidence of cocaine, marijuana, methadone, PCP, and opiates, using radioimmunoassay screening and gas chromatography/mass spectroscopy confirmation analyses.

Study Findings

Self reports. Juveniles were reluctant to report using drugs in the arrest or detention setting, even when they had been assured that an admission would not be held against them. If they reported anything, it was likely to be having used marijuana "at some point in their lives." The more recent the time frame queried, the more likely the juvenile was to deny use.

Cocaine and marijuana detection. Hair analysis identified higher drug prevalence for cocaine than did urinalysis—a finding consistent with the data reported in the original study. However, the findings for marijuana were inconsistent. In the Cleveland group, marijuana was detected in urine nearly four times as frequently as in hair. The opposite was true in St. Petersburg, where approximately 60 percent more marijuana use was detected by hair assays than by urinalysis. Few other drugs were detected in subjects at either site.

In many cases, cocaine was detected in an offender's hair but not his or her urine. Rarely was the reverse true, i.e., in almost no instance was a cocaine-positive urine test contradicted by a cocaine-negative hair assay. High levels of cocaine in hair indicated more chronic and high-dose cocaine use, which is more readily detected by urine testing. Persons who use cocaine infrequently or in very low doses (and who ought, therefore, to have low hair assay values) are likely to pass a urine screen.

COMPASS assessment. Virtually all subjects had high COMPASS scores relative to the general population norms for the instrument, showing clearly that youths at both sites were at risk for substance abuse. In this regard, the assessment instrument was successful. High risk was indicated without reference to either the bioassay or self-report outcomes. However, COMPASS did not finely differentiate among the juveniles in the sample.

Implications

Samples in both jurisdictions were small, quite different from one another, and perhaps not representative of the juvenile justice population. However, study findings generally affirm those reported in the earlier research. Both hair and urine assays detected more drug use than was reported in interviews. Cocaine use was substantially underreported—and substantially undercounted by urine assays: at both sites, hair analysis revealed much more cocaine use than did urine testing. This study suggests that a drug monitoring program using hair assays can be implemented in field settings, but very short hair styles may be a stumbling block. Although other body hair can be used, collecting specimens could prove awkward. Further research is needed to determine the accuracy and timeliness of hair testing methodology and the costs and benefits of hair testing relative to other technologies.

Notes

1. T. Feucht, R. Stevens, and M. Walker, "Drug Use Among Juvenile Arrestees: A Comparison of Self-Report, Urinalysis, and Hair Assays," *Journal of Drug Issues* 24 (1 and 2): 99-116, 1994.

2. The COMPASS is a 98-page self-report questionnaire on substance abuse designed for use with any adolescent or adult, regardless of sex, marital status, or ethnic background. Since October 1995, COMPASS has been known as MAPP (Multidimensional Addictions and Personality Profile).

—by Tom Mieczkowski, Ph.D.

Tom Mieczkowski is an Associate Professor of Criminology at the University of South Florida.

Chapter 42

Improved Testing for Carbon Monoxide and Cyanide

Traditional methods for detecting carbon monoxide and cyanide during postmortem examinations have proven cumbersome, time consuming, and prone to interference from putrefactive and other changes in the substances analyzed. Even relatively recent methods are often too expensive for routine use or too dependent on subjective interpretations.

Despite the foregoing difficulties, testing for the presence of carbon monoxide and cyanide in biological material is a critical task for forensic laboratories nationwide: knowledge of the presence or absence of those substances in the deceased often helps determine cause of death (murder, accident, natural causes, etc.)—or at least narrows the range of possibilities. For example, the absence of carbon monoxide in the charred remains of an apparent fire victim would suggest that death did not occur as the result of the fire—in which case the victim would likely have inhaled fire-generated carbon monoxide—but prior to it.

The importance and prevalence of testing for those substances motivated the National Institute of Justice (NIJ) to support development and evaluation of an improved postmortem method for detecting (1) hydrogen cyanide gas released from inorganic cyanide in biological material and (2) carbon monoxide gas found in fire gases or automobile exhaust.

From "Improved Postmortem Detection of Carbon Monoxide and Cyanide," by Barry K. Logan, Ph.D., in the U.S. Department of Justice, Office of Justice Programs publication, *NIJ Research Preview,* July 1996.

Lethal Effects of Carbon Monoxide and Cyanide

A colorless, odorless gas produced in the combustion of fossil fuels, automobile exhaust vapors, and poorly ventilated gas heating equipment, carbon monoxide is the best known example of an agent that can decrease the oxygen transport capability of blood and prevent oxygen from reaching body tissues in sufficient quantity. Exposure to very high concentrations can result in enough hemoglobin saturation to produce death by asphyxiation in minutes with almost no warning signs.

Cyanide, a common poison, is also a byproduct of the burning of many synthetic polymers and plastics. Cyanide blocks tissue utilization of oxygen and results in abnormally rapid or deep breathing. Cardiac irregularities are often noted, but the heart invariably outlasts the respirations. Death is due to respiratory failure and can occur within seconds or minutes of the inhalation of high concentrations of hydrogen cyanide gas. Because of slower absorption, death may be delayed after the ingestion of cyanide salts but the critical events still occur within the first hour.

Development of an Improved Detection Method

First proposed in 1988, a gas phase electrochemical (GPE) method for detecting and measuring carbon monoxide, although promising, permitted analysis of only a few samples per hour and required full-time attention of the equipment operator. The NIJ-sponsored project improved the GPE method, which involves freeing a sample of either carbon monoxide or cyanide gas from the material examined and introducing the sample into a GPE detection system. Among the advantages of this alternative GPE method:

- Automation of the technique allows speedy analysis so that large numbers of samples can be screened in a relatively short time. Rapid turnaround time (1 minute per sample versus several hours for other approaches) makes the method ideal for the analysis of numerous samples that accident and product-tampering investigations can generate.

- Tests demonstrated that the method was sensitive to concentrations in the range of interest for postmortem material and was free from interference by changes in the substances analyzed.

- Putrefaction of samples did not cause problems for the method, according to test results.

- The technique is applicable to a great variety of solid and semi-solid materials that are incompatible with other methods.

Illustrations of Method's Utility and Effectiveness

Two cases illustrate the utility and effectiveness of the improved GPE technique. In one instance, charred, decomposed remains of a suspected drug dealer were found in a burned trailer. The coroner wanted to determine whether the deceased had been dead before the fire started. Blood samples were not available. The only specimen available for testing was the victim's decomposed liver, which was unsuitable for spectroscopic testing for cyanide. However, the improved GPE method determined that the deceased had been breathing when the fire started, allowing the coroner to rule out foul play.

In another instance, the technology was applied to a wide variety of products suspected of having been targets of product tampering. Traditional testing methods would have required 4 hours for each product sample; the GPE method took minutes.

Such cases, among other evidence, indicates that the improved GPE methodology is a reliable and advantageous alternative to other techniques and promises to become even more so as the method is refined in the years ahead.

— by Barry K. Logan, Ph.D.,
Washington State Toxicology Laboratory,
Department of Laboratory Medicine,
University of Washington

Chapter 43

Gunshot Residue Analysis

Introduction

A procedure is presented that can be used for the analysis of residues generated by the combustion of ammunition and explosives prepared with smokeless gunpowder. The bases of the test are the qualitative and quantitative identification of characteristic organic components present in the post-combustion residues. The residues are collected by adhesive film lift and/or alcohol swabbing of hands, clothing, spent shell casings, and explosive debris, and analyzed using micellar electrokinetic capillary electrophoresis (MECE). The MECE technique provides identification of organic additives in the smokeless powder. The procedure described here may provide positive identification of the use of materials containing smokeless powder.

Purpose

The purpose is to provide evidence in crimes involving the use of firearms and improvised explosive devices (such as pipe bombs), based on the analysis of residues from fired smokeless powder collected from the hands of shooters, clothing, spent shell casings, or explosive remains.

Excerpted from *Smokeless Powder Residue Analysis by Capillary Electrophoresis* (NIJ Report 600-91), a U.S. Department of Justice, Office of Justice Programs publication, by David M. Northrop and William A. MacCrehan, February 1997.

Scope

The test is based on the compositional analysis of gunshot and explosive residues left on surfaces that (1) provide limited interferences from complex matrices such as soil, blood, sweat, etc., and (2) are easily sampled using adhesive film lifts or by swabbing with solvent. Quantitative compositional data on more than 100 commercially available smokeless powders provide the framework for a database for matching purposes. The possible occurrence of characteristic smokeless powder components that could result in false positive tests has been extensively evaluated. Samples were collected from 100 people in the general population to identify interfering components for the MECE analysis. Results obtained by the MECE method are compared to the results obtained by scanning electron microscopy/ energy dispersive x-ray analysis (SEM/EDX). Finally, this procedure is used to evaluate forensic casework samples for the presence and composition of gunpowder residues. MECE analysis of residues left on the hands of a suspect may provide a link to a shooting. The composition of these residues may also provide a link to a weapon.

Definitions

Adhesive film lift. A method used for the collection of gunshot residues from surfaces, such as skin, and clothing. This method uses an adhesive tape to collect the residue. Residues are recovered from the tape by physical removal of visible particles with tweezers, or solvent extraction for microscopic residues.

Capacity factor. An indexing term that allows normalization for random variations in migration times for a given component in multiple MECE analyses. The capacity factor, k, is defined by the following equation:

$$k = \frac{t_r - t_0}{t_0(1 - t_r/t_m)}$$

where t_r is the migration time of a solute, t_o is the migration time for ethanol, which migrates with the electroosmotic flow, and t_m is the migration time for dibutylphthalate (DBP—a compound that moves with the micellar agent).

Capillary electrophoresis (CE). An analytical technique in which chemical compounds are separated based on their relative movement through a conductive liquid (buffer) in a small diameter capillary tube under the influence of a high voltage electric field. Compounds separate as a result of differences in size and positive or negative charge.

Characteristic residue components. These are smokeless powder additives that are good markers for the MECE identification of gunshot residues. These compounds are typically present in amounts greater than 0.1 percent in the unfired powder, can be detected by optical absorbance, and occur in many types of ammunition powders. These may include, but are not limited to, nitroglycerin, dinitrotoluene isomers, diphenylamine, and ethyl centralite. Although alkyl phthalate esters are present in most smokeless powders, they are also present in many plastic and adhesive materials. Therefore the phthlate esters are not suitable for consideration as characteristic components of gunshot residue.

Electroosmotic flow. The bulk flow of buffer towards the detector end of the capillary, caused by electrostatic interactions of the buffer with the charged walls of the capillary under the influence of the high voltage field.

Explosive residue. Traces of material that remain on fragments of an explosive device and/or are deposited on other objects as a result of the detonation of such a device. The sources of these materials are the propellants, stabilizers, and plasticizers used in the explosive device as well as the compounds formed from the decomposition of these materials as a result of detonation.

False positive result. Erroneous identification of characteristic residue components in a sample that by definition should not contain any of these components.

Gunshot residue. Traces of material that remain after the use of a firearm using smokeless gunpowder ammunition. The major sources of these materials are the primer, propellant and associated stabilizers, and plasticizers that are used in ammunition, as well as any decomposition products of these materials formed during detonation.

Micellar electrokinetic capillary electrophoresis (MECE). A CE method in which electrically neutral compounds, not possessing a positive or negative charge, may be separated based on differences in their interaction with a charged micellar agent (such as sodium dodecylsulfate—SDS) added to the buffer. See Figure 43.1.

Micellar Electrokinetic Separation

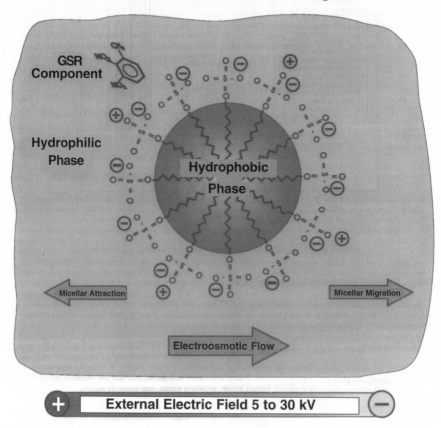

Figure 43.1. *Schematic of MECE Separation*

Migration time (t_m). Unique time required for the electrophoretic movement of a single organic component to travel from the beginning of the capillary to the detector. Using current MECE instruments, small variations in the migration time for a given component occur from test to test as a result of system instability. Computing capacity factors and normalizing to an internal standard substantially eliminates these variations.

Plasticizers in smokeless powders. Organic materials added during manufacture of propellant and explosive mixtures to aid in their fabrication. These materials may include, but are not limited to, short chain aliphatic phthalic acid esters, of which dibutylphthalate is the most common.

Primers. Devices used to initiate the propellant in ammunition, and may consist of a single component or a mixture of various inorganic and organic materials. Primer ingredients may include, but are not limited to, lead azide, lead styphnate, tetracene, diazodinitrophenol, barium nitrate, strontium nitrate, and antimony sulfide.

Propellant components of smokeless powder. Smokeless powder propellants are organic materials that undergo rapid combustion when initiated with a primer. In smokeless gunpowder, the bulk material is nitrocellulose (NC). Propellant materials found in double- and triple-base smokeless gunpowders may also include, but are not limited to, nitroglycerin (NG), nitroguanidine (NGU) (rare in small arms propellants), and the isomers of dinitrotoluene (DNT).

Residue extract. Prepared by taking either an adhesive film lift or collection swab and extracting with an organic solvent to remove the residue.

Scanning electron microscopy/energy dispersive x-ray (SEM/EDX) analysis. SEM is an analytical technique that uses an electron beam to examine microscopic particles. In the SEM/EDX technique, an x-ray detector provides additional information of the chemical composition of selected particles. This technique has been used to identify gunshot residues based on the selective detection of primer compounds containing lead, and/or barium, and/or antimony.

Stabilizers. Organic materials that are added to propellants and explosives to retard their decomposition during storage. These materials may include, but are not limited to, diphenylamine (DPA) and ethyl centralite (EC). Both decomposition and combustion of the propellants result in the formation of nitrated stabilizer derivatives such as N-nitrosodiphenylamine (N-nDPA), 2-nitrodiphenylamine (2-nDPA), and 4-nitrodiphenylamine (4-nDPA).

415

Test Equipment and Analytical Procedures

Residue Collection and Preparation

The MECE test relies on preparing a liquid extract of the fine particles that remain following the use of ammunition and explosives. Both adhesive film lift and swabbing methods can be used for residue collection. Gloves and tweezers rinsed with alcohol are used to handle all materials.

Adhesive lift method. The adhesive material used for sample collection should be a masking-type tape with an adhesive that does not dissolve in alcohol. The tape should be precleaned using methanol in an ultrasonic bath to eliminate any alcohol-soluble material on the tape. Samples are collected by using a 2.5 cm x 2.5 cm section of masking tape held by tweezers and pressed onto the surface to be examined. This method can be adapted for analysis by both SEM/EDX and MECE by using a double-sided masking type adhesive tape placed on an aluminum SEM/EDX sample stub. Samples are then collected by holding the aluminum stub while pressing the adhesive onto the surface to be examined.

Samples from the hands of a suspected shooter should be collected using a separate adhesive lift for both back and palm of each hand. Samples from clothing should be collected using a separate adhesive film lift pressed onto the clothing near any bullet hole or area suspected of being exposed to gunshot residue. All samples are placed in capped vials and refrigerated until analyzed.

A blank sample also should be collected as a part of the crime scene protocol. A blank sample tests both the sample collection and preparation systems for interferences or contamination. To collect a blank sample, an adhesive film lift should be collected from the skin of a suspected shooter in an area that could not be exposed to gunshot residue, e.g., a foot, leg, back, etc. From clothing samples, the blank should be collected from an area of the clothing that could not have been exposed to any gunshot residue. The blank sample should then be tested in the same manner as evidence samples. The following protocols are used for MECE analysis.

Sample preparation for residue samples:

1. Place a 2 mm x 2 mm section of adhesive lift in $50 \mu L$ of methanol

2. Agitate in an ultrasonic bath for 15 min

3. Add 5 μL of ethylene glycol to prevent complete evaporation

4. Evaporate methanol under a stream of dry nitrogen

5. Reconstitute residue in 50 μL of MECE buffer

Sample preparation for unfired powder:

1. Place 0.050 g of powder in 5.00 mL of methanol

2. Agitate in an ultrasonic bath for 15 min

3. Add 5 μL of the methanol extract to 50 μL of MECE buffer

Swab residue collection method. Cotton used for swabbing is precleaned in an ultrasonic bath with high purity ethyl alcohol. Alcohol-cleaned cotton, moistened with ethanol and held with tweezers, is used for swab collection of residues from the surface to be sampled.

Samples are collected from shell casings or debris from improvised explosive devices by swabbing each surface of interest with a separate swab. The swabs are placed in capped glass vials and refrigerated prior to analysis.

As with the adhesive lift method, a blank sample also should be collected for the swab method. A swab should be made of a surface that could not have been contaminated with gunshot residue.

Samples for MECE analysis are prepared as follows:

1. Place swab in 500 μL of ethanol

2. Agitate in an ultrasonic bath for 15 min

3. Add 5 μL of ethylene glycol to prevent complete evaporation

4. Centrifuge sample through a 1 μm fluoropolymer filter

5. Evaporate ethanol under a stream of dry nitrogen

6. Reconstitute residue in 50 μL of MECE buffer.

Residue Generation

Controlled firing range studies were used to generate test residue samples for method validation. Eight handguns, varying from 22 to 45 caliber, with both revolver and semiautomatic mechanisms, were used to generate residues. The hands of the individual firing the weapons are thoroughly washed with soap and water and dried with paper towels before firing. A blank sample is then collected to verify that the hands are free of any residues prior to firing the weapon. This procedure is repeated before each test. Gunshot residues for this test are generated by firing three rounds of commercial ammunition from the test weapon. Examination of gunpowder composition before and after firing is achieved by analysis of unfired powder and the residues generated by firing a single round of commercial ammunition with the same powder through a 15 cm x 15 cm section of sterile 100 percent nylon cloth placed over a white paper target from a distance of about 20 cm (muzzle-to-target distance). These tests are repeated with each weapon and ammunition studied.

Residue Persistence and Component Aging

In casework, it is important to establish how long residues from a particular weapon will persist on the hands or clothing of a shooter after deposition. This persistence may be studied by firing ammunition from the weapon and collecting residues at hourly intervals. In this study, adhesive film lift samples were collected at hourly intervals

Capillary Electrophoresis Instrumentation

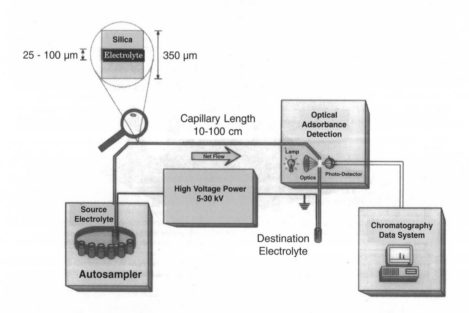

Figure 43.2. Schematic of Capillary Electrophoresis System

from 0 h to 6 h from hands used to fire three rounds from a semiautomatic handgun. Individuals were involved in normal activities during the time period of this study.

In order to simulate the effect of environmental exposure on gunpowder components, bulk gunpowder was placed in glass test tubes, positioned outside in direct sunlight, and sampled every hour for 28 h.

Capillary Electrophoresis Equipment

Commercially available apparatus for capillary electrophoresis, providing controlled voltage to 30 kV and using on-column ultraviolet absorbance detection, is required. A schematic of a typical capillary electrophoresis system is shown in Figure 43.2. The capability to select the exact detection wavelength is required. Wavelength programming or simultaneous multiwavelength detection is advantageous, permitting measurement of component spectra to enhance the certainty of component identification.

Chromatography Data Station

A chromatography data system, capable of precise measurement of peak retention time, peak height and peak area is required. The capability to edit graphically the peak measurements and to overlay multiple sample runs is desirable.

MECE Operating Conditions

The operating conditions used for the MECE analysis are as follows:

- SDS buffer: 10 mmol/L sodium tetraborate decahydrate (adjusted to pH 8.50 with boric acid), 25 mmol/L sodium dodecylsulfate (SDS)

- Sample preparation buffer: SDS buffer with 1x 10^{-4} mol/L 2-naphthol as an internal standard

- Sample injection: samples are injected using pressure injection at 300 Pa (30 mbar) for 1.5 s

- Separation column: 75 μm diameter capillary of 82 cm length with an extended path length optical cell

- Separation voltage: analyses are conducted at 30 kV

- Detection mode: diode array ultraviolet absorbance monitored at 200 nm

Discussion

In this work, the MECE method for use in forensic gunshot residue and explosive cases has been validated by collecting the following information:

1. a reliable and reproducible residue collection and sample preparation protocol has been developed;

2. the minimum detection limits of the characteristic smokeless powder components using the MECE apparatus have been determined;

3. the occurrence of false positive results in the general population was studied and was determined to be unlikely;

4. a database of the composition of more than 100 commercially available smokeless powders has been generated;

5. the persistence of characteristic residue components on sample surfaces and the loss of residues from the shooter's hands over time has been investigated;

6. changes in characteristic residue component composition resulting from environmental exposure have been determined;

7. multiple firings of two weapons were performed to determine if residues would be deposited each time a given weapon was fired;

8. MECE analysis of firing range samples was compared to those obtained using SEM; and,

9. casework samples were examined using both the MECE method and SEM/EDX.

Residue Collection and Sample Preparation

Adhesive film lifts, as evidenced by this study, provide a reliable method for sample collection of gunshot residues from the hands of individuals who have fired a weapon and from clothing. The adhesive used for the film lift must be evaluated for method interferences by extraction using the residue protocol and analysis by MECE before being used for collection.

Adhesives that do not dissolve in methanol must be used. Various commercially available solvent resistant masking tapes (both single- and

420

double-sided tapes) are most likely to meet these requirements. The double-sided tape may be used on a SEM/EDX sample holding aluminum stub so that gunshot residue samples can be collected for both MECE and SEM/EDX. This is the collection method of choice.

Alcohol swab collection can be used to recover residues from spent cartridges and bomb fragments. However, it was found that recovery of characteristic residue components from cotton swabs is less than 50 percent using solvent extraction. Swabbing is not suitable for residue collection from the bands since the alcohol recovers large quantities of fats and oils from the skin that can interfere with quantitative residue recovery and analysis.

Ultrasonic agitation of residues in methanol for 15 min was found to be sufficient to completely extract the characteristic residue components from gunpowder. This was determined by performing a second extract on all commercial gunpowders examined. Negligible quantities of the components were detected in the second extract. An evaluation of solvents found that methanol was more efficient than ethanol as a residue extraction agent. The addition of ethylene glycol, when used at a volume fraction of 5 percent, was found to prevent losses of the residue constituents during the evaporative concentration of the extract, and did not alter the quantitative analysis by MECE.

Minimum Detection Limits

The minimum detection limits for gunshot residue constituents using four commercially available CE instruments were found to be in the picogram mass range using the MECE method. Detection limits were approximately 1 pg to 2 pg for the components with aromatic functionalities and 4 pg for nitroglycerin. Future improvements in detection technology may improve the sensitivity of the test.

Interferences and False Positives

Using the outlined protocols and MECE analysis, no false positive tests for the characteristic residue components were found on the adhesive film lifts from the hands of 100 volunteers representing a wide variety of occupational backgrounds. The individuals sampled included law enforcement officers, mechanics, teachers, construction workers, farmers, chemists, secretaries, and many other professions. The sample group included men, women, right-handed, left-handed, employed, and unemployed individuals, as well as people with visibly clean hands and dirty hands. No peaks were identified with capacity factors that match any of the characteristic residue components.

All blank samples collected during this study were also found to be negative for the characteristic residue components. Hand washing with soap and water was determined to effectively remove all MECE-detectable residue components.

These results indicate that the identification of the characteristic residue components by MECE can only occur if an individual has been exposed to a recently fired weapon. False positive results because of occupational duties or environmental exposure were not found to occur.

Gunpowder Identification

In order to provide evidence to identify a gunpowder or its residues, including the type of propellant, manufacturer, and lot, it is necessary to identify and quantitate the characteristic components of both the residues and the unfired powder. In determining a match between a residue sample and unfired powder, it is also necessary to take into account any chemical compositional changes that may result from the firing of the gunpowder.

Factors to be considered in matching of smokeless powders. There are several factors that need to be considered in the identification of a smokeless powder or residue sample based on matching known and unknown materials. In a matching study of the residue composition of 17 smokeless powders before and after firing, clear matches were not always obtained. The matching criteria consisted of a qualitative test and a quantitative test. Both tests had to be satisfied for a match to be obtained. The qualitative test identified the characteristic residue components in the residue and compared them to the components in the unfired gunpowder. The quantitative test compared the measured value of each component in the residue to the measured value of those components in the unfired powder. For this exercise, a match was considered to be achieved if the relative amount of a component in the residue was within one standard deviation of the measured value of that component in the unfired powder. In this test, residues obtained from 5 of the 17 powders met this match criteria, while 12 of the powders did not. In addition, multiple subsamples from the same residue gave significantly different quantitative results. Therefore, there may be a number of factors that need to be considered in interpreting the results.

Some of the factors that should be considered in comparing pre- and post-firing composition are:

1. nonuniformity in the manufactured composition of the unfired powder;

2. nonuniformity in the individual residue particles collected;

3. nonuniformity resulting from changes in composition from burning or partial burning of the gunpowder;

4. nonuniformity from changes in composition that may result from environmental exposure; and,

5. nonuniformity resulting from the use of different ammunition in the same weapon.

The relative contribution of each of these 5 factors to the interpretation of matches between known and unknown materials has yet to be determined.

Persistence of Residues After Firing

The persistence of post-firing residues on shooters' hands was studied to evaluate the effect of normal activity on the MECE test results. The residues from a weapon discharged at a firing range were studied to examine residue persistence. Samples were collected immediately after the weapon was fired (time zero), and test samples were taken to correspond to hourly collections up to 6 h. One hour after firing, no residues were found on any of the subjects. Subsequent samples at 2 h to 6 h also were found to be negative for gunshot residues. Initial residues (at time zero) were at low concentrations, thus it is possible that weapons that deposit higher concentrations of residues may result in longer residue persistence. As discussed previously, all residues can be deliberately removed from the hands by washing with soap and water.

Based on this experiment, residues found on the hands of a suspect are a clear indication that a weapon has been fired or handled within a short period of time prior to the collection of the sample. These results also indicate that sampling for gunshot residues from the hands must occur as soon as possible. A suspect that is not captured until several hours after a shooting is not likely to be found to have residues present on his/her hands at that time, as determined by the MECE test.

423

Clothing was found to retain residues for a long period after firing. Residues may persist for days, weeks or months if the clothing is not washed or involved in significant frictional contact with other objects.

Environmental Exposure and Residue Decomposition

Changes in the chemical composition of a given gunpowder might be expected to occur over time, particularly when exposed to heat and/or light. However, when an unfired powder was exposed to direct summer conditions over a 28 h period, no significant change was found in the measured value of the following characteristic gunpowder components: NG, 2,4-DNT, DPA, N-nDPA, 2-nDPA, and 4-nDPA. Although unfired powder composition appeared to be unchanged in this simple experiment, the decomposition of the characteristic components when deposited as residues might be expected to be more rapid. We evaluated whether this compositional change could be used to provide an estimate of the time of firing.

Samples of post-firing residues on cloth targets obtained by point blank firing of a handgun were stored in the laboratory and examined over a 2-month period of time. Residue composition immediately after firing, in some cases, was different from the unburned powder and varied from sample to sample as determined by replicate analyses, as noted previously. Very slow loss of nitroglycerin was seen over the 2 months of the study. However, the measured variation in composition is similar in magnitude to the particle-to-particle variability both of unfired gunpowder particles and collected residue particles. Thus, a determination of when a weapon was discharged based on the change in residue composition does not appear to be possible. The decomposition rate is too slow relative to the measurement uncertainty.

Frequency of Residue Deposition

In cases where a positive MECE test for gunshot residues is obtained, it is a strong implication that the individual has been exposed recently to a discharged weapon. We evaluated the frequency of positive MECE test results by firing two weapons. Multiple firings were made using two different 9 mm semiautomatic weapons. Each weapon was fired multiple times with each hand. The first weapon, a Mac 9, has an ejection port on the right side of the weapon. The second weapon, a Walther P38, has an ejection port on the top of the weapon.

Samples collected from the Mac 9 were positive for gunshot residues 53 percent of the time when the weapon was fired with the right hand and 20 percent of the time when fired [with] the left hand. Samples collected from the Walther P38 were positive for gunshot residues 93 percent of the time when the weapon was fired with the right hand and 71 percent of the time when fired [with] the left hand.

These results indicate that, even in controlled conditions, detectable gunshot residues may not be deposited on the hands of the shooter every time the weapon is fired. Deposition may be dependent on the caliber of weapon, type of weapon (e.g., semiautomatic versus revolver, etc.), configuration of ejection port, mechanical condition of the weapon, how clean the weapon is, the ammunition composition, completeness of the ammunition combustion, wind conditions, perhaps weapon temperature, random trajectories of residue particles, and which hand the shooter used to fire the weapon. Thus, a negative residue test does not prove that a weapon was not fired.

MECE Analysis Versus SEM/EDX Analysis

If MECE analysis is to augment the current technology for gunshot residue detection, it is necessary to compare the results obtained by MECE to those obtained using SEM/EDX on the same sample. Firing range samples examined using both MECE and SEM/EDX were found to be positive for gunshot residues by both methods. Some samples found to be positive by SEM/EDX were found to be negative by MECE. However, all samples that were positive by MECE were positive by SEM/EDX. Some false positive SEM/EDX results were obtained on blank samples. Since multiple firings were conducted by the same volunteer, it was assumed that hand washing would remove the inorganic residues as efficiently as the organic residues. This was not always the case with all blank samples. The false negative MECE results obtained on these identical samples could be caused by a difference in the quantities of inorganic versus organic residues. However, the most important result is that no false positive results were obtained by MECE analysis, and SEM/EDX analysis confirmed the positive results.

Casework Results

MECE and SEM/EDX has been conducted simultaneously on samples collected from the hands of individuals suspected of having fired a weapon in seven criminal investigations. No gunshot residues were conclusively identified by MECE in any of these cases. However, SEM/EDX analysis has conclusively identified gunshot residues in two of these cases. MECE analysis in one of those cases suggested the presence of nitroglycerin, but at quantities too small to confirm. The negative MECE results for the five other cases were confirmed by SEM/EDX. This would indicate that the organic gunshot residues were either not deposited, or were not present at high enough concentrations to be detected.

MECE analysis has been performed on a total of 16 samples from two cases involving the examination of clothing for the presence of gunshot residues. Gunshot residues were conclusively identified in seven of the samples from these cases using MECE analysis. SEM/EDX analysis of the samples confirmed the presence of gunshot residues on five of these samples and three additional samples that were negative by the MECE method. The results on five of the samples were the same using both MECE and SEM/EDX analysis. However, three samples were positive by SEM/EDX and negative by MECE, and two samples were positive by MECE and negative by SEM/EDX.

Conclusion

The results of this research suggest that MECE analysis is a valid analytical method for gunshot residue analysis. MECE analysis has been achieved on adhesive film lifts from hands and clothing, and these same lifts are compatible for SEM/EDX of the inorganic residues. Risk of false positive tests from occupational exposure to characteristic residue components does not appear to be a concern. Positive MECE results are not always obtained when a weapon is fired. This could be due to a number of factors, including low efficiency of residue deposition, low residue persistence, and lack of sensitivity of the MECE test. Recoverable residues do not appear to persist on skin for more than an hour. Thus, residues must be collected immediately from skin. However, residues on clothing are stable for a long period of time. Quantitative analysis for the purpose of generating a "chemical fingerprint" to match residues to known gunpowders must be interpreted with great care. Compositional variations of unfired and fired gunpowder particles has been noted. However, the presence or absence of components may provide valuable information for the inclusion or exclusion of an ammunition type or manufacturer. Residue decomposition over time resulting from environmental exposure is slow compared to the time that residues persist on samples. Thus, time of firing information cannot be obtained from quantitative analysis of the residues.

Sample preparation and analysis can be achieved in about 2 h per case. Qualitative and quantitative information is generated concerning the characteristic organic constituents in gunshot residues. The cost of instrumentation is four to five times less than the cost of an SEM/EDX system. MECE analysis does provide a rapid and complementary analytical tool for gunshot residue analysis.

References

Northrop, D. M., D. E. Martire, and W. A. MacCrehan. "Separation and Identification of Organic Gunshot and Explosive Constituents by Micellar Electrokinetic Capillary Electrophoresis." *Analytical Chemistry* 63: 1038-42 (1991).

Northrop, D. M. Ph.D. thesis, Georgetown University, 1991.

Northrop, D. M., and W. A. MacCrehan. "Sample Collection, Preparation, and Quantitation in the Micellar Electrokinetic Capillary Electrophoresis of Gunshot Residues." *Journal of Liquid Chromatography* 15 (6): 1041-63 (1992).

Northrop, D. M., B. R. McCord, and J. M. Butler. "Forensic Applications of Capillary Electrophoresis." *Journal of Capillary Electrophoresis* 1 (2): 158-68 (1994).

— by David M. Northrop and William A. MacCrehan

David Northrop is employed by the Washington State Patrol Crime Laboratory in Kennewick, Washington. William A. MacCrehan is employed by the Chemical Science and Technology Laboratory, Analytical Chemistry Division, National Institute of Standards and Technology in Gaithersburg, Maryland.

Chapter 44

Condom Trace Evidence

In an age filled with potentially fatal sexually transmitted diseases, more and more individuals practice safe sex. Even perpetrators of sex crimes have begun to wear condoms.[1] It is not likely that a fear of disease prompts this behavior. Rather, just as a burglar dons gloves to avoid leaving fingerprints, sexual offenders now wear condoms to avoid depositing seminal fluids.

Forensic experts typically identify sexual assault offenders by examining seminal fluid residues for sperm, proteins, blood grouping factors, and DNA profile. When sexual assailants use condoms, however, assuming no leaks or spills, this valuable evidence gets trapped inside the condom, which investigators may never recover. The same can be said for any traces from the victim—including vaginal cells, blood, and saliva—that otherwise might have been transferred to the assailant's penis. Nevertheless, when assailants use condoms, they leave behind other valuable evidence.

Types of Condom Trace Evidence

Manufacturers produce condoms using a variety of materials, both natural and synthetic. Each manufacturer has its own formula, which may vary even among its different brands.

From "Condom Trace Evidence: A New Factor in Sexual Assault Investigations," by Robert D. Blackledge, M.S., in the FBI *Law Enforcement Bulletin,* May 1996.

Some condoms are made from lamb membranes, and one manufacturer recently introduced a model made from polyurethane plastic. Still, latex rubber condoms have, by far, the largest share of the market, perhaps because they cost considerably less. In addition to the basic materials they use to produce condoms, manufacturers also add other substances, known as exchangeable traces, which comprise particulates, lubricants, and spermicide.

Particulates

Condom manufacturers add finely powdered particulates to prevent a rolled-up latex condom from sticking to itself. Particulates found in different brands include corn starch, potato starch, lycopodium (a powder found in plants), as well as amorphous silica, talc, or other minerals. In the laboratory, forensic scientists use several different techniques to characterize these particles and compare them with those obtained from other condom brands.

Lubricants

Sexual assailants prefer lubricated condoms, probably for the same reason that they use petroleum jelly, that is, to facilitate their crimes.[2] Many condom brands contain a liquid lubricant, which may be classified as either "wet" or "dry."

Both types of condom lubricant have an oil-like consistency, but wet lubricants are water-based and/or water-soluble, while dry lubricants are not. Although many different manufacturers use the same dry lubricant, their viscosity grades sometimes differ. The forensic laboratory can recover these silicone oils easily from items of evidence and possibly associate them with a condom manufacturer.

Wet lubricants may contain either polyethylene glycol or a gel made from a combination of ingredients similar to those found in vaginal lubricants. Despite similarities to other products on the market, forensic examination can associate specific formulations with particular condom brands.

Spermicide

Both wet- and dry-lubricated condoms also may contain the spermicide nonoxynol-9. Its recovery and detection, along with lubricant ingredients and particulates, can help show condom use and indicate the specific brand.

The Value of Condom Trace Evidence

Condom trace evidence can assist investigators in several ways. It can help prove corpus delicti, provide evidence of penetration, produce associative evidence, and link the acts of serial rapists.

In Proving Corpus Delicti

Traces associated with condoms can help prove corpus delicti, the fact that a crime has occurred. This evidence can support the claims of either the victim or the accused. For example, the U.S. military can prosecute personnel diagnosed as HIV-positive for aggravated assault if they engage in unprotected sex, even if it is consensual. If service men accused of aggravated assault claim that they did in fact wear a condom but it broke or slipped off, condom trace evidence can support that claim.

In Providing Evidence of Penetration

Condom traces found inside a victim can provide evidence of penetration. In many jurisdictions, this evidence raises the charge to a higher degree of sexual assault.

In Producing Associative Evidence

Recovered condom traces may correspond to those found in a certain brand or used by a certain manufacturer. An empty packet of this particular brand found near the crime scene, especially if it bears the suspect's fingerprints, provides a strong association between the suspect and the crime. Unopened condom packages of this same brand found on the suspect, in his car, or at his residence also would help tie the suspect to the crime.

In Linking the Acts of Serial Rapists

People tend to be creatures of habit, and sexual criminals are no exception. A serial rapist likely will use the same brand of condom to commit repeated acts. Moreover, repeat offenders whose DNA profiles have been stored in a computer data bank may be likely to use a condom when committing subsequent crimes. Along with other aspects of his modus operandi, traces from the same condom brand or manufacturer found during several different investigations can help connect a suspect to an entire series of assaults.

431

Guidance for Evidence Collection

Investigators need not make any drastic changes in their usual procedures in order to include the possibility of condom trace evidence. The following guidelines will assist criminal investigators and medical examiners when collecting this valuable evidence.[3]

At the Crime Scene

First and foremost, investigators must wear powder-free gloves to protect themselves from bloodborne pathogens and to avoid leaving particulates that may be similar to those contained in some condom brands. After collecting the evidence, they should package the gloves separately and submit them with the evidence so that the forensic laboratory can verify that the gloves did not leave behind any particulates.

At the crime scene, investigators should make every effort to locate any used condom and its foil package. If a condom is recovered, the traces from the victim on the outside and the seminal fluids from the assailant on the inside would have the greatest evidentiary value.

If investigators find an empty condom packet, they first should try to recover any latent prints from the outside. The inside of the package probably will not contain prints, but may contain lubricant, spermicide, and particulate residues. Investigators should wipe the inside with a clean cotton swab. The traces on this swab will serve as the standard for comparison with traces recovered from the victim and the suspect.

During Medical Examinations

Examination kits. Most commercial sexual assault examination kits provide two cotton swabs for each type of examination, i.e., vaginal, penile, etc. In the past, before assailants began using condoms frequently, these two swabs proved adequate—one swab for immediate examination and a second in case the defense team requested another examination by its own experts or by an independent laboratory. With sexual offender's using condoms, however, forensic laboratories should use three swabs: One to save for the defense and two to conduct examinations.

With the potential for positively identifying a suspect, most laboratories first look for traces of seminal fluids, vaginal cells, blood, and the like. Unfortunately, the solvents used to conduct this examination also remove any condom traces present, thus losing potentially valuable evidence. Although examiners feasibly could divide each

432

swab in half, providing an additional swab in kits for each condom trace examination easily could solve the problem.

The gloves provided in commercial examination kits usually come powder-free. However, the medical personnel who examine sexual offenders and their victims frequently prefer the gloves they normally wear, which often contain the same powders (corn starch, amorphous silica, and talc) found on many condom brands. While medical staff members may insist that their collection procedures are above reproach, forensic examiners cannot guarantee the integrity of the condom trace evidence if the medical staff wears their own gloves. In short, investigators must persuade examining personnel to wear unpowdered gloves.

After the medical examinations, investigators should recover and separately package the used gloves. The forensic laboratory then can confirm that the gloves were powder-free.

Examination of victims. Victims of sexual assault may feel ashamed and may not want to disclose some of the more personal details of the crime. Although investigators should make every effort to spare victims any unnecessary discomfort or embarrassment, they must ensure a thorough investigation. This may mean asking victims embarrassing questions and then making sure that medical examiners obtain samples from any area of the victim's body where evidence may exist, including the vagina, the mouth, and the anus.

In addition to collecting traces from inside the victim's vagina, medical examiners should swab the external genitalia. Traces of water-soluble condom lubricants may have been absorbed or lost, and as a result, any traces found internally may be at a very low level. Thus, if the victim has not showered or bathed, swabs may recover undiluted traces present on the external genitalia. Although these traces would not indicate penetration, they at least would support the victim's assertion that sexual contact took place.

Moistening each swab with a few drops of isopropyl alcohol helps recover traces from external genitalia. To create control swabs for the forensic laboratory, investigators should moisten two unused swabs, allow them to air-dry, and then package them with the evidence. Examining these control swabs will confirm that any traces found on the victim did not come from the cotton swabs or the alcohol.

At the lab, forensic experts first examine the victim's swabs. If these swabs are negative for seminal fluids but show traces of condom evidence, examiners would then look for the same traces on the suspect's swabs.

Examination of suspects. If investigators identify and arrest a suspect only a few hours after the alleged assault, medical personnel should examine him promptly. If a suspect has not washed his penis, identifiable traces (either from a condom or from the victim) may be present. Examiners should moisten two swabs with two drops of isopropyl alcohol, then wipe the penis from the base to the tip. As they did when collecting evidence from the victim, examiners should prepare two control swabs.

Interviews

With the Victim

In addition to providing general information about the crime, victims may be able to supply valuable details about the condom and its wrapper. They may recall the brand itself or other important details, including the condom's color, shape, texture, odor, taste, and lubrication. After obtaining facts about the condom, investigators should ask victims about their sexual and hygienic habits, which might account for traces not attributable to the crime. A comprehensive interview would include the following questions:

- Has the victim recently engaged in consensual sex?

- If so, was a condom used? A vaginal lubricant? What brands?

- Does the victim use any external or internal vaginal products (anti-itch medications, deodorants, douches, suppositories, etc.)?

- If so, what brands?

These questions assume an adult female victim. Investigators must modify the interview to accommodate male or child sexual assault victims.

With the Suspect(s)

Investigators also should question the suspect about the condom. A cooperative, honest suspect can reveal the brand, tell where he purchased it, and describe how and where he disposed of both the condom and the empty packet. An uncooperative or deceitful suspect may claim he does not know or cannot remember, or he may name a popular brand but will not be able to describe the condom or the packet in detail.

Legal Considerations

When investigators know or suspect that a sexual offender used a condom, they must remember to list condoms on the warrant obtained to search the suspect's possessions. The search of a suspect's home may reveal intact condom packets, but if investigators have not listed condoms on the search warrant, they will not be able to seize this valuable evidence.

Conclusion

When sexual assailants wear condoms to commit their crimes, they attempt to protect themselves from disease and apprehension at the same time. Although these crimes become more difficult to solve, investigators should not overlook the evidentiary potential of condom traces. By considering the possibility of condom use while processing the crime scene, supervising medical examinations, and conducting interviews, investigators can ensure that this valuable evidence receives the attention it deserves.

Notes

1. In 80 sexual assault cases submitted to the Forensic Laboratory of the Las Vegas Metropolitan Police Department between 9/10/93 and 12/3/93, 19 victims reported that the assailant or one of several assailants had worn a condom during the assault or that a consensual sexual partner had used a condom within 72 hours preceding the incident. Eight additional victims believed that their assailant might have used a condom. Terry L. Cook, criminalist, Forensic Laboratory, Las Vegas Metropolitan Police Department, telephone conversation with the author, December 6, 1993.

2. R. D. Blackledge and L. R. Cabiness, "Examination for Petroleum Based Lubricants in Evidence from Rapes and Sodomies," *Journal of Forensic Sciences* 28: 451-62 (1983).

3. R. D. Blackledge, "Collection and Identification Guidelines for Traces from Latex Condoms in Sexual Assault Cases," *Crime Laboratory Digest* 21: 57-61 (1994).

— by Robert D. Blackledge, M.S.

Robert Blackledge is senior chemist at the Naval Criminal Investigative Service Regional Forensic Laboratory in San Diego, California.

Chapter 45

Integrated Automated Fingerprint Identification System

The Integrated Automated Fingerprint Identification System (IAFIS)—the new-generation system being developed to support the electronic capture, submission, processing, matching, and storage of fingerprints received by the FBI—will replace the current automated system known as Identification Automated Services (IDAS). Currently, IDAS supports the National Crime Information Center by searching the Interstate Identification Index (III) for criminals by physical and biographic data such as name, FBI number, and Social Security number; it also supports the current 10-print identification system.

IAFIS will provide five major services to local, state, and federal law enforcement and criminal justice agencies:

- *Ten-Print-Based Identification Services.* City-, county-, or state-level fingerprint data acquired as a result of an arrest or for employment and licensing will be electronically forwarded to a state or federal agency processing center; for most cases, it will then be electronically transmitted through the CJIS Wide-Area Network (WAN) to the FBI for processing by IAFIS. The results will be returned electronically to the originator. Ten-print cards received by mail will be scanned and converted to an electronic format for use in the IAFIS environment.

From "Integrated Automated Fingerprint Identification System: 21st Century Technology for Law Enforcement," by Kimberley Smith, in *The Police Chief,* May 1998, p. 14. Reprinted with permission.

- *Latent Fingerprint Services.* IAFIS will provide users with case investigation and image identification services. Latent prints, photos, and negatives will be electronically transmitted to and processed by IAFIS. Additionally, IAFIS will support the processing of hard-copy latent prints and evidence through the Latent Fingerprint Section.

- *Subject Search and Criminal History Services.* IAFIS will respond to requests to search the criminal history file for both known and unknown subjects and associated criminal history information based on the subject's name, date of birth, and other descriptive information. Searches of the criminal history file will determine whether one or more subjects meeting the search criteria have criminal records and will return appropriate responses to the user.

- *Document and Image Services.* IAFIS will support requests to update criminal history files, post disposition notices as a follow-up to arrest charges, purge data from a subject's record, and retrieve an individual's personal criminal history. Users may request images of fingerprints and photos stored in IAFIS to assist in their own subject identification process. Users may also submit fingerprint images that are candidates for upgrading a subject's fingerprint images stored in IAFIS files. Requests may be submitted electronically, as hard copy, or on machine-readable media.

- *Remote Search Services.* IAFIS will support electronically submitted images and features for 10-print and latent remote fingerprint search requests from local, state, and federal law enforcement users. IAFIS will automatically search the fingerprint features files for possible matches with the fingerprint features submitted in a remote search request. Possible candidates and images will be returned electronically to the requesting agency that will perform the fingerprint comparisons. Images of the top-ranked candidate will be returned with the request, as well as the FBI numbers for other possible candidates. Remote searches will not require intervention by FBI personnel and will be available 24 hours a day, seven days a week.

Scheduled to be implemented in 1999, IAFIS will provide enhanced system capabilities, improved reliability, and rapid response times. When fully operational, there will be a two-hour turnaround on electronically submitted criminal print search requests and a 24-hour turnaround on all other criminal and civil submissions.

IAFIS will support a paperless environment. Users will be able to submit requests electronically, via magnetic media or in hardcopy form (fingerprint cards). IAFIS will convert incoming fingerprint cards to digital images before processing. However, the ultimate goal is to move all fingerprint processing to an electronic environment as soon as possible. This includes beginning the process by capturing the fingerprints using a certified live-scan device. Local agencies are encouraged to begin preparing for this by procuring a certified live-scan device compatible with the state system through which they submit fingerprints. To support the electronic environment, national standards have been established for fingerprints, facial imaging, and transmission, and are listed below:

- Data format for the interchange of fingerprint information (ANSI/NIST-CSL 1-1993)

- Electronic Fingerprint Transmission Specification (EFTS)(CJIS-RS-0010 v6)

- IAFIS Image Quality Specifications (EFTS Appx. F) (CJIS-RS-0010 v6)

- Interim IAFIS Image-Quality Specifications for Scanners (EFTS Appx. G) (CJIS-RS-0010 v6)

- Wavelet Scalar Quantization Grayscale Fingerprint Image Compression Specification (IAFIS-IC-0110 v3 December 19,1997).

FBI/CJIS personnel are available to provide information on IAFIS to local, state, and federal law enforcement agencies. For additional information on IAFIS, please visit the FBI's Internet Home Page at www.fbi.gov.

—by Kimberley Smith, Management Analyst, FBI,
Criminal Justice Information Services Division,
Clarksburg, West Virginia.

Chapter 46

The Electronic Signature

With the growing dependence on computers to perform all types of laboratory tasks—from sample log-in to reporting—the issues surrounding the integrity, accuracy, and authenticity of electronic records and signatures and the ability to validate those data effectively have come to the fore.

The U.S. Food and Drug Administration (FDA) has been wrestling with the issue of electronic alternatives for handwritten records and signatures since computers first entered the laboratory. From the lab's perspective, stopping a task in mid-stride whenever data are being updated to print out a copy, sign that copy, file it manually, and then continue with the task adds needless paperwork, slows productivity, and defeats the purpose of computers. From FDA's perspective, personal computers are anything but personal, and electronic data can too easily be changed accidentally or intentionally, without the proper authority or audit trail for validation purposes.

In 1991, FDA created a task force called the Electronic Identification/Signature Working Group to determine how to accommodate paperless record systems under the current Good Manufacturing Practice (GMP) regulations. On 20 March 1997, the final rule on electronic records, signatures, and submissions—known as 21 Code of Federal Regulations (CFR), Part 11[1]—was signed. It became effective 20 August, five months after publication in the Federal Register.

Reprinted with permission from *Today's Chemist at Work,* Vol. 6, No. 10, pp. 15-16, 18-19, November 1997, "The Electronic John Hancock," by Helen Gillespie. © 1997 by the American Chemical Society.

Paper vs. Electronic

The central issues surrounding electronic records and signatures hinge on the validation of such data. Validation of a laboratory procedure, method, record, or data of any kind requires that several points be addressed, including the existence of a process definition, documentation, demonstration of fitness for use, and provision for maintenance. Simply stating that a person is authorized to change a record and having that person sign off on the change is inadequate. There are numerous differences between paper and electronic record technologies that must be addressed before an electronic system can be validated.

For instance, electronic records are culled from information databases. Such databases are dynamic. The content changes as new information is added; therefore, the electronic records contained in information databases are transient views rather than static entities. In addition, all database software is slightly different, in how it is programmed and in how it operates. Depending on the way the software is written, it is possible to misrepresent the database information when performing certain operations (e.g., similar queries can provide different answers). Worse, database elements can easily be changed at any time without evidence that a change was made and in a manner that destroys the original information.

Electronic signatures face similar issues. It is much more difficult to falsify a paper signature and easier to detect when this has happened than it is to falsify an electronic one. In addition, paper signatures cannot be borrowed or loaned, whereas an electronic one can. These issues do not arise in paper-based systems. Therefore, additional controls are necessary for electronic signatures.

The Final Rule

According to the FDA:[1]

> The final rule provides criteria under which FDA will consider electronic records to be equivalent to paper records, and electronic signatures equivalent to traditional handwritten signatures. Part 11 applies to any paper records required by statute or agency regulations and supersedes any existing paper record requirements by providing that electronic records may be used in lieu of paper records. Electronic signatures which meet the requirements of the rule will be considered to be equivalent to

full handwritten signatures, initials, and other general signings required by agency regulations.

The rule provides the additional controls necessary to ensure the integrity, accuracy, and authenticity of system operations and information stored in the systems. In particular, the issue of security was addressed. FDA is mainly concerned with control—not only of the data in the system, but also of the system and access to the system—and set forth certain stipulations. System access must be limited to authorized individuals. Operational system checks must be performed regularly. Database information must provide time- and date-stamped audit trails. Access to the database search software must be limited. The type of security required also depends on the type of system being used and whether that system is open or closed.

Security Factor

Electronic signatures are a significant factor in the security of the system. Hence, according to the rule,[1] the electronic signature must be backed up with documentation that includes:

> the printed name of the signer, the date and time the signature was executed, and the activity (such as review, approval, responsibility, and authorship) associated with the signature. In addition, electronic and handwritten signatures executed to electronic records must be linked to their respective records so that signatures cannot be excised, copied, or otherwise transferred to falsify an electronic record by ordinary means.

Because of these security concerns, electronic signatures must be unique. Unique signatures comprise more than just different usernames and passwords. The reuse or reassignment of electronic signatures to someone other than the original user must also be taken into consideration. In a forensic laboratory, for instance, officers may be assigned electronic signatures based on their badge numbers rather than their names. If an officer retires or a badge number is reassigned, the previous owner must not be confused with the current owner. The same criteria apply to any other laboratory.

Because electronic signatures can often be guessed easily, FDA included requirements to guard against this occurrence. Each signature must consist of more than just a password, and passwords must be unique. It is not acceptable for people to use passwords associated with their personal lives, such as the names of their children or pets. And passwords need to be changed frequently. FDA believes that without such precautions, the possibility of a password being compromised and of impersonation and/or falsification continuing as long as the password is valid is greatly increased. These parameters are more awkward than difficult to accommodate.

Despite the stringency of FDA requirements, any number of electronic signature technologies may be used so long as the conditions of the rule are satisfied. These technologies range from identification codes used in conjunction with manually entered passwords to more sophisticated biometric systems.

Biometric Devices

The final rule allows for the use of a wide variety of electronic record technologies—the most popular being biometric devices. Biometrics is the method of verifying an individual's identity based on measurement of physical features or repeatable actions that are unique to that individual. Biometric devices use one or more biometric parameters to identify the individual. These devices include palm-print readers, fingerprint readers, iris scanners, and retinal-pattern scanners. They are connected, usually by direct wire or network, to the system that requires authentication and are typically placed next to the computer. Biometric devices verify identification by comparing patterns presented by the individual at the time of verification with stored patterns obtained from the authorized user under controlled circumstances. Most of these devices are easily adapted to a variety of situations. For instance, iris scanners are already being used by Japanese banks to authenticate users of automatic teller machines.

When biometric devices are used for electronic signatures, the electronic signature must be designed in such a way that it cannot be used by anyone other than the genuine owner. Some devices integrate biometric signature capture with cryptographic technology that binds signatures with time and date stamps to documents. Some biometric-based electronic signature systems use dynamic signature verification with a parameter code recorded on magnetic-strip cards. These biometric devices are effective and meet the provisions set forth in the final rule, but they can be expensive, particularly when there are many system users.

Despite the complexity of the requirements, FDA does not establish numerical standards for levels of security or validation. This flexibility allows industry to determine what level is appropriate for a particular situation. Furthermore, although the rule requires operational checks, authority checks, and periodic testing of identifying devices, organizations have the flexibility to use any suitable method to accomplish these tasks. And, in situations in which the final rule calls for a particular control, such as periodic testing of identification tokens, organizations can determine the frequency.

Implementation

Laboratories that have implemented a laboratory information management system (LIMS) have already set the foundation for validating electronic records and signatures in accordance with Part 11, although industry manufacturers are modifying their products to conform to the final rule more precisely.

Instrument manufacturer Beckman Instruments (Allendale, NJ) recently announced the inclusion of electronic signature functionality that meets the requirements of Part 11 in a version 8.4 update for its LIMS and chromatography data systems. "It provides the ability to reidentify who the operator is at the workstation prior to a major operation being committed, such as updating something, validating results, or releasing a sample," states Bob Voelkner, worldwide tactical marketing manager for Beckman. "It confirms that the name in the database matches the operator who performs the function. The system administrator has the ability to configure where and when this confirmation takes place. Biometric devices can be used, but old-fashioned keyboard entry works well."

The R&D laboratory for the electronic materials division (EMD) of Morton International (Chicago) addressed electronic signatures through its document control system, which is connected to its LIMS. "FDA is concerned that someone walking by a desk could alter data in the system," remarks Phil Lofty, scientist at EMD. "Of course, anyone who did would be fired. However, FDA wanted to ensure that whenever data were changed they were approved 'contemporaneously'—their favorite word. This means that at the time you commit the data, there's a pop-up box that requires the username and password to be re-input in order for the change to take place."

Whether accessing such electronic signature functionality on or through the LIMS, most systems have yet to pass an FDA audit. Beckman Instruments worked closely with its customers to implement an electronic signature solution. "Our customers believe that they can defend it and that FDA will OK it," Voelkner emphasizes. "And, most importantly, this function can be validated," he adds.

SAP AG (Walldorf, Germany), a well-known developer of enterprise solutions, will be implementing an electronic signature solution in much the same way as Beckman Instruments has. With various industry players addressing the issue in similar ways, there's no doubt that such solutions will soon be commonplace.

What's Next

The newly effective 21 CFR Part 11 does not require, but rather permits, the use of electronic records and signatures, so the initial financial impact will be minimal because any company already in compliance with FDA regulations remains in compliance. However, the opportunity is now available for modifying certain electronic practices in ways that enhance productivity.

Indeed, there are many benefits to using validatable electronic records and electronic signatures in the lab. These benefits include increased speed of information exchange, reduced costs for storage space, reduced numbers of errors, streamlined manufacturing processes, and improved process control. In addition, there are advantages to using electronic systems over paper systems, including the ability to search a database for information; view information from multiple perspectives; determine trends, patterns, and behaviors easily; and avoid the potential for misfiled documents. In fact, these benefits and advantages are expected to offset any system modification costs required to achieve compliance.

However, these same benefits might not offset the costs of implementing biometric solutions. Originally, FDA was going to make biometric devices mandatory," recalls Voelkner, "but every PC would need one, and at $1,000-$2,000 a pop, it's too expensive." However, Voelkner points out that "smart cards may be used as the biometric device, and the capability to use these will become standard. Standard hardware will be coming out that includes smart-card ports just like floppy disk, CD-ROM, and modem ports. But it may be too easy to steal someone else's card, and FDA may not find them acceptable." Hence, FDA expects to issue supplements to the regulations as time goes on, depending on the issues that arise.

Industry can expect to see FDA criteria for electronic records and signatures spill over into other areas. These rules will most likely be viewed by other government agencies as a standard and may also strongly influence the direction of electronic record and signature technologies. What has affected the GMPs will no doubt also affect the GLPs, GCPs, GAMPs, and other government regulations as well as certain voluntary standards, such as ISO 9000 and ISO 14000. What form this influence will take remains to be seen.

Reference

1. Electronic Records; Electronic Signatures. *Code of Federal Regulations,* Part 11, Title 21, 1997; *Fed. Regist.* 62 (54): 1000-7 (1997).

—by Helen Gillespie

Helen Gillespie is editor/publisher of the LIMS/Letter and webmaster of the LIMSource. She can be reached at P.O. Box 935, Kenwood, CA 95452. Tel: 707-833-6885, Fax: 707-833-6865, E-mail: Webmaster@ LIMSource.com.

Part Six

The Courtroom

Chapter 47

Admissible Evidence—Who Decides?

A landmark Supreme Court decision concerning the use of scientific evidence in legal proceedings—although handed down a year ago—is still a subject of vigorous debate among scientists and legal scholars. Observers say that one clear effect of the drug-liability case, *Daubert et al.* v. *Merrell Dow Pharmaceuticals, Inc.*, has been to spur a crucial dialogue between the institutions of science and law, contributing to a number of cooperative initiatives now under way in several settings.

Also, they say, judges in subsequent cases are expressing a new appreciation for the values and methods of science.

At issue in *Daubert* was what the criteria should be for admissibility of scientific evidence into the courtroom, scientists and lawyers say. Should peer review—the gold standard within science—be the measure, or should more flexible standards be used in admitting such evidence? And, by inference, who should be charged with deciding what constitutes good science in court—scientists or judges?

"It's a question of institutional judgment," says David Kaye, a professor at the Center for the Study of Law, Science, and Technology at Arizona State University in Tempe, and editor of *Jurimetrics Journal,* a science-and-law publication affiliated with the American Bar Association (ABA). "Who's competent to decide what minimally acceptable science is?"

Excerpted from "Science in The Courtroom: What Evidence Is Admissible—And Who Decides?" by Franklin Hoke, in *The Scientist,* Vol. 8, No. 12, pp. 1, 4-5, June 13, 1994. © 1994 by The Scientist, Inc. Reprinted with permission.

451

Daubert exposed important tensions at the intersection of science and law, two powerful voices of authority in society. The case drew extraordinary attention from scientists, a number of whom were among the 22 parties who filed friend-of-the-court briefs on both sides. Scientists saw in the case a rare opportunity to weigh in directly, through the briefs, on the way their profession is represented in the courts.

In the *Daubert* case, two children, Jason Daubert and Eric Schuller, and their parents contended that Merrell Dow's anti-nausea drug Bendectin, taken by the mothers while pregnant, had caused the children's birth defects. Each side marshaled its experts to interpret research on the drug, but only the evidence put forth by Merrell Dow (now Marion Merrell Dow Inc., Kansas City, Mo.) was backed by peer review and publication. Noting, among other things, that the plaintiffs' scientific evidence was "unpublished," the United States Court of Appeals for the Ninth Circuit in San Francisco rejected their claim. The appeals court decision affirmed a U.S. District Court for the Southern District of California summary judgment for the drug maker, and prompted the plaintiffs to appeal to the Supreme Court.

In its June 28, 1993, decision, written by retiring Justice Harry A. Blackmun, the Supreme Court opted for the more "permissive" standard, remanding the case to the appeals court to be reargued. The Supreme Court also called on judges to play a more active, "gatekeeping role" in screening scientific evidence and, in doing so, for them to use only relevance and reliability as their guides.

Among the joint projects in progress to help judges fulfill the new, more active role the Court's decision would have them take is a reference manual for judges under development at the Federal Judicial Center in Washington, D.C., a research, education, and planning arm of the federal judiciary. The manual is designed to help judges manage scientific evidence effectively. In another effort, the National Conference of Lawyers and Scientists, a group sponsored by the American Association for the Advancement of Science and ABA, is exploring ways that judges could better use court-appointed scientific experts and individuals called special masters, who are designated by a judge to help assess evidence.

The Scientists' Stake

For the courts and society generally, the need for reliable scientific evidence in deciding cases that will affect people's lives is perhaps self-evident. Also, the number of cases involving scientific evidence continues to grow each year, focusing more attention on this need. But why should scientists concern themselves with the question of what constitutes good science in the eyes of judges? Observers say that scientists, in fact, have a strong investment in how science is represented in the courts.

"Maybe scientists should just stick to the laboratories and forget how their work is used or abused," says Dorothy Nelkin, a professor of sociology and law at New York University in New York City. "But that [view] is kind of passe these days, because science is a public endeavor."

Scientists have a socially responsible role to play, others agree, and monitoring the uses of their work in the courts is one aspect of this.

"Scientists have to become better citizens," says Daryl Chubin, director of the research, evaluation, and dissemination division in the education and human resources directorate of the National Science Foundation. "They have to develop a larger sense of what they're all about and the various arenas that they're asked to play in. Being a research scientist doesn't exempt you from other kinds of responsibilities."

"And even for self-interested purposes, scientific funding depends on how the public sees science," says Nelkin. "The legal appropriation of scientific information is one of the ways in which science is visible."

"The fact that there has not been research into birth control for many years is due in large part to a fear of litigation, for example," says Steven G. Gallagher, a senior staff associate with the task force on science and technology in judicial and regulatory decision-making of the Carnegie Commission on Science, Technology, and Government, which produced the March 1993 report *Science and Technology in Judicial Decision Making.* "More and more science is industry-funded now, and if industry is looking over its shoulder at liability, that's driving their [research] decisions."

Scientists and lawyers have often viewed each other with suspicion, too, some say, a situation that exacerbates the questions surrounding the admissibility of scientific evidence in courts. Scientific expert witnesses are sometimes seen by lawyers and other scientists as mercenaries whose views are for hire.

"The involvement of scientists as experts is generally belittled, denigrated, or unpleasant," says Gilbert S. Omenn, dean and professor at the school of public health and community medicine at the University of Washington, Seattle. "There's a legacy which has to do with the clash of cultures and clash of jargon between scientists and lawyers."

Lawyers, Omenn says, are invested in the adversarial system of arguing legal cases, a system that tends to polarize the viewpoints of opposing parties.

"Scientists, although they engage in this sometimes, like more to build consensus and to try to find common positions," he says.

Partly as a result, lawyers are often seen by scientists as having no understanding of or regard for scientific findings.

"Many people in this society take a fairly dim view of law," says Chubin, a sociologist and science-policy analyst. Scientists do that at their peril. If anything, we have to engage with other kinds of specialists who are linked to very powerful professions."

Omenn says that scientists who serve as experts in court are involved in important work, despite its negative reputation. He also feels that if courts were to increase their use of scientists as nonpartisan advisers, more scientists would be willing to enter the courts.

"We just don't see it as a truly professional activity for which there could be training and preparation, and it shows," Omenn says. "But scientists, I think, would respond well to the court asking them to be a court-appointed expert."

Assessing the Case

Immediately after the Supreme Court's decision, some scientists worried publicly that *Daubert,* by not relying on the peer-review standard for science, opened the way for substandard scientific evidence to enter the courts. But how, in fact, has the relationship between science and the law fared in the year since the *Daubert* opinion was handed down? Perhaps surprisingly, the purportedly lower standards for evidence have had less impact than the directive to judges to be more active, according to some scientists and lawyers.

"This phrase that Blackmun used—the gatekeeper—has really empowered judges and made them feel very comfortable that they can exclude so-called junk science," says Dan L. Burk, a molecular biologist and a visiting assistant professor of law at George Mason University, Arlington, Va.

"All of the DNA identification-testing cases that have come up have passed through with flying colors," Burk says. "Judges are accepting DNA evidence, which has a strong scientific basis. Other kinds of things, including some claims of cancer caused by exposure to cathode ray tubes on computer monitors, are being thrown out. So, the practical effect of *Daubert* seems to be what the scientific community would want, even if the language of *Daubert* may not be everything that [some members of] the scientific community asked for."

Others agree that the impact of the case has been substantial, even in some cases not directly citing *Daubert*.

"Courts have become more aware of peer review as a phenomenon," says Arizona's David Kaye. "Many judges didn't have much sense of what scientists do and what creates prestige in the field."

For example, Kaye says, the number of opinions using the phrase "peer review" has jumped dramatically since *Daubert*. "Even though the Supreme Court said peer review wasn't an absolute requirement [for admissibility], *Daubert* raised the consciousness of courts about the role of peer-reviewed articles in the scientific community."

The fact that the court named peer review as only one factor for judges to consider when assessing scientific evidence is entirely appropriate, according to some observers.

NSF's Chubin coauthored *Peerless Science* (State University of New York Press, Albany, 1990), a book critical of the peer-review process, and also helped write a friend-of-the-court brief on behalf of the plaintiffs. Some scientists' efforts to defend peer review in their court briefs, he says, were little more than "tradition for tradition's sake."

"The significance of *Daubert* is that peer review is not going to carry the day," says Chubin. "Peer review can only take us so far."

—by Franklin Hoke

Chapter 48

Science and Law in the Courtroom

The cultures of science and law both seek their own versions of truth. But their purposes differ in important ways, as do their methods. Partly as a result, interactions between the two historically have been fraught with misunderstandings and, at times, mutual suspicion. Today, however, a number of projects are under way to bring the scientific and legal professions into greater alignment. These projects seek to increase the insight members of both groups have into the processes of the other and to develop something like a shared vocabulary of ideas.

For example, a reference manual to help judges manage scientific evidence is being developed at the Federal Judicial Center in Washington, D.C., a research, education, and planning arm of the federal judiciary, with help from the Carnegie Corporation. Also, the National Conference of Lawyers and Scientists, a group sponsored by the American Association for the Advancement of Science (AAAS) and the American Bar Association (ABA), is working to identify mechanisms whereby the scientific community can identify potential candidates to serve as court-appointed scientific experts or so-called special masters, individuals designated by a judge to help assess the validity of scientific evidence.

Excerpted from "Scientists And Lawyers: Projects Aim to Bridge Gap between the Traditionally Contentious Professions," by Franklin Hoke, in *The Scientist,* Vol. 8, No.13, pp. 1, 4-5, June 27, 1994. © 1994 by The Scientist, Inc. Reprinted with permission.

The tasks are complex ones that attempt to bring closer the differing goals of these two groups, both of which are socially powerful.

"Although both scientists and the courts say they are looking for truth, what they mean by that is very, very different," says Dan L. Burk, a molecular biologist and a visiting assistant professor of law at George Mason University in Arlington, Va. "When a scientist says that she's looking for the truth or she's looking for an understanding of how the universe works, she's working inside a very definite kind of empirical and social framework. When the law says they're after truth, they're after something completely different, which is that they're trying to help people live together in society. They're trying to resolve conflicts.

"That may mean that the courts come to a decision that completely flies in the face of the scientific evidence," Burk adds. "The scientists have one particular worldview, and the lawyers really have a very different one. And each one is well adapted to what that community is trying to accomplish. But when you get on the interface between them, you're going to get some conflict of priorities."

That conflict was clearly drawn in the landmark Supreme Court ruling in *Daubert et al.* v. *Merrell Dow Pharmaceuticals,* a product-liability case originally decided in Merrell Dow's favor in the U.S. District Court for the Southern District of California in 1989. In the *Daubert* case, two children, Jason Daubert and Eric Schuller, and their parents contended that Bendectin, a drug marketed by Merrell Dow (now Marion Merrell Dow Inc., Kansas City, Mo.) and taken by the mothers while pregnant to avert morning sickness, had caused the children's birth defects.

The twin questions of what should qualify as minimally admissible scientific evidence and who should make that decision were at the heart of the case, scientists and lawyers say. In 1991, the U.S. Court of Appeals for the Ninth Circuit in San Francisco upheld the summary judgment in the case that the more stringent standards of the scientific community—in this case, reliance on peer-reviewed research—should outweigh other considerations in evaluating the admissibility of such evidence.

But in the Supreme Court's June 28, 1993, decision, written by Justice Harry A. Blackmun, the Court allowed for more judicial latitude and called on judges to take a more active, "gatekeeping role" in screening scientific evidence. In determining the admissibility of such evidence, the Court said, judges should use only relevance and reliability as their guides, rather than rely on the peer-reviewed status of the work, for example, as some scientists had advised.

The decision has led judges to a greater appreciation of the methods of science, scientists and legal scholars say, and, perhaps ironically, findings in cases since *Daubert* appear to conform at least as closely with scientific consensus views as before.

"The courts are very conscious of their role now," says Richard A. Meserve, a lawyer with the Washington, D.C.-based firm of Covington and Burling. Meserve, who holds a Ph.D. in applied physics and once served as clerk to Justice Blackmun, is also cochairman of the National Conference of Lawyers and Scientists. "The Supreme Court has told judges that their obligation is to police scientific evidence. They're supposed to look at these matters closely, and they're doing it."

"The *Daubert* opinion is saying to judges, `Don't let in junk science,'" says David Kaye, a professor at the Center for the Study of Law, Science, and Technology at Arizona State University, Tempe, and editor of *Jurimetrics Journal*, a science-and-law publication affiliated with ABA. "Be vigorous."

Scientific Advice to Judges

The purpose of the reference manual under development at the Federal Judicial Center is to help judges more effectively assess scientific evidence and to do so as early in the legal process as possible, according to project director Joseph A. Cecil.

"It is intended to advise on the management of expert testimony and the use of extraordinary procedures—like use of court-appointed experts and special masters—in cases that pose difficult science problems," Cecil says.

The manual, scheduled to be published in November 1995, will contain a series of "reference guides," or overview papers, in areas of science that have proved troublesome to the courts, according to Cecil. Information provided about such areas as epidemiology and toxicology will enable a judge to engage in a meaningful conversation with the attorneys and experts for each side about the basis of the expert opinions. Other areas to be covered in the manual are forensic analysis of DNA, survey research, inferential statistics, and multiple-regression analyses.

"The guides are written not to tell judges what evidence is admissible," Cecil says, "but to explain to judges how [scientists in] these disciplines go about determining their findings. For example, in the epidemiology paper, there's an explanation of case-control research designs and cohort research designs, so that when judges hear these terms, they'll understand exactly what kind of research design was used. In the toxicology paper, there's a discussion about in vitro and in vivo studies, and the issues that arise among toxicologists when discussing extrapolation of findings of animal research to humans."

Advice on what role peer review should play in deciding the admissibility of scientific evidence will be part of the handbook, too, according to Steven G. Gallagher, a senior staff associate of the task force on science and technology in judicial and regulatory decision making of the Carnegie Commission on Science, Technology, and Government, which produced the March 1993 report *Science and Technology in Judicial Decision Making*. The importance of peer review is not simply a matter of asking whether or not a study has been peer reviewed, he says. A more subtle approach to the question is needed.

"For example, how long has it been between the study or the other background work and its presentation to the court?" Gallagher says. "If the study was just done last year, there may not have been time for peer review. If the study was done 20 years ago and there's no peer review, then you might need to ask more questions."

Also, scientific journals differ in their level of scholarly credibility, Gallagher says.

"There are allegations that some people have set up journals just to publish and validate their studies," Gallagher says. According to Burk, publications in the area of clinical ecology might fit this description.

"Most members of the scientific community view clinical ecologists with a great deal of suspicion," Burk says. "These are people saying the immune system [can be] irreparably damaged by almost undetectable amounts of formaldehyde coming off the carpets and drapes."

The manual will strongly urge judges to make their assessments of scientific evidence at the pretrial stages of a case, according to Gallagher, a goal also emphasized by the Supreme Court in *Daubert*.

"Why go through three or four years of discovery, empanel a jury, start the expert testimony, and then have the testimony ruled inadmissible?" Gallagher asks. "If the testimony is going to be inadmissible, why not find that out earlier and save everybody heartache? If it is inadmissible, that then gives the plaintiff the opportunity to go back and try to find better evidence."

"The science community has long been critical of the kind of testimony that is presented in court," says Cecil. "And one of the consequences of the *Daubert* case is that federal judges, at least, are instructed to look into the scientific validity of the information. So, this manual will, to an extent, address what has been a long-standing complaint among scientists about the way information that they have developed is being used in a public-policy arena."

Finding Neutral Experts

Margaret A. Berger, associate dean and a professor at the Brooklyn School of Law in New York, is playing a central role in preparing materials for the Federal Judicial Center manual. Berger was also the primary author of the Carnegie Commission report.

Berger says that judges are reluctant to use court-appointed nonpartisan experts, despite existing powers that allow them to do so, even in cases with complex scientific or technical issues. Among the concerns of judges, Berger says, are ensuring neutrality of the expert and maintaining judicial independence, especially in areas in which their own expertise is likely to be limited. The judicial reference manual, she says, should encourage judges and give them guidance in how to use such court-appointed experts for help in understanding the methodology used by a given scientific expert, whether proffered by the plaintiff or the defendant, rather than for findings of fact.

"A court might be more willing to use an expert," Berger says, "if the expert were called upon to advise the court more on [questions such as]: How do you set up an epidemiological study correctly? Were the number of subjects adequate to reach the conclusions that were reached? Were confounding factors taken into account?"

Finding ways for judges to make better use of nonpartisan experts is also one of the aims of the National Conference of Lawyers and Scientists. The conference organized a November 1993 meeting of judges, attorneys, scientists, and others in Washington, D.C., to discuss establishing a demonstration project in which the professional scientific and engineering societies would create mechanisms to identify appropriate experts that judges could call on for help.

"The attitude of the judges was that this was something that they would only apply rarely," says Meserve. "It would be an extraordinary case in which they would be prepared to consider calling their own experts, chiefly because judges are accustomed to the adversarial system and want to have each party have the responsibility to present its case. But, then, they were prepared to believe that, in extraordinary cases, it might well be useful and were very interested in seeing how their ability to identify experts could be improved."

"Several of the judges said they would like their courts to be included in the demonstration project," says Deborah Runkle, associate staff officer for the conference and a senior program associate at AAAS. "We're going to try to have coordinating mechanisms that the federal judges can use when they would like to use a court-appointed expert in any of a number of capacities. We will work with, probably, the scientific and technical societies, but will not be limited to that. We might work with universities, for example, to help get experts in a timely fashion."

Some attendees at the conference say that judges' concerns over the impartiality of court-appointed experts are only one set of difficulties to be overcome.

"The judges were more interested than the attorneys [in introducing such experts]," says one meeting participant, speaking on condition of anonymity. "Attorneys who actually try cases are a little bit more wary, particularly—but not exclusively—the plaintiffs' [attorneys]. They don't see this working to their advantage."

One reason for this is that it is often the plaintiff's side that introduces novel scientific ideas of injury or disease causation by, for example, pesticides or electromagnetic fields.

"It is more often seen as being in the [defense's] interests to go with consensus or established science," this source says. "Also, who is neutral? Where do these scientists get their money? Who pays them? Where do they get their grants? Often the scientists who know the most about a particular thing work for industry. Who knows more about pesticides than the people who make them?"

If the process of selecting nonpartisan experts can be done in such a way that the concerns of judges and the attorneys who try cases can be answered, some observers see expanding roles for scientists in the courtroom.

"There may be more call on the scientific community, not to render ultimate opinions in the case about the issue that's being disputed, but rather to serve as experts who would advise the court about whether the opinions were reached in accordance with the scientific method," Berger says. "So, there might really be more of a role for scientists."

—by Franklin Hoke

Chapter 49

Exonerated by DNA

Commentary

Postconviction DNA exonerations provide a remarkable opportunity to reexamine, with greater insight than ever before, the strengths and weaknesses of our criminal justice system and how they bear on the all important question of factual innocence. The dimensions of the factual innocence problem exceed the impressive number of postconviction DNA exonerations listed in this report. Indeed, there is a strong scientific basis for believing these matters represent just the tip of a very deep and disturbing iceberg of cases. Powerful proof for this proposition lies with an extraordinary set of data collected by the Federal Bureau of Investigation (FBI) since it began forensic DNA testing in 1989.

Every year since 1989, in about 25 percent of the sexual assault cases referred to the FBI where results could be obtained (primarily by state and local law enforcement), the primary suspect has been excluded by forensic DNA testing. Specifically, FBI officials report that out of roughly 10,000 sexual assault cases since 1989, about 2,000 tests have been inconclusive (usually insufficient high molecular weight DNA to do testing), about 2,000 tests have excluded the primary suspect, and about 6,000 have "matched" or included the primary suspect.[1] The fact that these percentages have remained

Excerpted from *Convicted by Juries, Exonerated by Science*, National Institute of Justice report, publication no. 161258, June 1996, by Edward Connors, Thomas Lundregan, Neal Miller, and Tom McEwen.

constant for 7 years, and that the National Institute of Justice's informal survey of private laboratories reveals a strikingly similar 26 percent exclusion rate, strongly suggests that postarrest and postconviction DNA exonerations are tied to some strong, underlying systemic problems that generate erroneous accusations and convictions.

It must be stressed that the sexual assault referrals made to the FBI ordinarily involve cases where (1) identity is at issue (there is no consent defense), (2) the non-DNA evidence linking the suspect to the crime is eyewitness identification, (3) the suspects have been arrested or indicted based on non-DNA evidence, and (4) the biological evidence (sperm) has been recovered from a place (vaginal/rectal/oral swabs or underwear) that makes DNA results on the issue of identity virtually dispositive.

It is, of course, possible that some of the FBI's sexual assault exclusions have included false negatives. False negatives could occur, for example, because of (1) laboratory error, (2) situations where the victim of the assault conceals the existence of a consensual sexual partner within 48 hours of the incident *and* the accused suspect did not ejaculate (if the suspect ejaculated, the DNA should be identified along with the undisclosed sexual partner); or (3) multiple assailant sexual assault cases where none of the apprehended suspects ejaculated (the FBI counts the exclusion of all multiple suspects in a case as just one exclusion). Nonetheless, even with these caveats, it is still plain that forensic DNA testing is prospectively exonerating a substantial number of innocent individuals who would have otherwise stood trial, frequently facing the difficult task of refuting mistaken eyewitness identification by a truthful crime victim who would rightly deserve juror sympathy.

Without DNA testing, the prospects of wrongful convictions in these exclusion cases are evident. Even if one assumes half the normal conviction rate (state conviction rates for felony sexual assaults average about 62 percent), one would expect that hundreds of people who have been exonerated by FBI DNA testing in sexual assault cases over the last 7 years would have otherwise been convicted.

The Institute for Law and Justice report does not purport to be more than a quick survey, based primarily on press clippings and summary interviews, of postconviction DNA exoneration cases, and it does not undertake any systematic analysis of them. Since we have been, through the Innocence Project at Cardozo Law School, either attorneys of record or assisting counsel in the vast majority of these cases, we have attempted to investigate, with care and in detail, some of the factors that have led to the conviction of the innocent.[2]

Interestingly, in many respects the reasons for the conviction of the innocent in the DNA cases do not seem strikingly different than those cited by Yale Professor Edwin Borchard in his seminal work, *Convicting the Innocent* (Garden City Pub., 1932), which reviewed 65 cases, and more recently by Hugo Bedau and Michael Radelet in *In Spite of Innocence* (Northeastern University Press, 1992), which reviewed 416 erroneous convictions in death cases from 1900 to 1991. Mistaken eyewitness identification, coerced confessions, unreliable forensic laboratory work, law enforcement misconduct, and ineffective representation of counsel, singly and often in combination, remain the leading causes of wrongful convictions.

There are, however, historically unique aspects to the DNA exoneration cases. Most significantly, both the postconviction cases described in this report and the prospective sexual assault exclusions produced by the FBI and other laboratories create an opportunity for groundbreaking criminal justice research.

Take, for instance, just the FBI's sexual assault cases. One can confirm among these cases, with greater scientific assurance than is ordinarily provided by a trial verdict, which suspects charged were truly innocent and which suspects were truly guilty. We believe it crucial to identify, prior to any DNA testing, precisely what factors in the investigatory and charging process produced incorrect results in some of these cases and correct results in others. Are there systemic weaknesses that can be identified in eyewitness identification procedures, crime scene investigations, non-DNA laboratory tests (hair, fiber, etc.), police interrogation techniques, or other investigatory methods used by police and prosecutors that are conducive to false or true arrests and convictions? Perhaps there has never been a richer or more exciting set of cases for criminal justice researchers to explore in terms of shedding light on how law enforcement methods impact the crucial problem of factual innocence.

Finally, notwithstanding the research opportunities presented by the postarrest and postconviction DNA exoneration cases as to *how* wrongful accusations and convictions occur, the most significant implication of these cases is already apparent—the extent of factually incorrect convictions in our system must be much greater than anyone wants to believe. Postarrest and postconviction DNA exonerations have invariably involved analysis of sexual assault evidence (sperm), even if a murder charge was involved, that proved the existence of mistaken eyewitness identification. Since there does not seem to be anything inherent in sexual assault cases that would make eyewitnesses more prone to mistakes than in robberies or other serious

crimes where the crucial proof is eyewitness identification, it naturally follows that the rate of mistaken identifications and convictions
is similar to DNA exoneration cases.

The recently passed anti-terrorism bill contains a sweeping and un-
precedented curtailment of the right to obtain postconviction habeas
corpus relief in the Federal courts: Strict time limits (1 year in nondeath
cases, 3 months in death cases) have been set for filing the writ; state
court factual findings are "presumed to be correct"; state court misinterpretations of the United States Constitution are not a basis for relief
unless those misinterpretations are "unreasonable"; and all petitioners
must show, prior to obtaining a hearing, facts sufficient to establish by
clear and convincing evidence that but for the constitutional error, no
reasonable factfinder would have found the petitioner guilty. In short,
just as DNA testing, the most important technological breakthrough of
twentieth-century forensic science, demonstrates that the problem of
wrongful convictions in America is systemic and serious, Congress and
the President, in our view, have eviscerated the "great writ" that for two
centuries provided relief to those who were unjustly convicted. Hopefully,
before this century closes, as the ramifications of the DNA exoneration
cases become better understood, this triumph of political expediency over
America's traditional concerns for liberty and justice will be redressed.

Introduction

Background on Forensic Use of DNA Identification Testing

Perhaps the most significant advance in criminal investigation
since the advent of fingerprint identification is the use of DNA technology to help convict criminals or eliminate persons as suspects. DNA
analyses on saliva, skin tissue, blood, hair, and semen can now be
reliably used to link criminals to crimes. Increasingly accepted during the past 10 years, DNA technology is now widely used by police,
prosecutors, defense counsel, and courts in the United States.

An authoritative study on the forensic uses of DNA, conducted by
the National Research Council of the National Academy of Sciences,
has noted that:

> . . . the reliability of DNA evidence will permit it to exonerate
> some people who would have been wrongfully accused or con-
> victed without it. Therefore, DNA identification is not only a way
> of securing convictions; it is also a way of excluding suspects
> who might otherwise be falsely charged with and convicted of
> serious crimes.[3]

466

Forensic use of DNA technology in criminal cases began in 1986 when police asked Dr. Alec J. Jeffreys (who coined the term "DNA fingerprints"[4]) of Leicester University (England) to verify a suspect's confession that he was responsible for two rape-murders in the English Midlands.[5] Tests proved that the suspect had not committed the crimes. Police then began obtaining blood samples from several thousand male inhabitants in the area to identify a new suspect.[6] In a 1987 case in England, Robert Melias became the first person convicted of a crime (rape) on the basis of DNA evidence.[7]

In one of the first uses of DNA in a criminal case in the United States, in November 1987, the Circuit Court in Orange County, Florida, convicted Tommy Lee Andrews of rape after DNA tests matched his DNA from a blood sample with that of semen traces found in a rape victim.[8]

Two other important early cases involving DNA testing are *State v. Woodall*[9] and *Spencer v. Commonwealth*[10] In *Woodall,* the West Virginia Supreme Court was the first state high court to rule on the admissibility of DNA evidence. The court accepted DNA testing by the defendant, but inconclusive results failed to exculpate Woodall. The court upheld the defendant's conviction for rape, kidnaping, and robbery of two women. Subsequent DNA testing determined that Woodall was innocent, and he was released from prison.

The multiple murder trials in Virginia of Timothy Wilson Spencer were the first cases in the United States where the admission of DNA evidence led to guilty verdicts resulting in a death penalty. The Virginia Supreme Court upheld the murder and rape convictions of Spencer, who had been convicted on the basis of DNA testing that matched his DNA with that of semen found in several victims. In *Spencer,* the defendant's attack upon the introduction of DNA evidence was limited to the contention that its novelty should lead the court to "hold off until another day any decision . . . "[11] There was no testimony from expert witnesses that challenged the general acceptance of DNA testing among the scientific community.[12]

The first case that seriously challenged a DNA profile's admissibility was *People v. Castro;*[13] the New York Supreme Court, in a 12-week pretrial hearing, exhaustively examined numerous issues relating to the admissibility of DNA evidence. Jose Castro was accused of murdering his neighbor and her 2-year-old daughter. A bloodstain on Castro's watch was analyzed for a match to the victim. The court held the following:

- DNA identification theory and practice are generally accepted among the scientific community.

- DNA forensic identification techniques are generally accepted by the scientific community.

- Pretrial hearings are required to determine whether the testing laboratory's methodology was substantially in accord with scientific standards and produced reliable results for jury consideration.

The *Castro* ruling supports the proposition that DNA identification evidence of exclusion is more presumptively admissible than DNA identification evidence of *inclusion.* In *Castro,* the court ruled that DNA tests could be used to show that blood on Castro's watch was not his, but tests could not be used to show that the blood was that of his victims.

In *Castro,* the court also recommended extensive discovery requirements for future proceedings, including copies of all laboratory results and reports; explanation of statistical probability calculations; explanations for any observed defects or laboratory errors, including observed contaminants; and chain of custody of documents. These recommendations soon were expanded upon by the Minnesota Supreme Court, in *Schwartz* v. *State,*[14] which noted, ". . . ideally, a defendant should be provided with the actual DNA sample(s) in order to reproduce the results. As a practical matter, this may not be possible because forensic samples are often so small that the entire sample is used in testing. Consequently, access to the data, methodology, and actual results is crucial . . . for an independent expert review."[15]

In *Schwartz,* the Supreme Court of Minnesota refused to admit the DNA evidence analyzed by a private forensic laboratory; the court noted the laboratory did not comply with appropriate standards and controls. In particular, the court was troubled by failure of the laboratory to reveal its underlying population data and testing methods. Such secrecy precluded replication of the test.

In summary, courts have successfully challenged improper application of DNA scientific techniques to particular cases, especially when used to declare "matches" based on frequency estimates. However, DNA testing properly applied is generally accepted as admissible under *Frye*[16] or *Daubert*[17] standards.[18] As stated in the National Research Council's 1996 report on DNA evidence, "The state of the profiling technology and the methods for estimating frequencies and related statistics have progressed to the point where the admissibility of properly collected and analyzed DNA data should not be in doubt."[19] At this time, 46 states admit DNA evidence in criminal proceedings. In 43 states, courts have ruled on the technology, and in 3 states, statutes require admission (see Table 49.1.).

Table 49.1. DNA Evidence Admission in Criminal Trials by State

State	DNA Admitted	State	DNA Admitted
Alabama	Yes	Montana	Yes
Alaska	Yes	Nebraska	Yes
Arizona	Yes	Nevada	Statute
Arkansas	Yes	New Hampshire	Yes
California	Yes*	New Jersey	Yes*
Colorado	Yes	New Mexico	Yes
Connecticut	Yes	New York	Yes
Delaware	Yes	North Carolina	Yes
Florida	Yes	North Dakota	No
Georgia	Yes	Ohio	Yes
Hawaii	Yes	Oklahoma	Statute
Idaho	Yes	Oregon	Yes
Illinois	Yes*	Pennsylvania	Yes
Indiana	Yes	Rhode Island	No
Iowa	Yes	South Carolina	Yes
Kansas	Yes	South Dakota	Yes
Kentucky	Yes	Tennessee	Statute
Louisiana	Yes	Texas	Yes
Maine	No	Utah	No
Maryland	Yes*	Vermont	Yes
Massachusetts	Yes	Virginia	Yes
Michigan	Yes	Washington	Yes
Minnesota	Yes	West Virginia	Yes
Mississippi	Yes	Wisconsin	Yes
Missouri	Yes	Wyoming	Yes

* Decision by Intermediate Court of Appeals

Study Findings

Findings pertaining to characteristics of the 28 DNA exculpatory cases identified during the study are discussed first. The chapter concludes with the results of the telephone survey of DNA laboratories.

General Characteristics Shared by Many Study Cases

The 28 cases in this study were tried in 14 states and the District of Columbia. The states are Illinois (5 cases), New York (4 cases), Virginia (3 cases), West Virginia (3 cases), Pennsylvania (2 cases), California (2 cases), Maryland, North Carolina, Connecticut. Kansas, Ohio, Indiana, New Jersey, and Texas. Many cases share a number of descriptive characteristics, as noted below.

Most cases mid- to late 1980s. Most cases involved convictions that occurred in the 1980s, primarily mid to late 1980s, a period when forensic DNA technology was not readily accessible. The earliest case involved a conviction in 1979, the most recent in 1991.

In each of the 28 cases, a defendant was convicted of a crime or crimes and serving a sentence of incarceration. While in prison, each defendant obtained, through an attorney, case evidence for DNA testing and consented to a comparison of the evidence-derived DNA to his own DNA sample. (In *Nelson,* the prosecutor conducted the tests.) In each case, the results showed that there was not a match, and the defendant was ultimately set free. Table 49.2. presents an overview of the study cases.

Sexual assault the most frequent crime. All 28 cases involved some form of sexual assault. In six (*Bloodsworth, Cruz, Hernandez, Linscott, Nelson,* and *Vasquez*), assailants also murdered their victims. All alleged assailants were male. All victims were female: most were adults, others teenagers or children. All but one case involved a jury trial. (The nonjury case, *Vasquez,* involved a guilty plea from a defendant who had mental disabilities.) Of the cases where the time required for jury deliberations was known, most had verdicts returned in less than 1 day, except for *Kotler,* which required 2 days.

Prison time served. The 28 defendants served a total of 197 years in prison (an average of almost 7 years each) before being released as a result of DNA testing. The longest time served was 11 years, the shortest 9 months. For a variety of legal reasons, defendants in several cases continued to remain in prison for months after exculpatory DNA test results. In *Green,* DNA testing was performed after conviction, but prior to sentencing.

Many defendants also qualified for public defenders or appointed counsel. Most defendants appealed their convictions at least once; many appealed several times. Most appeals focused on trial error (e.g., ineffective assistance of counsel) or new evidence. For example, in some cases, the victims recanted their defendant identification testimony.

Prior police knowledge of the defendants. Police knew 15 defendants prior to their arrests, generally through criminal records. It is not known whether, in some cases, that may have influenced police to place suspects in photo spreads and lineups shown to victims and other eyewitnesses.

Evidence Presented during/after Trial: Common Attributes

The 28 cases shared several common themes in the evidence presented during and after trial.

Eyewitness identification. All cases, except for homicides, involved victim identification both prior to and at trial. Many cases also had additional eyewitness identification, either placing the defendant with the victim or near the crime scene (e.g., in *Bloodsworth,* five witnesses testified that they had seen the defendant with the 9-year-old victim on the day of the murder).

Many defendants presented an alibi defense, frequently corroborated by family or friends. For example, Edward Honaker's alibi was corroborated by his brotber, sister-in-law, mother's housemate, and trailer park owner. The alibis apparently were not of sufficient weight to the juries to counter the strength of the eyewitness testimony.

Use of forensic evidence. A majority of the cases involved non-DNA-tested forensic evidence that was introduced at trial. Although not pinpointing the defendants, that evidence substantially narrowed the field of possibilities to include them. Typically, those cases involved comparisons of nonvictim specimens of blood, semen, or hair at the crime scene to that of the defendants. Testimony of prosecution experts also was used to explain the reliability and scientific strength of non-DNA evidence to the jury.

Table 49.2a. (continued in Table 49.2b.) Overview of DNA Study Cases

Case Name/Location	Primary Charges	Date Convicted	Sentence/Served
Alejandro, Gilbert Uvalde, TX	Sexual assault	October 1990	12 yrs/4 yrs
Bloodsworth, Kirk Baltimore, MD	Murder, rape	March 1985	Death, later reduced to life/Almost 9 yrs
Bravo, Mark Diaz Los Angeles Co., CA	Rape	December 1990	8 yrs/3 yrs
Brison, Dale Chester County, PA	Rape, kidnaping	June 1991	18–42 yrs/3½ yrs
Bullock, Ronnie Chicago, IL	Aggravated sexual assault	May 1984	60 yrs/10½ yrs
Callace, Leonard White Plains, NY	Sodomy, sexual abuse	March 1987	25–50 yrs/Almost 6 yrs
Chalmers, Terry Leon White Plains, NY	Rape, sodomy	June 1987	12–24 yrs/8 yrs
Cotton, Ronald Burlington, NC	Rape (2 counts)	January 1985 November 1987 (second trial)	Life+54 yrs/10½ yrs
Cruz, Rolando Chicago, IL	Murder, kidnaping, rape	March 1985	Death/11 yrs
Dabbs, Charles Westchester Co., NY	Rape	April 1984	12½–20 yrs/7 yrs
Davis, Gerald Wayne Kanawha Co., WV	Kidnaping, sexual assault (2 counts)	May 1986	14–35 yrs/8 yrs
Daye, Frederick Rene San Diego, CA	Rape (2 counts), kidnaping	August 1984	Life/10 yrs
Dotson, Gary Chicago, IL	Rape, aggravated kidnaping	July 1979	25–50 yrs/8 yrs
Green, Edward Washington, DC	Rape	July 1989	Never sentenced/9 months
Hammond, Ricky Hartford, CT	Sexual assault, kidnaping	March 1990	25 yrs and 3 yrs probation/2 yrs
Harris, William O'Dell Charleston, WV	Sexual assault	October 1987	10–20 yrs/7 yrs, then 1 yr home confinement

Table 49.2b. (continued from Table 49.2a.) Overview of DNA Study Cases

Case Name/Location	Primary Charges	Date Convicted	Sentence/Served
Hernandez, Alejandro Chicago, IL	Murder, kidnaping, rape	March 1985	Death/11 yrs
Honaker, Edward Nelson County, VA	Rape, sexual assault, sodomy	June 1985	3 life terms+34 yrs/10 yrs
Jones, Joe C. Topeka, KS	Rape, aggravated kidnaping	February 1986	Life+10–25 yrs/6½ yrs
Kotler, Kerry Suffolk County, NY	Rape (2 counts)	February 1982	25–50 yrs/11 yrs
Linscott, Steven Cook County, IL	Murder, rape	November 1982	40 yrs/3 yrs in prison; 7 yrs out on bond
Nelson, Bruce Allegheny Co., PA	Murder, rape	September 1982	Life/9 yrs
Piszczek, Brian Cuyahoga Co., OH	Rape	June 1991	15–25 yrs/4+ yrs
Scruggs, Dwayne Indianapolis, IN	Rape	May 1986	40 yrs/Over 7½ yrs
Shephard, David Union County, NJ	Rape	September 1984	30 yrs/Almost 10 yrs
Snyder, Walter (Tony) Alexandria, VA	Rape, sodomy	June 1986	45 yrs/Almost 7 yrs
Vasquez, David Arlington Co., VA	Murder, rape	February 1985	35 yrs/5 yrs
Woodall, Glen Huntington, WV	Sexual assault, kidnaping	July 1987	2 life terms+203–335 yrs/4 yrs, then 1 yr under electronic home confinement

Alleged government malfeasance or misconduct. Eight cases, as reported by defense attorneys and reflected in some judges' opinions, involved allegations of government misconduct, including perjured testimony at trial, police and prosecutors who intentionally kept exculpatory evidence from the defense, and intentionally erroneous laboratory tests and expert testimony admitted at trial as evidence. For example:

- In *Honaker,* the defendant's attorney alleged that the government intentionally kept exculpatory evidence from the defense, including information that two of the government's witnesses were secretly hypnotized to enhance their testimony and that the prosecution's criminalist was never told that Honaker had a vasectomy (and could not have been the source of the sperm in the victim).

- In *Cruz,* a supervising officer in the sheriff's department admitted, during the third trial, that he had lied about corroborating the testimony of his deputies in the earlier trials. This testimony focused on Cruz's "dream visions" of the murder.

- In *Kotler,* the government's serologist reportedly lied about his qualifications. In addition, Kotler's attorneys alleged that the government intentionally withheld exculpatory evidence from the defense. For example, police reports stated that the victim did not actually positively identify the defendant's picture, but described him only as a "look-alike." Furthermore, as recorded in police reports, the victim's description of the defendant was inaccurate for age, height, and weight. The defense was never informed about those reports.

- In cases involving defendants Glen Woodall, William O'Dell Harris, and Gerald Wayne Davis (and his father), the perjured testimony of Fred Zain, a serologist then with the West Virginia State Police, was in large part responsible for the wrongful convictions that ensued. The West Virginia Supreme Court of Appeals, in a special report on Zain's misconduct in more than 130 criminal cases, stated that such behavior included " . . . overstating the strength of results; . . . reporting inconclusive results as conclusive; . . . repeatedly altering laboratory records; . . . ."[20] The report also noted that Zain's irregularities were "the result of systematic practice rather than an occasional inadvertent error." In addition, the report stated that Zain's "supervisors may have ignored or concealed complaints of his misconduct."[21]

- In *Alejandro,* the defendant was also wrongfully convicted by expert testimony from Fred Zain, who had moved from West Virginia to Texas and worked for the Bexar County crime laboratory. In July 1994, a Uvalde County grand jury indicted Zain for perjury, tampering with government records, and fabricating evidence. As of early 1996, charges of tampering and of fabricating evidence had been dropped, leaving three charges for aggravated perjury in effect, for which Zain reportedly seeks dismissal on statute of limitations grounds.

Evidence discovered after trial. In most of the cases in this study, DNA test results represented newly discovered evidence obtained after completion of the trials. States have time limits on filing motions for new trials on the basis of newly discovered evidence. For example, in Virginia, new evidence must be presented by motion within 21 days after the trial.[22] Thus, the *Honaker, Snyder,* and *Vasquez* cases required a pardon from Virginia's governor to release the defendants from prison.

In some of the study cases, prosecutors waived time limits when presented with the DNA exculpatory results. However, prosecutors also have contested defendants' attempts to release evidence for DNA testing.

States also differ in the legislation and procedures pertaining to postconviction appointment of counsel and to authorization to pay for the DNA testing. Many cases involved indigents.

DNA testing. The DNA testing phase of these cases also has common characteristics. Nearly all the defendants had their tests performed by private laboratories. The tests were conducted using blood from defendants, blood or blood-related evidence from victims, and semen stains on articles of the victims' clothing or on nearby items (a blanket was tested in one case). In over half the cases, the prosecution either conducted a DNA test totally independent of that of the defense or sent test results obtained by the defendant's laboratory to a different one to determine whether the laboratory used by the defense interpreted test results properly.

Eight laboratories used Restriction Fragment Length Polymorphism (RFLP) DNA testing, 17 conducted Polymerase Chain Reaction (PCR) testing, and 2 used both tests. For one case, the type of DNA test conducted is unknown.

Preservation of evidence. In some cases, evidence samples had deteriorated to the point where DNA testing could not be performed. In *Brison,* the laboratory could not test cotton swabs from the rape kit but, instead, tested a semen stain from the victim's underwear. In *Daye*, after the appellate court affirmed the defendant's conviction and the State Supreme Court denied certification, the evidence was about to be destroyed when Daye's attorney filed to stay the destruction in order to conduct DNA testing.

The chain of custody in some of the cases also demonstrated a lack of adherence to proper procedures. Authorities on the subject note that the "mishandling of real evidence affects the integrity of the factfinding process."[23] In *Dabbs,* the defendant's attorneys reported that the defense was initially advised by the prosecution that the evidence (victim's underwear that contained a semen stain) had been destroyed (a conclusion based on failure of authorities to find the evidence in police or court custody). Eventually, the defense found the evidence at the county crime laboratory.

Results of DNA Laboratory Survey

Conducted in June 1995, the nationwide telephone survey of 40 public and private laboratories that performed DNA tests sought answers to such questions as: From the time the laboratories began DNA testing, how many cases have they handled? Of that number, what percentage yielded results that excluded defendants as sources of the DNA evidence or were inconclusive?

The 40 surveyed laboratories yielded 19 whose available data were sufficient for the purposes of this study. The 19 included 13 at the state/local level, 4 in the private sector, an armed forces laboratory, and the FBI's laboratory.

Most of the laboratories had initiated DNA testing only within the previous few years. Twelve began testing between 1990 and 1992. Three of the four private laboratories began in 1986 or 1987, while the FBI started DNA testing in 1988.

Seven of the laboratories reported using RFLP testing; four, PCR testing, and eight, both types of tests.

The 19 laboratories reported that, since they began testing, they had received evidence in 21,621 cases for DNA analysis, with the FBI accounting for 10,060 cases. Three of the 4 private laboratories averaged 2,400 each; the state and local laboratories averaged 331 each.

In about 23 percent of the 21,621 cases, DNA test results excluded suspects, according to respondents. An additional 16 percent of the cases, approximately, yielded inconclusive results, often because the test samples had deteriorated or were too small. Inconclusive results aside, test results in the balance of the cases did not exclude the suspect.

The FBI reported that, in the 10,060 cases it received, DNA testing results were about 20 percent inconclusive and 20 percent exclusion; the other 18 laboratories (11,561 cases) reported about 13 percent and 26 percent, respectively.[24]

Unfortunately, the laboratories were unable to provide more details. They did not maintain data bases that would permit categorization of DNA test results by type of offense and other criteria. What happened to the suspects who were excluded through DNA testing also cannot be determined. Were they released, or were they charged on the basis of other evidence, for example?

Thus, only the most general information is known about the results of DNA testing by laboratories. To obtain more detailed information would require a comprehensive research project.

Policy Implications

The 28 cases examined by the study raise issues that have policy implications for the criminal justice system. The most significant are presented below.[25]

Reliability of Eyewitness Testimony

In the majority of the cases, given the absence of DNA evidence at the trial, eyewitness testimony was the most compelling evidence. Clearly, however, those eyewitness identifications were wrong. In one of the clearest examples of eyewitness testimony overwhelmingly influencing the jury, the Pennsylvania Intermediate Court of Appeals commented on the evidence in the Dale Brison case:

> The Commonwealth's evidence consisted primarily of the victim's identification testimony. However, the victim's stab wounds in addition to the weather and reduced visibility may well have affected the victim's ability to accurately view her assailant, and thus, she may have been prompted to identify appellant merely because she remembered seeing him in the neighborhood. Moreover, the victim did not specifically describe any of her assailant's facial characteristics to the police. There was also no conclusive physical evidence, aside from a single hair sample which may have been consistent with any male of [A]frican-[A]merican descent, linking appellant to the crime.[26]

477

This points conclusively to the need in the legal system for improved criteria for evaluating the reliability of eyewitness identification.

In *Neil* v. *Biggers*,[27] the U.S. Supreme Court established criteria that jurors may use to evaluate the reliability of eyewitness identifications. However, the reliability of eyewitness testimony has been criticized extensively in the literature.[28] In a recent interview, Dr. Elizabeth Loftus, one of the best-known critics of the reliability of eyewitness identification, commented on the role of DNA testing in exonerating innocent persons who served time in prison. Dr. Loftus noted that a significant factor is the potential susceptibility of eyewitnesses to suggestions from police, whether intentional or unintentional. As reported, Dr. Loftus stated that there is "pressure that comes from the police [who] want to see the crime solved, but there is also a psychological pressure that is understandable on the part of the victim who wants to see the bad guy caught and wants to feel that justice is done."[29]

Dr. Loftus has recommended more open-ended questioning of victims by the police to avoid leading questions. In addition, Dr. Loftus and others have recommended use of expert testimony regarding the pros and cons of relying on eyewitness testimony.[30]

Reliability of Non-DNA Analyses of Forensic Evidence Compared to DNA Testing

In many of the study cases, according to documentation examined and those interviewed, scientific experts had convinced juries that non-DNA analyses of blood or hair were reliable enough to clearly implicate the defendants. Scientific conclusions based on non-DNA analyses, however, were proven less discriminating and reliable than those based on DNA tests. These findings point to the need for the scientific community to take into account the reliability of non-DNA forensic analyses vis-à-vis DNA testing in identifying the sources of biological evidence.

In a recent habeas corpus hearing in a murder case, a U.S. district court held that expert testimony on microscopic hair comparisons was inadmissible under the *Daubert* standard.[31] The court cited studies documenting a high error rate and found that there are no accepted probability standards for human hair identification. The court ruled that in this case the expert's hair testimony was "imprecise and speculative, and its probative value was outweighed by its prejudicial effect."[32]

Competence and Reliability of DNA Laboratory Procedures

One of the lasting effects of the O. J. Simpson case will likely be greater scrutiny by defense lawyers of the prosecution's forensic DNA evidence presented in criminal cases. In the Simpson case, the defense, in essence, put the crime laboratory on trial. The National Research Council (NRC) report entitled *DNA Technology in Forensic Science* states: "There is no substantial dispute about the underlying [DNA] scientific principles. However, the adequacy of laboratory procedures and the competence of the experts who testify should remain open to inquiry."[33]

The NRC report recommends some degree of standardization to ensure quality and reliability. The report recommends that each forensic laboratory engaged in DNA testing must have a formal, detailed program of quality assurance and quality control. The report also states:

> Quality assurance programs in individual laboratories alone are insufficient to ensure high standards. External mechanisms are needed to ensure adherence to the practices of quality assurance. Potential mechanisms include individual certification, laboratory accreditation, and state or federal regulation.[34]

As recently reported by the American Society of Crime Laboratory Directors, 32 public DNA laboratories have been accredited. In addition, one private laboratory is accredited.[35]

Whether laboratories that conduct DNA tests possess the requisite qualifications has significant cost implications for the criminal justice system in terms of reducing the number of redundant DNA tests. In many cases in this study, both prosecution and defense obtained independent DNA tests of the biological stain evidence. Although independent examinations are common in areas that are more open to interpretation (e.g., mental fitness for trial), DNA testing, for exculpatory purposes, should be performed in a qualified laboratory, and the results, if they exculpate the suspect, should be accepted by both parties. Such acceptance would seem more likely if DNA tests were performed by laboratories that all parties agreed were qualified.

Preservation of Evidence for DNA Testing

In some states, sentenced felons may experience difficulty obtaining access to evidence for DNA testing. With an increasing volume of criminal cases, some police agencies destroy evidence when defendants have exhausted their appeals. Even when defendants obtain access to the evidence, it may be too deteriorated for DNA testing. In some of the study cases, insufficient evidence prevented laboratories from conducting Restriction Fragment Length Polymorphism (RFLP) testing, but Polymerase Chain Reaction (PCR) testing was still possible.

Preserving biological stain evidence and maintaining the proper chain of custody of the evidence are essential for successful DNA testing.[36] At the trial stage, however, the U.S. Supreme Court has ruled that unless a criminal defendant can show bad faith on the part of the police, failure to preserve potentially useful evidence does not constitute a denial of due process of law.[37] After a defendant's conviction, prosecutors are not required by constitutional duty to preserve evidence indefinitely. As noted earlier in *Daye,* the evidence was about to be destroyed when his attorney filed to stay the destruction to conduct what turned out to be an exculpatory DNA test.

Training in DNA Forensic Uses

The introduction of DNA technology into the criminal trial setting is likely to create uncertainty, spawned in part by the complexity of the technology, and also to possibly generate unrealistic expectations of the technology's power in the minds of some or all of the players: prosecution, defense, judges, and jurors. The scientific complexities of the technology may influence all parties to rely more heavily on expert testimony than on other types of evidence.

As the use of DNA technology becomes more widely publicized, juries will come to expect it, like fingerprint evidence. This will place more pressure on prosecutors to use the technology whenever possible, especially as the cost decreases. Prosecutors must be trained on when to use the technology and how to interpret results for the jury.

When the prosecution uses DNA evidence, the defense will be forced to attack it through expert testimony. The defense must rebut the persuasiveness of the evidence for the jury. As stated in the NRC report, "Mere cross examination by a defense attorney inexperienced in the science of DNA testing will not be sufficient."[38] Thus, defense counsel as well as the prosecution and judiciary must receive training in the forensic uses of DNA technology.

Third-Party Consensual Sex Sources

The primary objective of the defense in using DNA testing in rape cases is to show that the defendant is excluded as the source of the semen evidence. Even when exclusion is established, the prosecution may be motivated, as in *Davis,* to eliminate as suspects any and all consensual sex partners as sources of semen in rape cases. During the first trial of Gerald Wayne Davis, the prosecution contended that the semen in the victim came from Davis. After DNA testing had excluded Davis as the source of the semen, the prosecution contended, in the second trial, that Davis could have still raped the victim but not ejaculated and that the semen in the victim could have come from the victim's fiance just prior to the rape. The prosecution never obtained a blood sample from the fiance because he died before the second trial.

A question under the law is whether third parties can be compelled to provide biological evidence for DNA testing. In some cases, the government refused to release defendants after exculpatory DNA results until third parties were located and tested. Kerry Kotler was held for an additional year after his exculpatory DNA test so the government could test the victim's husband. Edward Honaker was held for an additional 9 months after his exculpatory DNA test so the government could test the victim's boyfriend and "secret lover."

Multiple-Defendant Crimes

The DNA technology used to analyze biological evidence from crime scenes must not be oversold as an exculpatory tool—it does have limitations. Multiple-suspect crimes present a particular problem for use of DNA identification as a crime-solving tool. In multiple-suspect sexual assaults without eyewitnesses, such as a rape-murder, it is possible that only one of the suspects ejaculated in, or even raped, the victim. In such cases, DNA testing of semen would seem likely to exculpate one or more of the suspects. This type of situation presents a real dilemma for police and prosecutors. Because of exculpatory DNA tests on semen and possibly other exculpatory evidence (e.g., an alibi, lack of other physical evidence), pressure mounts on prosecutors to release one or more of the suspects. The only other evidence against them may be the testimony of a suspect who is matched to the crime by DNA analysis.

In *Dabbs,* for example, the victim testified that she was dragged into an alley and raped by one man while two other men held her down. The police arrested Dabbs on the basis of identification of him by the victim, a distant cousin. The other alleged assailants were never identified or arrested. The DNA test showed that the semen evidence from the victim did not match Dabbs. One theory of the case, however, was that Dabbs participated in the crime but was not the rapist. The prosecutor ultimately dismissed the original indictment against Dabbs because of the DNA results and the reluctance of the victim to testify at a new trial.

Posttrial Relief

Most states have a time limit on presenting evidence newly discovered after trial, conviction, and sentencing. The reason for limiting the time to file appeals based on new evidence is to ensure the integrity of the trial process and jury verdicts. Many DNA issues in the study cases were not raised until the postconviction stages. Absent constitutional issues, many state procedures, as in Virginia,[39] may preclude consideration of new exculpatory DNA evidence at postconviction stages. Some of the study defendants, after receiving exculpatory DNA results, were released only by agreement of the prosecutor, sometimes they needed a pardon by the governor.

Some states, such as Oregon, permit judges to use discretion to waive new-evidence rules and set aside verdicts or order new trials.[40] Thus, some states may allow an out-of-time motion for a new trial when newly discovered evidence clearly serves the interests of justice.[41]

At postconviction stages, appointment of counsel and payment for DNA testing become issues for indigents. While some appeals courts have ordered state-paid DNA testing for indigents where justified (e.g., where the overall case against the defendant is weak), other court rulings deny such relief, especially where the exculpatory value is speculative.[42] As DNA testing to exculpate convicted persons becomes more widespread, states need to consider these issues.

Future DNA Forensic Uses

The momentum is growing, spurred in part by the public's education from the Simpson trial, for DNA testing in criminal cases. Juries may begin to question cases where the prosecutor does not offer "conclusive" DNA test results if the evidence is available for testing. More defense attorneys in courtappointed cases may file motions for DNA testing and request the state to pay for the tests (this issue may also be raised as a *Brady* motion for the prosecutor to conduct the tests).

The shift will be for more DNA testing in pretrial stages. Prosecutors should find that DNA testing is as helpful to them as to the defense in excluding suspects early in the investigation. This will enable the police and prosecution to save money in the long run by focusing investigations in more fruitful directions.

In Britain, mass DNA screening in search of suspects has, in recent years, produced arrests in several highly publicized cases. The most recent case involved the rapemurder of a 15-year-old South Wales girl.[43] The South Wales constabulary obtained saliva swab samples from over 2,000 men who lived in the vicinity of the murder. Police went door-to-door inviting men to a makeshift laboratory to submit the samples. The saliva samples were used to develop DNA profiles to compare to the DNA profile obtained from the assailant's semen.

British law does not permit compulsory sampling, but the police made it clear that anyone who refused would become the subject of intense police investigation. A 19-year-old resident of the victim's neighborhood was arrested when his saliva sample was the only one of the thousands taken that could not be eliminated.

Such DNA dragnet methods, while employed sparingly in Great Britain, may increase as the ease and affordability of DNA testing improves. It is unlikely that such mass-testing methods would gain favor in the United States. Constitutional protections against self-incrimination and unreasonable searches and seizures, as well as the American public's zealous protection of privacy rights, would preclude such DNA dragnet practices from being implemented in this country.

Notes

1. Although there is no sure way to determine what the results would have been on the inconclusive tests if results had been obtainable, it seems a fair assumption, given the strong trends over a 7-year period, that the percentages of exclusions and inclusions of the primary suspect would have run about the same as the cases where results were obtainable. Indeed, since most of the FBI's cases since 1989 involved RFLP tests, which require greater amounts of sample than PCR-based testing, it would be interesting to test this hypothesis by performing PCR tests on some of the old inconclusive cases where primary suspects were either acquitted or convicted.

2. While we would be the last to discount the possibility of laboratory error in any DNA testing case, be it an exclusion or an inclusion, great pains have been taken in the postconviction DNA exoneration cases to minimize this factor. First, it must be stressed that these cases, even if involving a homicide, have invariably involved analysis of sperm from swabs (vaginal, oral, or anal) or from clothes worn by the victim. Thus, the chance of inadvertently cross contaminating the samples with someone else's sperm is remote. Secondly, sexual assault evidence provides an intrinsic redundancy, or internal control,

in that the DNA profile from epithelial cells found in samples can be cross-checked against the known DNA profile of the victim. Finally, before convicted prisoners have been released, either through postconviction court orders or clemency grants from governors, the prosecution has insisted upon independent testing of samples by their own experts and elimination samples from other possible sperm donors (husbands or boyfriends) even if it was the prosecution's position at trial that the sperm came from the perpetrator.

3. National Research Council, National Academy of Sciences, *DNA Technology in Forensic Science* (Washington, D.C.: National Academy Press, 1992:156). (Cited as NRC report.) Another reference source is Judith McKenna, J. Cecil, and P Coukos, "Reference Guide on Forensic DNA Evidence," *Reference Manual on Scientific Evidence* (Federal Judicial Center, 1994). This guide has a useful glossary of terms at p. 323.

4. Alec J. Jeffreys, Victoria Wilson, and Swee Lay Thein, "Hypervariable 'Minisatellite' Regions in Human Nature," *Nature* 314: 67 (1985); "Individual-Specific 'Fingerprints' of Human DNA," *Nature* 316: 76 (1985).

5. The first reported use of DNA identification was in a noncriminal setting to prove a familial relationship. A Ghanaian boy was refused entry into the United Kingdom (U.K.) for lack of proof that he was the son of a woman who had the right of settlement in the U.K. Immigration authorities contended that the boy could be the nephew of the woman, not her son. DNA testing showed a high probability of a mother-son relationship. The U.K. Government accepted the test findings and admitted the boy. See K. F. Kelly, J. J. Rankin, and R. C. Wink, "Methods and Applications of DNA Fingerprinting: A Guide for the Non-Scientist," *Criminal Law Review* 105, 108 (1987); Note, "Stemming the DNA Tide; A Case for Quality Control Guidelines," *Hamline Law Review* 16: 211, 213-14 (1992).

6. Peter Gill, Alec J. Jeffreys, and David J. Werrett, "Forensic Application of DNA Fingerprints," *Nature* 318: 577 (1985). See also Craig Seton, "Life for Sex Killer Who Sent Decoy to Take Genetic Test," *The Times* (London): 3 (January 23, 1988). A popular account of this case, *The Blooding,* was written by crime novelist Joseph Wambaugh (New York, N.Y.: William Morrow & Co., Inc., 1989).

7. Bureau of Justice Statistics, "Forensic DNA Analysis: Issues," Washington, D.C.: U.S. Department of Justice, Bureau of Justice Statistics, June 1991, at 4, note 8.

8. The admissibility of the DNA evidence was upheld by the intermediate appeals court, which cited the uncontroverted testimony of the state's expert witnesses. *State* v. *Andrews,* 533 So.2d 841 (Dist. Ct. App. 1989). See also Office of Technology Assessment, Congress of the United States, *Genetic Witness: Forensic Uses of DNA Test* (Washington, D.C.: July 1990).

9. 385 S. E. 2d 253 (W. Va. 1989).

10. 384 S. E. 2d 775 (1989). Additional court appeals by Spencer were rejected by the Virginia Supreme Court at 384 S. E. 2d 785 (1989); 385 S. E. 2d 850 (1989); and 393 S. E. 2d 609 (1990).

11. Supra note 10 at 783.

12. Id., at 797.

13. 545 N. Y. S. 2d 985 (Sup. Ct. 1989). Castro's case was never tried. He pleaded guilty to the murders in late 1989.

14. *Schwartz* v. *State,* 447 N. W. 2d 422 (1989).

15. Id., at 427. The Minnesota Supreme Court further held that the use of statistical probabilities testimony should be limited because of its potential for prejudicing the jury. Id., at 428. The opinion was later modified in *State* v. *Bloom,* 516 N. W. 2d 159 (1994).

16. *Frye* v. *United States,* 293 F. 1013 (D.C. Cir. 1923). The test for the admissibility of novel scientific evidence enunciated in this case has been the most frequently invoked one in American case law. To be admissible, scientific evidence must be "sufficiently established to have gained general acceptance in the particular field in which it belongs."

17. *Daubert* v. *Merrell Dow Pharmaceuticals, Inc.,* 113 S. Ct. 2786 (1993). The Supreme Court used this civil case to articulate new standards for interpreting the admissibility of scientific evidence under the Federal rules of evidence. This standard, while encompassing *Frye,* allows a court to expand its examination to include other indicia of reliability, including publications, peer review, known error rate, and more. The court also should consider

factors that might prejudice or mislead the jury. For the application of *Daubert* to DNA technology, see Barry Sheck, "DNA and *Daubert*," *Cardozo Law Review* 15: 1959 (1994).

18. This brief overview is not a treatise on DNA evidence admissibility in criminal cases. For more authoritative articles, see, Thompson, supra note 3; D. H., Kaye, "The Forensic Debut of the National Research Council's DNA Report: Population Structure, Ceiling Frequencies and the Need for Numbers," *Jurimetrics Journal* 34 (4): 369-82 (1994); Comments, "Admissibility of DNA Statistical Data: A Proliferation of Misconception," *California Western Law Review,* 30: 145-178 (1993).

19. National Research Council, National Academy of Sciences, *The Evaluation of Forensic DNA Evidence* (prepublication copy) (Washington, D.C.: National Academy Press, 1996:2.14).

20. Matter of West Virginia State Police Crime Laboratory, 438 S. E. 2nd 501, 503 (W. VA. 1993).

21. Id., at 504.

22. Virginia Supreme Court Rules, Rule 3A: 15(h).

23. Paul Giannelli, "Chain of Custody and the Handling of Real Evidence," *American Criminal Law Review* 20 (4): 527-68 (Spring 1983).

24. If inconclusive cases were omitted, the exclusion rate for the FBI would be approximately 25 percent and the average exclusion rate for the other 18 laboratories would be about 30 percent.

25. This report does not discuss the issue of government misconduct because it is not particularized to the use of DNA technology. Beyond the limited instances noted in this report, enough examples of government misconduct in the criminal justice system exist in the popular media for government officials to be well aware of the problem.

26. *Commonwealth* v. *Brison,* 618 A.2d 420,425 (Pa. Super. 1992).

27. *Neil* v. *Biggers,* 409 U. S. 188, 199-200 (1972) (factors include accuracy of the witness' prior description of the defendant, opportunity to view the defendant at the time of the crime, level of certainty demonstrated, witness's degree of attention, and time between the crime and the confrontation).

28. Elizabeth Loftus, and D. Fishman, "Expert Psychological Testimony on Eyewitness Identification," *Law and Psychology Review* 4:87-103 (1978) (lack of reliability on cross-racial identification); Elizabeth Loftus and W. Wagenaar, "Ten Cases of Eyewitness Identification: Logical and Procedural Problems," *Journal of Criminal Justice* 18: 291-319 (1990) (witnesses can be induced to point to the suspect after subtle suggestion on the part of the investigator); and Brian Cutler, et al., "The Reliability of Eyewitness Identification: The Role of System and Estimator Variables," *Law and Human Behavior* 11 (3): 233-58 (1987) (level of stress experienced during crime may affect identification).

29. "DNA Testing Turns a Comer as Forensic Tool," *Law Enforcement News* 10 (October 15, 1995).

30. Elizabeth Loftus and N. Schneider, "Judicial Reactions to Expert Testimony Concerning Eyewitness Reliability," *UMKC Law Review* 56 (1): 145 (1987); and Roger Handberg, "Expert Testimony on Eyewitness Identification: A New Pair of Glasses for the Jury," *American Criminal Law Review* 32 (4): 1013-64 (Summer 1995).

31. *Williamson* v. *Reynolds,* 904 F. Supp. 1529 (E. D. Okl. 1995).

32. Id., at 1558. The National Research Council report, *DNA Technology in Forensic Science,* notes that, in contrast to microscopic hair comparison, with the advent of DNA technology, the use of hair as an individual identifier will become more common. National Research Council, National Academy of Sciences, *DNA Technology in Forensic Science* (Washington, D.C.: National Academy Press, 1992:158).

33. *DNA Technology in Forensic Science,* supra note 32, at 145-6.

34. Id., at 16. In its 1996 DNA report, *The Evaluation of Forensic DNA Technology* (National Academy Press, Washington, D.C.), the National Research Council reaffirmed this position (page 3.12). The DNA Identification Act of 1994 (Public Law 103-322) also provides for a DNA advisory board to set standards for DNA testing.

35. Telephone conversation with Manuel Valdez, treasurer, American Society of Crime Laboratory Directors, March 8, 1996. (More than 100 public laboratories perform DNA tests.)

36. See "Oops! We Forgot to Put It in the Refrigerator: DNA Identification and the State's Duty to Preserve Evidence," *The John Marshall Law Review* 25 809-36 (1992).

37. *Arizona* v. *Youngblood,* 109 S. Ct. 333, 337 (1988). The Supreme Court also stated that "police do not have a constitutional duty to perform any particular tests."

38. Supra note 33 at 160.

39. Virginia Supreme Court Rules, Rule 3A: 15(b).

40. An Oregon judge recently released Laverne Pavlinac and John Sosnovske from prison, where they had served 5 years after being convicted of murdering a young woman. The judge set aside their convictions because Keith Hunter Jesperson, a convicted serial killer, pleaded guilty to the murder for which the couple was convicted. See *The New York Times*: 28 (November 28, 1995)

41. *Tufflash* v. *State,* 878 S. W. 2d 197 (Tex. App. 1994). This case involved perjured trial testimony from Fred Zain, the state's forensic serologist.

42. See *State* v. *Thomas,* 586 A. 2d 250 (N.J. Appl. Div. 1991); and *Commonwealth* v. *Brison,* 618 A. 2d 420 (Pa. Super. 1992). Compare to *People* v. *Buxon,* 593 N.Y. S. 2d 87 (App. Div. 1993).

43. "Crime-Solving by DNA Dragnet," *The Washington Post*: A21 (February 2, 1996).

—by Edward Connors, Thomas Lundregan,
Neal Miller, and Tom McEwen;
commentary by Peter Neufeld, Esq., and Barry C. Scheck.

The authors of this report are staff members of the Institute for Law and Justice, Alexandria, Virginia. Barry Scheck is professor of law and director of clinical education, Benjamin N. Cardozo School of Law, New York, New York.

Chapter 50

Effective Expert Testimony

Types of Testimony

To present effective testimony, an expert witness (analyst, entomologist, chemist) must be able to accumulate the scientific evidence
necessary to prove a point. He/she is presumably educated to do this
by academic courses and experience. He/she must also, however, be
able to convey his/her findings to a judge or to a jury of 12 people,
usually laypersons, in language that they can easily understand.

The scientist is trained by experts in this chosen field. He/she reads
professional journals and converses with his/her colleagues. A very
large portion of his/her conversations or communications, though
meaningful to his/her associates, may be difficult or impossible for the
layperson to understand. Therefore, the scientific witness must
present his/her findings in such a way that all lay members of the
jury, as well as judges and attorneys, can easily grasp their significance. Technical expressions must be clearly and carefully explained.
A jury knows very little, if anything, about the laws of science, the
cumulation of evidence, precautions taken to avoid error, statistical
interpretation, etc.

Witnesses presenting scientific testimony fall into two categories.
There are witnesses of facts and expert witnesses. The fact witness,
even though he/she may have scientific training, can testify only to

Excerpted from "Court Testimony," Chapter 18.5.3, of the *FDA Laboratory
Procedures Manual*, [Online] undated. Available: http://www.fda.gov/ora/
science_ref/lpm. Produced by the FDA Office of Regulatory Affairs.

matters of fact that he/she has witnessed. He/she cannot give opinions. The expert witness is one who, by special study, practice, and experience, has acquired special skill and knowledge in relation to some particular science, art, or trade. Obviously, therefore, a fact witness must do only what his/her oath charges, namely, to tell the truth, the whole truth, and nothing but the truth. As an example, an inspector could testify, that he/she saw numerous insects crawling over the surface of stored-food packages in a warehouse. He/she could not be forced to venture an opinion as to whether the insects constituted a threat to the health of an individual who ate the foods. Such an opinion would have to be founded on the above-mentioned special study, practice, experience, etc. In other words, he/she would have to qualify as an expert in sanitation, public health, medicine, or some related scientific discipline. He/she could, however, offer the layperson's opinion that he/she found the observed conditions revolting.

Qualifying as an expert involves an examination of the individual's academic credentials and the duties connected with his/her career, past and present. This includes various professional achievements, such as the publication of original scientific papers. The possession of a bone fide degree from a state university, or employment of some duration by a state or federal agency in the scientific field covered by the testimony, practically assures that the judge will admit a person as an expert. If a state's educational system trains a person and presents him/her with a diploma, the state's judicial institutions cannot deny these credentials without good cause. Previous expert testimony also helps to qualify a person as an expert witness.

The main reason for expert testimony is to interpret difficult-to-comprehend facts to the jury. The judge will usually explain this fact to the jury and say that the court will permit the expert to evaluate the evidence and explain its significance to the case under examination. Even though an expert witness is entitled to give opinions, usually more than a mere statement of opinion is required to achieve maximum impact. Expert witnesses should know or conclude that certain conditions or findings prove the statements they make.

In most instances, witnesses are excluded from the courtroom during trial. If this is the case, then the witness will be required to give opinions regarding hypothetical questions.

Procedure in the courtroom is very formalized, and is probably quite unfamiliar to the average scientist. There are rigid rules of evidence designed to protect the rights of the accused. Also, all evidence must be presented in the form of answers to questions asked by the attorneys. A trial is an adversary proceeding in which the two sides have separate witnesses, each of whom will be questioned first by his/ her attorney (direct examination) and then by the opposing attorney (cross examination). The attorneys screen the evidence carefully, eliminating all that is irrelevant; they take extreme care not to omit any item pertinent to the case. Each tries to find inconsistencies in the testimony by the opposition or discredit the witness, and bring this to the attention of the court and jury.

The presiding judge is the ultimate authority in any given trial. His/her requests must be obeyed. In general, when it comes to evaluating evidence, the judge makes decisions on points of law, and the jury decides on matters of fact.

The jury is composed of 12 people of varied backgrounds. The conclusion of each one is of equal importance, and their verdict must be unanimous. The witness must speak loudly enough so that each juror can hear, and slowly and carefully enough so that each can remember as much as possible (jurors are forbidden to take notes). It is advisable to always address one's answer to the jury, or to the judge if no jury is present, rather than to the lawyer who asked the questions. Careful attention to the facial expressions of the jurors will make the witness aware of any lack of comprehension in time to simplify an explanation or expand upon it.

Effective Testimony

With this brief orientation to the courtroom scene, these suggestions about how to sharpen abilities as a witness should be read:

1. Think before speaking. A deliberate short pause before each answer, especially on cross examination, will prevent the expert from being stampeded into a poor answer.

2. Be frank. If a mistake or contradiction is made, admit it; don't try to cover it up.

3. Remain calm. Be polite to the interrogator even if he/she is insulting.

4. If a categorical answer can't be given, do not give such an answer; remember you swore to tell the whole truth. If forced to do so by the judge (only he can force you), say yes or no "with reservations." Similarly, do not answer any question that is not specifically asked.

5. If an answer is not known, admit it.

6. Avoid wisecracks. If you are given a "golden opportunity," remember that the attorney may be playing you for a fool. Injection of humor into a dry proceeding may be tempting, but should be done only if you are absolutely sure of the entire situation.

7. If not qualified as an expert witness, remember that the analyst can testify only to facts. Confine replies to matters of personal knowledge.

8. It is not enough only to tell the truth; appear to be telling the truth. The credibility of a witness often is judged very subjectively by the jury. These judgments often have their origin in the appearance and general demeanor of the witness, including clothes, posture, inflections of voice, and attitude towards the attorneys.

9. Be inconspicuous when not on the stand. You may prejudice yourself or the Government if you focus attention upon yourself.

10. Avoid conversations with principals or witnesses for the opposition. If conversations cannot be avoided, confine remarks to the weather, etc. If the defense attorney approaches you before trial, do not give him/her any information regarding what you know about the case. He/she has all of the information about you and your testimony before the trial.

11. Be sure the entire question is understood; do not hesitate to ask for it to be repeated if you cannot follow it completely. The attorney may try to make fun of your slowness and thereby try to discredit you. But this is much less damaging than having him/her get you thoroughly confused, and then proceed to show that you did not understand his/her question. Similarly, a multiple question should be broken down into its components, and each one answered completely.

12. Try to speak with the same speed and inflections when being questioned by either the Government's or the defendant's attorneys. A witness, especially an expert witness, is not supposed to be partial. The witness should maintain the poise and dignity of a professional person. Calmness or dignified reserve will inspire confidence in the speaker's integrity.

13. Don't answer any question objected to by either side until the court has ruled on the objection. If the witness has started his

answer, he should stop if any objection is raised, and should not continue until either the judge or one of the counsels so indicates.

14. A lawyer is not sworn in, so he/she is capable of deception in an effort to fish for perjury or equivocation. Be careful if the lawyer asks for a comment on a book or document. Before answering, request to see the documents he/she read from. He/she may be reading out of context or misquoting. Similarly, opposing counsel may ask if you regard certain persons in your field as recognized authorities. This is preparatory to asking you whether you agree with certain statements made by them. If you answer no (that is, you do not recognize them as authorities), then that line of cross examination cannot be pursued. Unless you definitely do consider a person a recognized authority, and are personally familiar with his/her publications, do not expose yourself by saying that you so recognize that person.

15. Avoid entrapment into detailed explanations of methods, equipment, etc. State that the method or equipment is widely accepted for use by federal and state laboratories. If directed by the judge or counsel to explain, then do so to the jury in the simplest, clearest way possible, stating that AOAC methods are recognized as the official methods of analysis.

16. Do not be afraid. "Stage fright" of a mild sort is natural. Remember that when you testify to facts, you "saw it happen." When you have qualified as an expert in your field, you will know more about the subject than any attorney, and as much as any other similarly educated expert. Therefore, you will understand what the attorneys are asking, unless they try to confuse you with trick questions or double-talk. You should recognize such maneuvers in time to protect yourself. There are times that you can stop cross examination by correcting the defense attorney.

17. If in doubt as to how to cope with a complex or misleading question, it is always proper to ask the clerk to repeat it, and answer each part separately. If you are flustered, or if for a moment you do not remember whether you are permitted to ask the attorney a question, you may say "If the court pleases, I should like to ask one or two questions of Mr./Ms" (whoever is questioning you). You will then be directed by the judge to

request your clarification, or to answer the question as asked. By then you will probably have regained your composure.

18. The opposing attorney may attempt to test your abilities by requesting you to identify certain materials. The first thing to remember is that, obviously, the identification on which your case rests was not made in "two minutes." Therefore, identification of the "test" material must take place by comparison with authentic identified examples, probably aided by instruments of various sorts. Counsel for the government should object on the grounds that the "test" material is not pertinent to the case. If the expert is directed to respond (something that a fact witness could avoid simply because it is beyond his purview), you may offer an offhand or superficial opinion in which he/she can speculate on similarities and dissimilarities of appearance. He/she then can state to the best of his/her knowledge, under the present circumstances, [what] the material is. When thus confronted, indicate that you do not advocate nor voluntarily indulge in giving "curbstone" opinions and state that upon authorization by the court you will make an in-depth study of the material and report your conclusions. If the judge approves the study, be sure that you are allowed as much time for your new assignment as was used to prepare your data for the case before the court.

19. Notes may be taken while on the witness stand but these are subject to inspection by the defense. Remember, anything taken to the stand can be examined by the defense. Be prepared to take notes if hypothetical questions are asked. This type of question is usually very lengthy and sometimes confusing. Notes will help to give categorical answers to the questions.

Typical Testimony

The following is typical testimony (on direct examination) of witness presenting analytical evidence in a food and drug filth case:

Q: State your name and address.

A: John A. Doe . . .

Q: What is your occupation and by whom are you employed?

A: I am a _ at the _ District of the Food and Drug Administration.

Q: How long have you been employed by the Food and Drug Administration?

A: I have been employed continuously since 19_ , about _ years.

Q: What are your education qualifications?

A: Degrees, graduate work, training courses, etc., as applicable.

Q: Do you belong to any scientific societies? Have you received any honors?

A: Enumerate professional scientific societies, such as AOAC, ARPE, etc.; fellow, associate referee, committee memberships, etc.

Q: Have you published any papers in your professional field?

A: State total number in current scientific journals and general subject area covered. Name a few. Emphasize subject matter specifically applicable.

Q: What are the duties of your position with FDA?

A: State general nature of duties including any supervisory and training activities, as applicable.

Q: In the course of your work with FDA, have you made analyses of products for filth?

A: Yes.

Q: Approximately how many such analyses have you made?

A (Give an approximate number).

Q: I call your attention to sample No. 12345A. Have you had occasion to receive and analyze this sample?

A: Yes, I have.

Q. From whom did you receive sample 12345A; what was the condition of the sample when you received it?

A. I received the sample from _; the sample was sealed with an official FDA seal identified "Sample No. 12345A; Date; and Signature." The sample was in a carton and consisted of cans labeled "_ ." Each can bore the Sample No. 12345A, date, and initials.

Q: What did you do with the sample?

A: I analyzed cans by method AOAC 440K, which is a determination of extraneous matter or filth in products as found in the "Official Methods of Analysis" of AOAC International.

Q: Is this method a published, standard, recognized method for determining filth in products?

A: Yes. The method I used is contained in the AOAC book of methods. All methods in this book are acceptable as official methods only after study and testing in different laboratories to show they are suitable for the intended analytical purpose and give uniform and reproducible results.

Q: Will you give the results of your analysis of sample 12345A?

A. (Ask for analytical results sheet.) The findings or results of analysis for each can are as follows: Can 1 contained rodent hair fragments of rat or mouse origin, and feather barbules; Can 2 contained _.

Q. Did you identify any of the insect material found in the sample as to type of insect?

A. Yes, I did. About one-quarter of the fragments were identified as being from the saw-toothed grain beetle; six fragments were from a dermestid beetle; four fragments were identified as being from Indianmeal moth larval form.

Q. Did anyone else examine the sample?

A. Yes, Mr. _ examined hair fragments isolated from the sample and identified them, as well as confirmed my identification of insect filth. My assistant, Mr. _, opened the cans, weighed out sample portions, and otherwise helped with the analysis.

Q. Did Mr. _, your assistant, work under your supervision or independently?

A. Mr. _ worked under my supervision during the entire analysis.

Chapter 51

Expert Testimony and the Standard of Care

Introduction

Malpractice lawsuits affect most physicians at some point in their career. Proving that malpractice has been committed is based on substantiation of a variety of elements, including that the patient was rendered care that was "below the standard" of care. While many physicians believe that the "standard" will be judged objectively on the basis of published scientific sources and accepted conventions, the standard is established rather by the testimony of expert witness(es). It is the expert testimony that sets the standard and is proof of the standard. The testimony is open for acceptance or rejection by the judge or jury for a variety of nonscientific reasons. We review what the defendant doctor might expect regarding proof required to establish breach of the standard of care and what the prudent expert should be obliged to demonstrate.

In the current, rapidly evolving medicolegal environment, risk management has become a byword for hospitals and insurers. To the practicing physician, a major risk to be managed is the threat of medical malpractice litigation. Despite the fact that >75% of the cases that actually reach court are found in favor of the physician/defendant,[1] the ultimate verdict does not diminish the physician's anxiety or sleepless nights, effects on self esteem, or the need to perpetually list on hospital or insurance applications any pending or prior malpractice actions initiated, even if they are subsequently resolved in the physician's favor.

This situation may also lead to practice patterns such as "defensive medicine" in the general medical community. The threat of awards for what are considered by some to be astronomical figures, and the undue consumption of time preparing for and attending a trial, often lead a physician/defendant to consider cutting the potential losses and consent to an out-of-court settlement, even when that physician believes no malpractice has occurred.

If ~1% of hospitalizations result in adverse events because of potential physician negligence[2] and that figure is extrapolated to the ~33.5 million hospitalizations that occur in the United States annually, then each year there are ~330,000 potential cases of malpractice[3] arising out of the hospital environment alone. There are also numerous outpatient encounters that can lead to malpractice claims. While 90% of patients who have an adverse outcome due to negligence do not file a malpractice suit,[4] numerous suits are filed annually.

Establishing the Standard of Care

The essence of many malpractice suits is that the physician allegedly rendered medical attention that was below the "standard of care or practice" and was therefore negligent. Assuming that it is also found that that negligence was a substantial factor in causing injury to the patient, then the doctor could be held liable for the consequent damages.

Most physicians expect that the standard of care applied in a case will be gathered from the scientific literature, from the textbooks and journals of the specialty that apply to a situation, and from the honest opinions of expert witnesses regarding the usual standard applied to similar cases treated by similarly trained colleagues. However, those expectations are not likely to be fulfilled, because of the sentiments and misconceptions of the public, the incentives for biased testimony, and the relative lack of sanctions for lack of integrity.

One of the primary problems is that the public (patients and juries) are often discouraged by modern health care and appear to expect more than medicine can reasonably offer. Often, patients seem to expect certainty of outcome in any individual case and are often disappointed by the inability of doctors to provide clear-cut answers and assurances.[3, 5] The divergence between such expectations and reality may result in consideration of a malpractice suit. Furthermore, one study of reasons for filing malpractice suits surprisingly found that 27% of patients who considered claims did so because of "explicit recommendations by health care providers to seek legal counsel."[3] Casual remarks by colleagues and righteous indignation thus fuel the medicolegal malpractice fire. In addition, there has been increasing disconnection between scientific findings and research results on the one hand, and the law as it is applied to cases on the other hand, in large part because of the use of expert testimony.[5]

The essential elements of a claim may vary from state to state, but in general, in order to prevail, the plaintiff/patient must establish that the care that was given was beneath the level that would have been provided by the majority or a respectable minority of physicians practicing under similar circumstances. Generalists and specialists are held to different standards,[6] unless a generalist attempts to treat a specialized problem that would ordinarily call for a referral.[7, 8] In that case, the generalist will be held to the standard of the specialist.

The plaintiff must also show that failure to meet the standard of care caused, or was a substantial factor in causing, the damage (the definition of legal causation may vary from state to state, but the concept is generally the same). This is the basic rule of "no harm, no foul." The patient must be able to prove that actual damage did occur as a result of the negligence.

Adapting the Basic Rule

While physicians are generally required to exercise the degree of skill and competence ordinarily possessed by fellow practitioners ("peers") under similar circumstances, there are numerous situations in which this basic rule can be applied, and the analysis of compliance with the standard of care must be adapted for each variation. For example, the nonspecialist may be held liable for medical malpractice for failing to call in a specialist.[9] The nonspecialist could be held liable if it were proven to a judge or jury that a majority of nonspecialists under the same circumstances would normally have called in a specialist. This rule applies to the ordering of diagnostic tests, the interpretation of test results, the institution of therapy, or the withholding of therapy. Again, one must still prove causation for this element to be of significance.

There are circumstances where the proof of negligence does not require expert testimony. In instances where the negligence would be obvious, even to the layperson, such as a surgeon who cuts off the wrong leg, or an injection with a dirty needle, then there need not be expert testimony to establish this element. The doctrine of *res ipsa loquitur* might apply. More specifically, that doctrine applies when a layperson can conclude without the assistance of medical testimony that (a) a result would not have occurred in the absence of negligence, (b) the instrumentality or agency of injury was within the exclusive control of the defendant doctor, and (c) the patient did not contribute to the injury by any voluntary act (e.g., falling out of a gurney).

In the context of a legal case, the standard of care, i.e., proof of what a reasonable doctor would or would not have done under given circumstances, is thus usually "proven" by "expert testimony" of another physician chosen by either the plaintiff's attorney or the defendant's attorney. Medical experts are usually well paid by the attorneys who engage them and may be selected by the attorneys on the basis of the positions they will likely take on any given issue. In the United States, the qualifications of experts are presented by the attorneys for whom they testify and the criteria for expertise are inexact, vague, and usually very liberal. Rather than excluding such testimony for lack of qualification, generally the judge simply instructs a jury that they may take information on qualifications into account in weighing the testimony—determining its value relative to other testimony.

There are notable exceptions. For example, in California there is a specific legal requirement that in order to qualify to testify as an expert in emergency room medicine, one must have had substantial experience in an acute care hospital within the preceding 5 years.[10] However, such requirements are the exception rather than the rule. So, the expert may or may not have significant experience in the same specialty or have seen similar patients, may or may not have done any research in the area under examination, and may or may not be considered an expert by his/her peers. The expert's credentials may be cross-examined by the opposing attorney on the same basis, but a well-prepared witness (and usually there are preparatory sessions before a trial) can often overcome such obstacles, at least in the mind of the jury. The credentials of expert witnesses and their depositions are available before the trial according to the rules of discovery (the process of investigating the facts before the trial).

Many physicians assume that these experts will produce concrete (as concrete as medicine gets, that is) guidelines generated from textbooks, published peer-reviewed articles, or local customs for evaluating the actions of the doctor accused of malpractice. Even in this context, however, it is well known that medicine is not an exact science, and there are a number of gray areas in terms of appropriate diagnosis and treatment. So, the law recognizes that there are often alternate methods of treatment, all of which may be acceptable.

For example, the California jury instructions[11] state "Where there is more than one recognized method of diagnosis or treatment, and not one of them is used exclusively and uniformly by all practitioners of good standing, a physician is not negligent if, in exercising his or her best judgment, he or she selects one of the approved methods, which later turns out to be a wrong selection, or one not favored by certain other practitioners." Note, however, that there may be an obligation to inform the patient that other members of the medical profession might render a different diagnosis based on a contrary recognized school of thought.[12]

However, experts need not rely on such evidence to support their testimony, "even when there are relevant studies in peer-review journals"[5] previously published. The testimony supplied by experts is the "proof," and their opinions are the evidence. Ignoring such authority is made all the easier given "widespread distrust and misunderstanding of science in American society and the view by jurors that medical research is irrelevant," as related in a recent article about breast implants.[5] Selection of jurors and their prior experiences and biases may have far more to do with the verdict than the scientific evidence presented. The courts also have compounded this problem "by ignoring the rules of science and handing down verdicts which fly in the face of evidence."[5]

The court may also impose its own view of the standard of care on physicians.[13] In a highly publicized decision in 1974, the court held that while it was not customary for ophthalmologists to perform screening tonometry on patients <30 years old because of the low incidence of disease in that population, the test should have been done for a 29-year-old patient who developed glaucoma because it was simple and easily performed and the disease has disastrous consequences if not recognized. In this case the court disregarded the usual physician's practice and imposed its own values.

Since the standard of care is generally established by expert witness testimony as subjectively interpreted by the judge or jury, verisimilitude can be a matter of the effectiveness of an attorney's presentation, the expert witness's demeanor or style or image, or how well the expert withstands cross-examination (which, in turn, usually depends on his legal experience at least as much as his medical experience). Ultimately, it is then what the jury believes regardless of any generally accepted medical doctrine that usually determines the standard of care in any case. Even the United States Supreme Court's finding[14, 15] that required federal judges to review expert testimony and set limits on admission based on reliability and relevance is often only loosely applied. State courts are sometimes under the same injunction.

The Statistics and Demographics of Malpractice

Under the current system, some interesting data have been accumulated about malpractice cases. A review[16] of 8,231 closed cases of medical malpractice that occurred in New Jersey between 1977 and 1992 found that in the 62% of cases that were considered defensible, the plaintiff received payment 21% of the time. However, of the 21% of cases considered indefensible and the 13% of cases with "unclear" defensibility, payment to the plaintiff occurred in 91% and 59% of cases, respectively. It was also noted that severity of injury was related to payments in cases with early settlements but was not related to "the likelihood of payment" in cases that required a jury verdict.[16]

Another study[17] noted that male physicians were more likely to be sued than female physicians and that the rate of claims varied with the physician's age and peaked at ~age 40. There was no association of claims filed and physician's country or site of training, or with the type of medical degree (e.g., D.O. vs. M.D.) of the practitioner; board-certified physicians had a slightly increased risk of being sued. Internists had a history of 0.13 claims per physician per year compared to that for "all physicians," which was 0.19 claims per physician per year. No data were given for the medical subspecialties such as infectious diseases.

Summary

All of these findings raise serious questions as to what are and should be the duties and obligations of an expert witness and, as a corollary, what can be done, if anything, to assist in establishing fairness and scientific reason in a malpractice case. In order to ensure that an expert witness would impartially review the case records, give advice to the attorney based on reasonable care guidelines, and not be influenced by the attorney's strategy and position, there are several possible avenues: (1) Reduce the monetary incentive to shade one's opinions, perhaps by putting a limit on compensation for such services and requiring doctors to devote a minimal number of hours per year to consultations and testimony; (2) Enact more legislative requisites to determine qualifications for testifying; (3) Require preliminary hearings in each case, wherein the judge would determine whether the witness is truly an expert, with adequate, current experience and training; (4) Allow more liberal use of treatises, practice guidelines, and journals; (5) Exert more peer pressure on those who become "professional" witnesses; and (6) Have professional societies qualify and provide listings of acknowledged experts in a given discipline.

References

1. R. R. Bovbjerg, "Medical Malpractice: Folklore, Facts and the Future," *Annals of Internal Medicine* 117: 788-91 (1992).

2. T. A. Brennan, L. L. Leape, N. M. Laird, et al., "Incidence of Adverse Events and Negligence in Hospitalized Patients: Results of the Harvard Medical Practice Study I," *New England Journal of Medicine* 324: 370-6 (1991).

3. M. I. Huycke and M. H. Huycke, "Characteristics of Potential Plaintiffs in Medical Malpractice Litigation," *Annals of Internal Medicine* 120: 792-8 (1994).

4. A. R. Localio, A. G. Lawthers, T. A. Brennan, et al., "Relationship between Malpractice Claims and Adverse Events Due to Negligence III," *New England Journal of Medicine* 325: 245-51 (1991).

5. "Angell M. Shattuck Lecture—Evaluating the Health Risks of Breast Implants: The Interplay of Medical Science, the Law and Public Opinion," *New England Journal of Medicine* 334: 1513-8 (1996).

6. *Quintal v. Laurel Valley Hospital* (1964), 62 Cal. 2d 154.

7. *Sanson v. Ross-Loos* (1961), 57 Cal. 2d 549.

8. *Valentine v. Kaiser* (1961), 194 Cal. App. 2d 282.

9. *Bickford v. Lawson* (1938), 27 Cal. App. 2d 416.

10. California Health and Safety Code, sec. 1799.110.

11. *California Jury Instructions—Civil (BAJI)*, 7th ed. (St. Paul: West Publishing, 1966) 6.03.

12. *Jamison v. Lindsay* (1980), 108 Cal.App.3d 223.

13. *Helling* v. *Carey,* 519 P.2d 981 (Wash. 1974) (en banc).

14. *Daubert* v. *Merrell Dow Pharmaceuticals, Inc.* (1993), 125 U.S. 469 Lawyer's Edition 2nd.

15. 113 Supreme Court Reporter 2786.

16. M. I. Taragin, L. R. Willett, A. P. Wilczek, R. Trour, and I. L. Carson, "The Influence of Standard of Care and Severity of Injury on the Resolution of Medical Malpractice Claims," *Annals of Internal Medicine* 117: 780-4 (1992).

17. M. I. Targan, A. P. Wilczek, M. E. Karns, R. Trout, and I. L. Carson, "Physician Demographics and Risk of Medical Malpractice," *American Journal of Medicine* 93: 537-42 (1992).

—by Gregg J. Gittler and Ellie J. C. Goldstein

From Gittler, Wexler and Bradford, Los Angeles, and R. M. Alden Research Laboratory, Santa Monica—UCLA Medical Center, Santa Monica, California.

Chapter 52

The Non-Physician Expert Witness

Medical malpractice litigation is an interesting and challenging field for the biomedical scientist. It offers the opportunity to apply his specialized knowledge and experience in the legal arena by participating in the defense of a doctor unjustly accused of injuring a patient, or in supporting the claim of a patient who has been harmed by the negligence of a physician.

Medical malpractice litigation revolves around the theory of negligence. To prove negligence the plaintiff must establish: a) a duty owed to the patient by the treating physician; b) a breach of that duty; c) injury or damage; and, d) proximate cause. Breach of the duty owed to the patient requires proof of the acceptable standard of care, a standard that has been defined as "what the reasonable person of ordinary prudence would do under like circumstances" (498 S.W. 2nd 388,391).

With the possible exception of limited circumstances that are self-evident, known as *res ipsa loquitor,* an expert witness is required to define for the court the appropriate standards of care, and possibly testify as to how the defendant physician's actions conformed or deviated from these standards.

Federal Rule of Evidence 702 states: If scientific, technical, or other specialized knowledge will assist the trier of fact to understand the evidence or to determine a fact in issue, a witness qualified as an expert

From "The Non-Physician Expert in Medical Malpractice Litigation," by Paul D. Ellner, Ph.D., in *The Expert & the Law,* Vol. 14, No. 1, January 1998, pp. 2, 4. © 1998 by the National Forensic Center. Reprinted with permission.

by knowledge, skill, experience, training, or education may testify in the form of an opinion or otherwise.

Expert witnesses asked to testify in medical malpractice cases are usually physicians who specialize in a medical discipline related to the case. However, biomedical scientists who are not physicians can often provide cogent and relevant information and/or testimony. Qualifications to be accepted as an expert witness usually include a doctoral degree in a basic medical science, teaching experience in a medical facility, publications in scientific journals, and membership in professional societies. Clinical chemists, pharmacologists, physiologists, microbiologists, immunologists, and others may furnish valuable input by acting *as a testifying expert* or as a *litigation consultant*.

The testifying expert plays an active role in the legal controversy. He will be examined by the opposition at deposition and possibly later at trial. All of the expert's activities relating to the case, as well as his work products, are discoverable. His effectiveness as a witness during trial will be as much determined by his demeanor and presentation in court as by his factual material.

Since 1993, many courts have adopted the *Daubert* standard which holds that scientific testimony must be screened by the trial judge to assure its relevance and reliability. The Federal Judicial Center's *Reference Manual on Scientific Evidence,* intended as a guide for judges, lawyers, and experts, asks a fundamental question: Is the expert qualified?

The opposition will try to negate or at least lessen the impact of the expert's testimony by raising the question of his/her qualifications. A serious attempt will be made to disqualify the non-physician expert on the basis of a lack of clinical experience, training, or education.

The litigation consultant who is not called as an expert witness is immune from these challenges. Like a coach at an athletic event, he does not participate in the contest but remains on the sidelines advising and counseling. The consultant is not subject to examination by the opposition, and his activities and work products such as reports to the attorney, are not subject to discovery.

The following three cases illustrate how a non-physician expert effectively functioned as a consultant in malpractice actions:

Case 1. The plaintiff cut his leg on a fence while chasing his horse. The emergency room physician treated the wound and sent him home. He returned several hours later in great pain, and was again treated by the physician. The following day the plaintiff consulted a surgeon who admitted him to the hospital and performed an extensive operation on the man's leg. The surgeon remarked that the emergency room physician had not properly cleaned and drained the wound. The patient sued the emergency room physician for malpractice. Acting as a consultant for the defense, the non-physician expert, familiar with minor surgical procedures, reviewed the emergency room physician's and nurse's notes, and was able to advise the defense attorney that the treatment provided by the physician conformed to or exceeded the standard of care in such cases. The expert relied upon several textbooks of surgery.

Case 2. A woman fell and injured her knee. Following treatment by a physician in the emergency room of the local hospital, she subsequently developed a severe infection that over the course of several years involved the bones of her leg. The non-physician expert acting as consultant for the plaintiff's attorney, was able to suggest that the treating physician closed the wound prematurely which predisposed to the infection. The consultant's opinion was based upon his review of the standards of care as published in several textbooks of surgery.

Case 3. An infant developed severe seizures several hours after delivery, and the obstetrician was sued for permitting prolonged labor that compromised the oxygen supply to the fetus resulting in brain damage. The non-physician expert, acting as consultant for the defense, reviewed the mother's prenatal history and advised the defense attorney that the infant's seizures could have been caused by a specific infectious disease contracted by the mother during her pregnancy.

In the first two cases, the consultant dealt with the standard of care; the third case was concerned with proximate cause.

An expert's opinion may be based upon his personal experience, experiments that he has conducted that directly relate to the case, or on scientific articles published by others (F.R.E. 703). In some instances, standards of care have been published by professional organizations, and the non-physician expert may refer to and rely upon such sources. The Hearsay Rule (F.R.E. 803) exempts material from learned treatises relied upon by the expert witness in direct examination. The rule notes that "statements contained in published treatises, periodicals, or pamphlets on a subject of . . . medicine, or other science or art, established as a reliable authority by the testimony or admission of the witness . . . may be read into evidence . . . ."

Non-physician biomedical scientists explaining aspects of anatomy, biochemistry, pharmacology, immunology, microbiology, pathology, or other basic medical sciences can be very effective as testifying experts for either plaintiff or defense. It is the writer's opinion that for psychological rather than legal reasons, it is easier for a non-physician expert to defend or justify a physician's actions than to disparage or criticize a doctor's treatment. Hence, non-physician experts dealing with questions relating to standards of care, especially when working for the plaintiff's attorney, may be more useful as litigation consultants.

—by Paul D. Ellner, Ph.D.

Chapter 53

Forensic Graphics

Litigators are profoundly aware of the need to use visual images in the modem courtroom. As our culture shifts its focus from verbal to visual communications, judges and juries demand that the facts be presented and illustrated quickly and clearly.

[Forensic graphics specialists understand] the unique need of the legal community to communicate concepts effectively and efficiently for strategy and case arguments. By concentrating on key issues and nonlinear (hyper-linked) graphics, [they] provide a flexible presentation system that builds agreement toward favorable settlement. . . .

Computer multimedia demonstrative evidence is a powerful and dramatic means by which to illustrate expert opinions. The forensic graphics specialist should also be involved with the primary investigative team, working closely with police, fire, and medical professionals and insurance adjusters to photograph and document the loss as well as protect and preserve the integrity of all evidence. Case progress can then be monitored through a careful and selective iterative approval process of expert witness graphics at all stages of investigation and presentation, from initial sketches to final trial exhibits.

Excerpted from "Forensic Graphics for Attorneys and Expert Witnesses," [Online] 1995. Formerly available: www.west.net/~arteng/. © 1995 by The Art Engineering Company. Produced by Michael Bloomenfeld, Legal Arts Multimedia, LLC, 444 High St., Ste. 244, Palo Alto, CA 94301. For complete contact information, please refer to Chapter 56, "Resources." Reprinted with permission.

The Investigation Begins

In the initial stages, the graphics investigator should accompany the primary investigators (engineers, police, fire, medical and insurance examiners) to the disaster site and begin a visual and photographic survey of the entire building or facility footprint. Using measuring (and data acquisition) equipment, the primary dimensions of the post-incident structure, machine, or site are determined.

Background

The graphic investigation specialist should be technically oriented and have a good basic engineering and construction background in order to understand how a structure or building facility goes together. He should be familiar with CADD (Computer Aided Design and Drafting) and optical field survey equipment. For example, he should be able to work safely at a post-fire site without disturbing evidence and, if necessary, help direct personnel and equipment to uncover and document evidence and arrangements around the origin area much like an archeological excavation. It is important to locate datum's or semipermanent reference markers which will be useful for offset measurements and show up in photo records

Creating the Field Notes File

The preliminary plan or field sketch can include such data as measured lengths, widths, heights, north bearing, distances, marks, witness locations, discolorments, furnishings, appliances, machinery, and burn or explosion behavior patterns. Doors, windows, vents, valves, and switch positions are noted. Electrical and HVAC (heating, ventilating, air conditioning) systems as well as clock and instrument dials are also documented.

Using the Field Notes File

In all, a good field notes file is created which can provide adequate reference information permitting the drafting board work at the office to be completed simultaneously with the investigation reports.

At the office, under the direction and coordination of the project's chief investigator, various approaches and types of drawings are created. For simple reports, a horizontal floor plan sketch showing the cause or origin location may be all that is required. In most of the hundreds of small residential and commercial fires and accidents encountered, this is all that is required.

In the more complicated or subrogated cases, more details are required. We try to stay with very basic orthographic diagrams such as simple schematic line drawings and intentionally expose only as much information as required to eliminate distraction or confusion. These flat, one-dimensional maps are sometimes enhanced with careful use of color or shading.

From Field Notes to Working Drawings

The next phase may be twofold. Initially, a slightly more complicated drawing may be required to illustrate the failure in question. These may include vertical plane elevation views, a three-dimensional pictorial or a CADD model (as will be discussed later). Also, the engineering staff may require measured or technical drawings for fuel load quantities or char studies, for example.

These "working" drawings are executed in the typical drafter's language, a kind of visual shorthand that would be confusing and tedious for most people to read but provide useful and organized information. In essence, we may be recreating the construction prints of the destroyed building or failed object. Facilities or apparatus may be designed as required for innovative or standard testing procedures.

Field Office Investigation and Research

The second phase begins by establishing an on-site field office in a trailer or site facility to continue the research and investigation. All pre-incident plans and diagrams of the subject structure or device need to be collected. This may include contacting the owner, renter, facility management, local, or regional building departments for codes and permits, Sanborn tax assessment maps, and old pre-incident photos or videos (local news media may be helpful here). Remodeling or alteration drawings and specifications with addendums and change orders may be available as well as fire police reports which may have relevant sketches. Surveyed plot plans, aerial and satellite photogametry, inspection reports, equipment maintenance schedules, assembly drawings and catalogs, etc., may also be used. The operation may include specimen and sample recovery, tagging and storing evidence, and site security.

If a case is to be litigated, depositions and interrogatories may have helpful witness exhibits such as descriptions, photographs, and diagrams.

Architectural and engineering plans and specifications that describe the "as built" condition of the property with code and profession stamps are very important information sources to review.

Reading the Plans and Drawings

Once the information has been gathered from such sources, an analysis to sift through the data is required. In order to perform this, the graphics investigator should be familiar with all the conventional symbology of many disciplines. He should be able to read any visual shorthand that is the language of the drafter's and designer's work.

The style and handwriting may indicate the degree of professionalism gone into the project. The layout and organization of the plans may indicate how much thought and planning preceded construction.

Finding When and Where Things Go Wrong

Today, with fast track management and construction techniques, projects (especially very large ones) are being assembled in the field by subcontractors concurrent with code agency approvals. This increases the possibility of defective apparatus arrangements or installations that fail.

For example, some safety systems may preclude or nullify others. The earthquake seismic separations in the MGM Hotel towers transmitted dangerous toxic smoke to the rooms resulting in horrendous loss of lives. Inadequate shop drawing reviews permitted the bolt failures of the concrete "skyways" at the Kansas City Hyatt—again with large loss of lives. The Cypress Freeway collapsed because of marginal seismic design.

Effectively Reviewing All the Documents for Facts

The process of examining plans and drawn documents as evidence demands skill and patient exactitude. I tend to review the complete set quickly to get the feeling for the project and then return to the first sheet for in-depth study.

The title block (if there is one) contains much valuable information on who made the drawings and when they were executed. It is important not to confuse pre-incident remodeling or alteration drawings with post-incident remodel drawings and looking for who and when on approvals and revision as well as checker's comments. Find out what professional registration or code agency approval stamps are present or required (i.e., sprinklers not approved for high stacked or combustible fluids). Also, we must know if the drawing had been reduced, thus changing the scale. Even the blueprint, diazo, or copying process may give us a clue as to the age of the structure.

For example, an aging and complicated inner-urban retail and commercial structure had been remodeled and subdivided numerous times since 1909. Some remodels even restored the original configuration but changed the type of interior structural wall system. Using ancient building department inspector records, plans and permits, we were able to create an evolutionary series of drawings which showed how the fire spread and pinpointed ownership responsibility.

Distributing Working Preliminary Drafts

This example also brings up the importance of accessibility: drawings and illustrations must be made available for client and staff review as the case develops. Certainly, the expression "a picture is worth a thousand words" is applicable here. "Progress print" or "preliminary" copies should be stamped, dated, and displayed for client conferences. As a communication tool, these drawings save many hours of unnecessary meetings. CADD generated drawings must be cataloged and time dated. I never mind having my shoulder looked over at a daily "mini-drafting board" meeting which keeps jobs flowing smoothly.

Developing More Detailed Pictorials

Once the data gathering has been accomplished and the analysis performed, the forensic graphic specialist must develop multi-dimensional pictorials which clearly illustrate the information requested by the legal consultant and determined by scientific staff. Implementing a CADD model may be appropriate.

There are several types of pictorials which are common and applicable to investigative procedures. Because of the interesting and very important information which crystallizes through the graphic process, the graphic investigator should understand the skills and theory of "how we see" or the biomechanics and psychology of visual perception.

Investigation and the Classes of Pictorial Graphics

The first type or primary group of pictorials are the paralines. These are simply drawings that project surface planes to indicate depth. These are called axonometric drawings and are very useful because they can be shaded and scaled and are quite simple to construct. They provide accurate information and with minimal shading are easy for most people to read.

The most popular is the 30 degree isometric. Often used as "exploded assembly" drawings that "float" out walls or parts to separate objects, they give an immediate visual sense of where and what is happening without confusing dialogs and minimal texts. This technique is also good for details and cross sections.

One caution here is to remember isometrics only mimic reality, and it is a geometric exercise which does not exist as we see. (Nature abhors straight and parallel lines.) Without properly weighted line work at edge surfaces or shading, the drawings may reverse or turn themselves inside out or cause other uncomfortable spatial illusions which often confuse observers.

Oblique projections are similar to the axonometrics and are useful because one may work directly and rapidly from an existing plan or orthographic to create a bird's-eye view of the action. Obliques tend to excessively elongate wall surfaces but are good for quick trace studies of arrangements. Again, one must use care that the drawing is absolutely clear and does not become a meaningless abstraction. Confusing a client or viewer must not be permitted.

Another class of pictorials are the perspectives. They are far more realistic than the axonometrics or obliques because they show things as the eye would see them. This would seem ideal but experience shows that objects seen in perspective may cover, block, foreshorten, and otherwise distort and distract from useful information.

The main elements of perspective contain unique, interesting, and valuable information for forensic graphic work. It is of utmost importance to have a working familiarity with the rules of perspective.

What the Witness Observes

Witness views can be created that can accurately determine what was or was not seen. Photographs can be analyzed as per location, distance, sun time, and point of view. CADD models may be examined using observer station points and clipping paths.

There are three types of perspectives: one point parallel, two point oblique and three point angular. The simplest "one point" type will be considered to demonstrate the kind of information and problems which will appear.

The (witness or even fictitious) observer's location is determined and called the station point. A cone of vision of 60 degrees is created for the observer's direction with a field of view along the line of sight. A picture plane frames the object or scene. A horizon line gives the altitude of view and vanishing points are established to which all receding lines converge.

We now have the basic elements that provide measured data that can be manipulated geometrically or mathematically to create a dimensioned grid. Objects can now be introduced on the grid in extended height, width, or depth. The developing appearance of the picture is analogous to knowing the "right questions" to ask in problem solving.

As the various types of forensic illustrations develop, materials and arrangements can be identified. Distortion can be controlled better than with lens photography. The structural skeleton or hidden objects can be revealed or prominently displayed. The scene can be recreated very closely to the time of the incident. Ultimately, well thought out presentation graphics can be a powerful tool in an engineering investigation, court judgement, or successful marketing decision.

—by Michael Bloomenfeld

Chapter 54

Digital Imaging Tools on Trial

Digital imaging tools, such as digital cameras, photo CD discs, and image handling software, can be important assets to the police department as it gathers and presents evidence. But as with any other tools, you must have standard operating procedures (SOPs) in place to ensure that evidence you gather and present will be accepted by courts of law.

Standard operating procedures governing the use of digital imaging technology need to incorporate five key elements.

1. Images must be recorded in an unalterable, archival form soon after the records are created.

A digital imaging technology that supports this requirement is a writable CD. Writable CDs are CD-ROM discs using CD writers and read using standard CD-ROM computer drives.

Writable CDs are ideal for storing images or information about evidence because they are a nonerasable medium. You can append data to writable CDs as long as sufficient space remains. However, it is not possible to remove or write over images that are already on the discs. Writable CD images are created by permanently altering the disc's dye layer with a laser light beam. CD writers cannot undo previous laser marks.

From "Ensure Admissibility of Digital Images," by Richard Kammen and Herbert Blitzer, in *The Indiana Lawyer*, Vol. 6., No. 15, November 1-14, 1995 [Online]. Available: http://www.engr.iupui.edu/ifi/articles/indlaw.html. © 1996 by Indiana University and Purdue University, Indianapolis (IUPUI). Reprinted with permission.

Some CDs have engraved serial numbers as well, which eliminates the possibility that altered discs might be substituted for originals.

Writable CDs are being used today in law enforcement to archive images and to display them in court.

2. The images should include information regarding their creation.

This requirement is also supported by today's digital imaging technology. For example, some digital cameras generate a uniquely written data file each time an image is captured. The file records information such as the camera's make, model and serial number, camera settings, and the date and time the image was captured. When you save the image, the data file can be stored as well.

If you write the image and data to a writable CD soon after the image capture and prior to any image enhancement, you will have created an archival reference copy.

3. The agency must control custody of all image records at all times.

This requirement ensures someone can testify about who had access to any images used to support testimony as evidence.

There are a number of procedures you can put into place to satisfy this requirement. For example, determine which computer or computers will be used for medium- or long-term storage of image files. Then password-protect sensitive computer files stored on those computers. Keep the computers and any archival media, such as CDs, in secure locations.

The use of unalterable media for storage, along with a separately managed index for each unit, helps ensure the integrity of information.

You should also establish procedures for the management of any files stored temporarily on portable computers. For example, you may want to specify how frequently those files will be removed from the portables and archived.

4. All agency personnel who prepare exhibits for court should be trained in digital image processing and should understand which images might require a special notation to show that the changes are not prejudicial.

Certain procedures for enhancing digital imaging files are analogous to using basic darkroom techniques to enhance film images. They are applied generally to an entire image. Digital imaging software can, for example, be used to control the contrast of images or to enlarge them.

Other digital processing procedures are potentially more problematic. These are applied to certain parts of an image. For example, you can use software to "morph" an image of a person's face to show how the person would look if he or she were older or several pounds heavier. In these cases, it may be necessary for the staff to document how the changes were made.

There is also a gray area between these two types of image processing. Selective color removal or fast Fourier transformation can be used to clean up the background or a latent fingerprint. Special procedures should be established to support expert witnesses as they testify concerning any of these image processing techniques.

In some cases, you can implement image processing SOPs using computer-based tools. For example, it is possible to record the keystrokes used to perform a computer operation in a file called a "macro". When a macro is replayed, it will re-execute the keystrokes in their original sequence. This technique could be used to document how a particular image alteration was accomplished.

5. The agency must establish rigorous procedures for entering work-in-progress into proper file systems.

Digital technology can help agencies document how and when images were captured, processed, or stored. However, additional procedures must be used to create a complete audit trail of how the computer files have been managed. Uniquely identifiable, unalterable media can make this much easier.

Digital imaging technology has brought new tools to law enforcement. Today, digital images appear in courts with increasing frequency, and the uncertainty about how they may be used is dwindling. In fact, in some ways, digital images may prove more secure than conventional images.

For example, using today's technology, it is relatively easy to alter an image scanned from a roll of film, create a new roll that includes the phony image, and then replace the original with the altered roll. However, if you use writable CDs which come with embedded serial numbers, and if you record an index of disc contents along with their serial numbers as part of your standard operating procedures, it would be virtually impossible to replace originals with altered discs.

The key is to select technology carefully and to put standard operating procedures into place that are derived from an understanding of operational requirements and the technology.

—by Richard Kammen and Herbert Blitzer

Richard Kammen is a partner at McClure, McClure and Kammen in Indianapolis. Herbert Blitzer is manager of the law enforcement segment at Eastman Kodak Company.

Part Seven

Additional Help and Information

Chapter 55

Forensics Glossary

Following the glossary is a list of acronyms used in this book.

A

accelerant: In arson investigation, refers to a volatile agent used to speed the ignition and rate of spread of fire. The accelerants most commonly used, gasoline, kerosene, mineral turps, and diesel, are complex mixtures of hydrocarbon molecules.

acute: Characterized by sudden onset, sharp rise, and short course (as in disease).

aliphatic: Organic compound having an open-chain structure.

alleles: Alternate gene forms or variations, which are the basis of DNA testing.

amino acid: Amphoteric organic acid containing the amino group NH_2.

This chapter includes definitions excerpted from "Hidden Evidence: Latent Prints on Human Skin," in *FBI Law Enforcement Bulletin,* April 1996; "FDA's Forensic Center: Speedy, Sophisticated Sleuthing," in *FDA Consumer* magazine, July-August 1995; "Who Wrote It?" in *National Institute of Justice Journal,* September 1997; "Automated DNA Typing: Method of the Future?" in *NIJ Research Preview,* February 1997; *Convicted by Juries, Exonerated by Science,* National Institute of Justice publication no. 161258; "Improved Postmortem Detection of Carbon Monoxide and Cyanide," in the U.S. Department of Justice,

(continued on next page)

antemortem: Before death; term used in relation to corpse during death investigation.

anthropometric: Relating to the study of human body measurements on a comparative basis.

antigen: Any biological substance that can stimulate the production of, and combine with, antibodies. Variances in human antigens can be used to identify individuals within a population.

arson: A fire that is not the result of an accident, but has been deliberately lit, often with the help of an accelerant. Motives for arson include vandalism, fraud revenge, sabotage, and pyromania.

arthropod: Any of the phylum of invertebrate animals (as insects, arachnids, and crustaceans) that have a segmented body and jointed appendages, a chitinous exoskeleton molted at intervals, and a dorsal anterior brain connected to a ventral chain of ganglia.

assay: Analysis to determine the presence, absence, or quantity of one or more drugs.

atomic spectroscopy: Determination of elements based on the emission or absorption of electromagnetic radiation (for example, ultraviolet and visible light) by atoms.

autopsy: Procedure utilized to study the corpse. It is primarily a systematic external and internal examination for the purposes of diagnosing disease and determining the presence or absence of injury. In modern times chemical analysis of body fluids for medical information as well as analysis for drugs and poisons should be part of any autopsy on a dead body coming under the jurisdiction of the medical examiner or coroner.

Office of Justice Programs publication, *NIJ Research Preview,* July 1996; "New Reagents for Development of Latent Fingerprints," in *National Institute of Justice Update,* September 1995; "Toxicology Tutor I," by the National Library of Medicine; "Bite Marks in Forensic Dentistry: A Review of Legal, Scientific Issues," © 1995 by American Dental Association; "Forensic Psychiatry and Medicine," by Harold J. Bursztajn, M.D.; "Forensic Entomology," © 1998 by Jason H. Byrd, Ph.D.; "An Introduction to Forensic Firearms Identification," © 1996-97 by Jeffrey Scott Doyle; "The Forensic Sciences Foundation, Inc., Career Brochure," The Forensic Sciences Foundation, Inc.; "The Role of Criminal Profiling in the Development of Trial Strategy," © 1997 by Knowledge Solutions, LLC, for Brent Turvey, M.S.; "Overview of Instrumental Analysis (Chemistry)," by Karen L. Kwek, Forensic Chemist; "Clinical Forensic Nursing: A New Perspective in the Management of Crime Victims from

(continued on next page)

B

bioassay: Method of determining the relative strength of a drug by comparing its effect on a test organism with that of a standard preparation.

biological profile: In forensic anthropology, it includes the age, sex, race, stature, and osseous anomalies or pathologies of human remains.

biometrics: Method of verifying an individual's identity based on measurement of physical features or repeatable actions that are unique to that individual. Biometric devices use one or more biometric parameters to identify the individual. These devices include palm-print readers, fingerprint readers, iris scanners, and retinal-pattern scanners. They are connected, usually by direct wire or network, to the system that requires authentication and are typically placed next to the computer.

C

cadaver: Corpse intended for dissection.

caliber: Term used to indicate the diameter of a bullet [manufactured in the United States] in "hundredths of an inch." Firearms and ammunition of European origin use the metric system and would refer to a 32 caliber bullet as an 8mm bullet.

calipers: Metric devices used by forensic anthropologists that take measurements of bones (sliding calipers); the cranium (spreading calipers); and the tooth crown and alveolar shapes (dial calipers).

capillary electrophoresis: Separation of chemicals by movement through a glass capillary tube in a solution under the influence of an electric field.

carbon monoxide: Colorless, odorless gas produced in the combustion of fossil fuels, automobile exhaust vapors, and poorly ventilated gas heating equipment, it is the best known example of an agent that can decrease the oxygen transport capability of blood and prevent oxygen from reaching body tissues in sufficient quantity. Exposure to very high concentrations can result in enough hemoglobin saturation to produce death by asphyxiation in minutes with almost no warning signs.

cause of death: The injury, disease, or combination of the two responsible for initiating the sequence of disturbances that produce the fatal termination. The important word is "initiating;" note that causes may not be immediately fatal, such as carcinoma or a stab wound.

chain of custody: Proper documentation, collection, and preservation of evidence at a crime scene investigation to ensure the integrity of the evidence, and safeguard against subsequent allegations of tampering, theft, planting, and contamination of evidence.

chromatography (thin-layer, gas, liquid, and ion): Separation of complex mixtures based on physical and chemical interaction with a solid adsorbent material (for example, activated carbon, alumina gel, or silica gel) on a plate or in a column.

chronic: Characterized by long duration or frequent recurrence (as in disease); not acute.

clavicle: Synonym for "collarbone."

colposcopic: Relating to colposcopy, an examination of the vagina and cervix by means of an endoscope.

comparison microscope: Two microscopes mounted side by side, connected by an optical bridge; used by firearms examiners to compare one specimen to another.

coroner: A public official, appointed or elected, in a particular geographic jurisdiction, whose official duty is to make inquiry into deaths in certain categories (accidents, homicides, suicides, undetermined).

corpus delicti: (From Latin) Fundamental fact necessary to prove the commission of a crime.

cortex: Outer layer of gray matter of the cerebrum and cerebellum.

costochondral: Relating to the costal (rib) cartilage.

cranial sutures: Line of union between the bones of the skull.

criminalistics: Analysis, comparison, identification, and interpretation of physical evidence. The main role of the criminalist is to objectively apply the techniques of the physical and natural sciences to examine physical evidence, and thereby prove the existence of a crime or make connections. The criminalist provides information to investigators, attorneys, judges, or juries. This information is helpful in determining the innocence or guilt of the suspect.

cyanide: A common poison, also a byproduct of the burning of many synthetic polymers and plastics. Cyanide blocks tissue utilization of oxygen and results in abnormally rapid or deep breathing. Cardiac irregularities are often noted, but the heart invariably outlasts the respirations. Death is due to respiratory failure and can occur within seconds or minutes of the inhalation of high concentrations of hydrogen cyanide gas. Because of slower absorption, death may be delayed after the ingestion of cyanide salts but the critical events still occur within the first hour.

cytochrome: Intracellular hemoprotein respiratory pigment, an enzyme functioning in electron transport as carrier of electrons.

D

***Daubert* v. *Merrell Dow Pharmaceuticals, Inc.*:** 1993 U.S. Supreme Court case which resulted in major changes in the way that expert testimony is admitted as scientific evidence. chemistry. The Court listed some of those characteristics: empirical testing, known or potential rate of error, standard procedures for performing a technique, peer review and publication, as well as general acceptance in the scientific community.

decedent: Deceased person.

dentition: The number, kind, and arrangement of a set of teeth.

deposition: Testimony taken down in writing under oath before a court.

diatoms: Aquatic unicellular plants that represent the most abundant single source of oxygen producers in the biosphere. The most distinctive feature of this unicellular organism is its extracellular coat or frustule, which is composed of silica. The postmortem identification of these frustules in human bone marrow may confirm that a corpse was the victim of drowning.

DNA: Deoxyribonucleic acid, the primary carrier of genetic information in living organisms, consists of a very long spiral structure, the "double helix," that has been likened to a "twisted ladder." The hand-rails of the ladder string together the ladder's "rungs," which are called bases. Bases, composed of four varieties of nucleic acid, combine in pairs called "nucleotides." The sequence of these base pairs constitutes the genetic coding of DNA.

DNA profiling: The process of testing to identify DNA patterns or types. In the forensic setting, this testing is used to indicate parentage or to exclude or include individuals as possible sources of body fluid stains (blood, saliva, semen) and other biological evidence (bones, teeth, hair).

DQ alpha (DQa): An area (locus) of DNA that is used by the forensic community to characterize DNA. Because there exist seven variations (alleles) of DNA at this locus, individuals can be categorized into 1 of 28 different DQ alpha types. Determination of an individual's DQ alpha type involves a Polymerase Chain Reaction-based test.

E

electromagnetic spectrum: The colors that are visible to the eye represent only a small portion of the light spectrum. Visible light, or white light, is a combination of all the visible colors. The visible region of the light spectrum ranges from 400 to 700 nanometers (nm) in wavelength.

electrophoresis: A technique by which DNA fragments are placed in a gel and separated by size in response to an electrical field.

endochondral: Relating to ossification of cartilage and deposition of lime salts in the cartilage matrix followed by secondary absorption and replacement by true bony tissue.

energy dispersive X-ray (EDX): An X-ray detector system which analyzes X-rays generated by the electron imaging beam in the scanning electron microscope (SEM).

epiphysial: Relating to bone that ossifies separately and later unites with the main part of the bone.

epithelial cells: Membranous tissue covering most internal surfaces, organs, and outer surface of the body.

etiology: Cause or origin of a disease or abnormal condition.

exclusion: A DNA test result indicating that an individual is excluded as the source of the DNA evidence. In the context of a criminal case, "exclusion" does not necessarily equate to "innocence."

exemplar: A typical or standard specimen used for comparison in cases of questioned documents.

F

facial reconstruction: Used as an investigative tool when no dental records, fingerprints, or comparative photographic material is available; it may either be three-dimensional from a skull or skull model or two-dimensional from radiographs and photographs of skulls. The three-dimensional facial image may be reconstructed by either building muscle and other soft tissues onto a skull or plaster cast using clay or plasticine and then adding facial features, or by means of a computer-aided facial reconstruction technique.

fantasy behaviors: Those committed to serve the offender's fantasies, and psychological and/or emotional needs. Fantasy behaviors are also called signature behaviors, are thematic in nature, and tend to be more stable over time.

femur: Also known as "thighbone."

fibula: The outer of the two bones between the knee and ankle in humans.

forensic: (From the Latin) Used in courts of judicature or in public discussion and debate.

forensic medicine: Application of medicine to the just resolution of legal issues.

forensic science: Application of scientific principles and technological practices to the purpose of justice in the study and resolution of criminal, civil, and regulatory issues.

Fourier transform infrared spectroscopy (FTIR): The theory of infrared spectroscopy is based upon differential absorption of infrared radiation by different molecules. A graph of energy absorbed versus frequency is the absorption spectrum of the sample. The spectrum is characteristic of the particular molecule and its molecular motions.

Frye test: In 1923, the justification for admitting scientific evidence was established as a standard that would become known as the "Frye test." This requirement for admissibility has three components: the principle must be demonstrable; it must have been sufficiently established; it must have gained the general acceptance of experts working in the particular scientific field(s) to which the evidence belongs.

G

gas chromatography/mass spectrometry (GC/MS): The instrument of choice for the detection of drugs since it has very high sensitivity and gives the identification of the compound from its mass spectral fragmentation pattern. It is also used in arson investigations, explosives cases, lacrimator cases (including pepper spray, tear gas, and mace), and paints and plastics analyses.

gene: A segment of a DNA molecule that is the biological unit of heredity and transmitted from parent to progeny.

genome: Each nucleated cell (with the exception of sperm and egg cells) usually contains the full complement of an individual's DNA, called the "genome," that is unvarying from cell to cell. The genome consists of approximately 3 billion base pairs, of which about 3 million actually differ from person to person. However, the base pairs that vary represent a virtually incalculable number of possible combinations.

genotype: The genetic makeup of an organism, as distinguished from its physical appearance or phenotype.

glabella: Smooth prominence between the eyebrows.

glass refractive index measurement (GRIM): The measure of how light bends as it passes through the glass, and is dependent upon the chemical composition and thermal history of the glass.

glue fuming (also known as "cyanoacrylate fuming"): Most successful technique for developing identifiable latent prints when used in conjunction with regular magnetic fingerprint powder. Similar to iodine/silver transfer, this method involves heating glue and directing the fumes onto the skin, then applying fingerprint powder to reveal the latent prints.

Greiss test: A test to detect the presence of nitrite residues. Nitrite residues are a particulate by-product of burned gunpowder.

gunshot residue: Combination of materials emitted from firearms during the firing process. These include unburned gunpowder particles, burned gunpowder particulate, vaporous lead, and particulate lead.

H

Haversian canals: Vascular canals that run longitudinally in the center of haversian systems of compact bony tissue.

headspace: Volume above a liquid or solid in a closed container. In arson investigation, the headspace is tested by various techniques to detect the presence of an accelerant among the debris.

hospital autopsy: Often performed on individuals in whom the disease causing death is known. The purpose of the autopsy is to determine the extent of the disease and/or the effects of therapy and the presence of any undiagnosed disease of interest or that might have contributed to death. The next of kin must give permission for the autopsy and may limit the extent of the dissection (for example the chest and abdomen only, excluding the head).

hyoid: Relating to a complex of bones at the base of the tongue that supports the tongue and its muscles.

I

immunoassay: Identification of a protein based on its capacity to act as an antigen.

inclusion: A DNA test result indicating that an individual is not excluded as the source of the DNA evidence. In the context of a criminal case, "inclusion" does not necessarily equate to "guilt."

inconclusive: The determination made following assessment of DNA profile results that, due to a limited amount of information present (e.g., mixture of profiles, insufficient DNA), prevents a conclusive comparison of profiles.

independent possession: Trait in good detector dogs that relates to how well a dog remains motivated to play a game that's used in training.

infrared (IR) photography: A region of the light spectrum invisible to the human eye extending from 700 nm (nanometers) and higher. The range of infrared light close to the visible spectrum is photographically reactive. Therefore, it is possible to produce images that may only be observed using photography.

interpupillary: Refers to the area between the pupils of the eyes.

L

lacrimator: An agent (such as tear gas) that irritates the eyes and produces tears.

lamella: Thin sheet, such as occurs in compact bone.

larva: Immature wormlike form that hatches from the egg of many insects, passes through several molts, and is finally transformed into a pupa from which the adult emerges.

larynx: Upper part of the trachea that, in humans, contains the vocal cords.

livor: Black and blue or gray discoloration of the skin on the dependent parts of the corpse.

M

malpractice: Failure to exercise an accepted degree of professional skill or learning by one (as a physician) which results in injury, loss, or damage.

mandibulometer: Metric device used by forensic anthropologists to take measurements of the mandible.

manner of death: The fashion or circumstance in which the cause of death arose. In the United States, there are five: natural, accident, homicide, suicide, or undetermined.

marker: Gene with a known location on a chromosome and a clear-cut phenotype (physical appearance or functional expression of a trait) that is used as a point of reference in the mapping of other locations.

mass spectrometry: Identification of chemical structures and quantitative elemental analysis based on the mass of ionized (charged) molecules, ionized fragments of molecules, and ionized elements.

maxillary: Relating to the upper jaw.

meatus: Natural body passage or channel.

mechanical fingerprint: Unique mark left on a bullet by an imperfection on the surface of the gun barrel.

mechanism of death: The physiologic derangement or biochemical disturbance incompatible with life initiated by the cause of death.

medical examiner: A physician who is charged, within a certain geographical jurisdiction, with the investigation and examination of persons dying a sudden, unexpected, or violent death.

medicolegal: Pertaining to law and medicine.

medicolegal (forensic) autopsy: Ordered by the coroner or medical examiner as authorized by law with the statutory purpose of establishing the cause of death and answer other medicolegal questions. The next of kin do not authorize and may not limit the extent of the autopsy.

metabolite: Product of metabolism.

metabolize: Chemically change within the body.

metalinguistic awareness: Ability to think consciously and talk about language itself (rather than the message language conveys).

microhabitat: Microenvironment in which an organism lives.

microscopy (light and electron): Production of magnified images of objects using light or electrons.

mitochondrion: Cellular organelles found outside the nucleus, which generate energy for the cell through cellular respiration.

MO (modus operandi) behaviors: Those committed by the offender during the commission of the crime which are necessary to complete the crime. MO behaviors are unstable across offenses, and may alter as the offender gains confidence or experience.

morphology: Form and structure of an organism or its parts.

N

necrophageous: Feeding on corpses or carrion.

ninhydrin: A common reagent found to be particularly helpful in developing latent fingerprints.

O

orbit: Bony socket of the eye.

osseous anomalies: Unusual bony developments that are present in a fraction of the population and include such things as a sternal foramina (a hole in the breast bone), bifurcated rib ends, or an extra rib, vertebra, or tooth.

osseous pathologies: Healed fractures and alterations to the bone resulting from disease processes which may include, but are not limited to osteoporosis, arthritis, endocrine disorders, and nutritional deficiencies.

ossification: Natural process of bone formation or hardening into a bony substance.

osteometric board: Metric device that takes measurements of long bones and pelvic bones.

osteon: Central canal containing blood capillaries and concentric osseous lamellae around it occurring in compact bone.

osteophytic: Relating to a bony outgrowth.

oxidative phosphorylation: Formation of high energy phosphoric bonds from the energy released by the flow of electrons to O_2 and the dehydrogenation of various substrates.

P

parietal: Relating to the upper posterior wall of the head.

PCR-STR (polymerase chain reaction-short tandem repeat): PCR is a technique used to replicate DNA quickly. STR refers to the region on a DNA strand where a sequence of three, four, or five nucleotides is repeated a different number of times in different people— the so-called STR loci.

peer review: Research proposals, manuscripts, or abstracts submitted for presentation at a scientific meeting, and judged for scientific merit by other scientists in the same field.

peptide: Inorganic compound derived from a combination of the amino group of one acid with the carboxyl group of another; usually obtained by partial hydrolysis of proteins.

perineal: Relating to the perineum, the area between the anus and the posterior part of the exterior genitalia.

petechiae: Pin-point hemorrhages over the whites of the eyes, and about the forehead and cheeks, and internally, over the surfaces of the heart and lungs, indicating rapid anoxial death.

philtrum: Groove in the midline of the upper lip.

poisons: Toxicants that cause immediate death or illness when experienced in very small amounts.

postcranial: Relating to the part of the body caudal to the head.

postmortem: After death; term used in relation to corpse during death investigation. Also refers to the autopsy, the examination of the body after death.

post-traumatic stress disorder: Psychological reaction to a stressful event, marked by depression, flashbacks, and recurrent nightmares.

protease: Enzyme that hydrolyzes proteins; classified according to the most prominent functional group at the active site.

pyrolysis: Chemical change due to the action of heat.

pyromania: Irresistible impulse to start fires.

Q

questioned document examiner: An expert in analyzing the authenticity of legal documents (checks, wills, contracts, deeds, etc.) in civil and criminal cases.

R

radiographic: Relating to an X-ray or gamma ray photograph.

radioimmunoassay: Immunoassay of a substance that is radioactively labeled.

rapid anoxial death: Death due to a rapid lack of oxygen as seen in deaths from suffocation, choking, strangulation, carbon monoxide or cyanide poisoning, and drowning.

reagent: Substance used because of its chemical or biological activity.

RFLP-VNTR (Restriction Fragment Length Polymorphism-Variable Number of Tandem Repeats): Highly reliable technology used in DNA profiling with the drawback of requiring abundant and clean specimens.

rifling: A system of spiral grooves in the surface of the bore of a gun causing a projectile when fired to rotate about its longer axis.

rigor mortis: Stiffening of the body, from one to seven hours after death, due to hardening of the muscular tissues. It disappears when decomposition begins.

S

scanning electron microscope (SEM): Utilizes a focused beam of electrons in an evacuated sample chamber to image samples of material (magnification range from 5X to 100,000X). The SEM has the advantage of producing images with great depth of field which allows one to examine surface morphology.

scanning electron microscope/energy dispersive X-ray (SEM/ EDX): The technique employed for the detection and identification of gunshot residue (GSR) particles (consisting of trace amounts of barium, lead, and antimony formed by the vaporized bullet and primer materials.

secretor: Person who secretes the ABH antigens of the ABO blood group in saliva and other body fluids.

serologist: Forensic scientist who specializes in biological fluid analysis.

sexual dimorphism: Skeletal differences between males and females.

signature behaviors: See fantasy behaviors.

skull-photo superimposition: Method of identification which involves superimposing a life size, front on, antemortem photograph of the decedent (preferably smiling) on the skull of the unidentified individual. This is accomplished utilizing computers or audiovisual equipment. Numerous points on the face and cranium are compared to verify correspondence between the photograph and the skull.

sniffer: Portable gas detector used to detect gas leaks or, as in the case of arson investigation, to detect the presence of accelerants.

sodium rhodizonate test: Test to detect the presence of lead residue (from the firing of a gun).

spalling: In fires, the breaking up or reducing as if by chipping with a hammer, especially of concrete or stone.

special masters: Court-appointed scientific experts and individuals who are designated by a judge to help assess evidence.

supracilliary arches: Relating to the region of the eyebrow.

symphysial: Grown together; fused.

T

Tardieu's spots: Large hemorrhages evident in the corpse of a hanging victim that has been suspended for more than three to four hours, due to the bursting of blood vessels after death by the effects of gravity.

target organs/tissues: Toxicants may affect only specific organs or tissues while not producing damage to the body as a whole. These specific sites are known as the target organs or target tissues.

tibia: The inner of the two bones between the knee and ankle in the lower limb of humans.

toluidine blue: A dye that will stain the nucleated squamous cells in deep layers of exposed epidermis to document microtrauma resulting from forced sexual activity, helping to rule out or confirm evidence of sexual abuse.

tool marks: In the case of forensic anthropology, distinctive marks inflicted on the human skeleton by knives, swords, axes, or saws.

tort: Wrongful act for which relief may be obtained in the form of damages or an injunction.

toxicants: Substances that produce adverse biological effects; may be chemical or physical in nature; may be of various types (acute, chronic, etc.).

toxins: Specific proteins produced by living organisms (mushroom toxin or tetanus toxin); most exhibit immediate effects.

U

ultra-trace elemental analysis: Technique using inductively coupled plasma/mass spectrometry to find contaminants in amounts as small as parts per trillion.

ultraviolet (UV) photography: Region in light spectrum invisible to the human eye extending below violet from 200 to 400 nm (nanometers). It is reactive with photographic materials. Therefore, it is possible to produce images that may only be observed using photography.

urinalysis: Chemical analysis of urine.

V

victimology: Study of victims and victimization.

W

wound characteristics: Detailed documentation of the appearance of a wound which may be the identifying factor in determining the type of weapon used to inflict the injury. Wound characteristics constitute evidence that may be obscured by emergency trauma care.

X

x-ray diffraction (XRD): Unlike other techniques that allow only the analysis of elemental composition, XRD gives the identification of the sample based on its crystal structure which allows conclusive identification of compounds.

xenobiotic: Term that is used for a foreign substance taken into the body. It is derived from the Greek term *xeno* which means "foreigner." Xenobiotics may produce beneficial effects (such as a pharmaceutical) or they may be toxic (such as lead).

Acronyms Used in This Book

AAAS: American Association for the Advancement of Science

AAFS: American Academy of Forensic Sciences

ABA: American Bar Association

ABC: American Board of Criminalists

ABFO: American Board of Forensic Odontology

ADA: Americans with Disabilities Act

ALAS: Automated Linguistic Authentication System

AOAC: Association of Official Analytical Chemists

ASCLD: American Society of Crime Lab Directors

ASFO: American Society of Forensic Odontology

ATF: Bureau of Alcohol, Tobacco, and Firearms

CADD: Computer-Aided Design and Drafting

CDC: Centers for Disease Control and Prevention

CD-ROM: Compact Disc-Read Only Memory

CE: Capillary Electrophoresis

CFR: Code of Federal Regulations

DBP: Dibutylphthalate

DEA: Drug Enforcement Administration

DEP: Diethylphthalate

DFO: 8-diazaflourenone

DNA: Deoxyribonucleic Acid

DNT: Dinitrotoluene

DOD: U.S. Department of Defense

DOJ: U.S. Department of Justice

DPA: Diphenylamine

DUF: Drug Use Forecast

EC: Ethyl Centralite

EEOC: Equal Employment Opportunity Commission

EMIT™: Enzyme Multiplied Immune Test

EMS: Emergency Medical Services

EMTALA: Emergency Medical Treatment and Active Labor Act

ERISA: Employee Retirement Income Security Act

FAA: Federal Aviation Administration

FBI: Federal Bureau of Investigation

FDA: U.S. Food and Drug Administration

FSF: Forensic Sciences Foundation, Inc.

FTIR: Fourier Transform Infrared Spectroscopy

GMP: Good Manufacturing Practices

GPE: Gas Phase Electrochemical

GRIM: Glass Refractive Index Measurement

GSR: Gunshot Residue

HIV: Human Immunodeficiency Virus

HMO: Health Maintenance Organization

HVAC: Heating, Ventilating, Air Conditioning

IAFIS: Integrated Automated Fingerprint Identification System

IBIS: Integrated Ballistic Identification System

IDAS: Identification Automated Services

III: Interstate Identification Index

IR: Infrared

JCAHO: Joint Commission on Accreditation of Health Care Organizations

LIMS: Laboratory Information Management System

MAPP: Multidimensional Addictions and Personality Profile

MC: Methyl Centralite

MECE: Micellar Electrokinetic Capillary Electrophoresis

MO: Modus Operandi

NAME: National Association of Medical Examiners

NASA: National Aeronautics and Space Administration

NC: Nitrocellulose

NCFS: National Center for Forensic Science

NCJRS: National Criminal Justice Reference Service

NCMEC: National Center for Missing and Exploited Children

nDPA: Nitrodiphenylmnine

NEIC: National Enforcement Investigation Center

NG: Nitroglycerin

NGU: Nitroguanindine

NIJ: National Institute of Justice

NIST: National Institute of Standards and Technology

NLECTC: National Law Enforcement and Corrections Technology Center

N-nDPA: N-nitrosodiphenylamine

NSF: National Science Foundation

OJP: Office of Justice Programs

OLES: Office of Law Enforcement Standards

OLETC: Office of Law Enforcement Technology Commercialization

OPO: Organ Procurement Organizations

OSHA: Occupational Safety and Health Administration

OTC: Organ Transplant Coordinator

PCR-STR: Polymerase Chain Reaction-Short Tandem Repeat

ppb: parts per billion

QDE: Questioned Document Examination

R&D: Research and Development

RFLP-VNTR: Restriction Fragment Length Polymorphism-Variable Number of Tandem Repeats

RGDAA: Royal Guide Dogs Associations of Australia

SART: Sexual Assault Response Team

SDS: Sodium Dodecylsulfate

SEM: Scanning Electron Microscopy

SEM/EDX: Scanning Electron Microscopy/Energy Dispersive X-Ray Analysis

TWGDOC: Technical Working Group on Documents

UCF: University of Central Florida

UV: Ultraviolet

WAN: Wide Area Network

WNS: Western Nurse Specialists, Inc.

XRD: X-Ray Diffraction

Chapter 56

Resources

For additional help, this chapter lists in alphabetical order contact information for some of the government agencies, professional organizations, and individual specialists involved in forensic medicine and related sciences.

Government Agencies

The following list features some of the public sector agencies engaged in crime investigation and prevention, law enforcement, evidence collection, lab analysis, criminal profiling, research, and education.

Centers for Disease Control and Prevention (CDC)
1600 Clifton Rd. NE
Atlanta, GA 30333
Phone: (404) 639-3286; (800) 311-3435
Fax: (404) 639-7394
http://www.cdc.gov

Drug Enforcement Administration (DEA)
801 I St. NW
Washington, D.C. 20001
Phone: (202) 305-8500
http://www.usdoj.gov/dea

Federal Bureau of Investigation (FBI) Laboratory
935 Pennsylvania Ave. NW
Washington, DC 20535-0001
Phone: (202) 324-3000
http://www.fbi.gov

Food and Drug Administration (FDA)
HFE-88
Rockville, MD 20857
Phone: (800) 532-4440
E-mail: execsec@oc.fda.gov
http://www.fda.gov

National Criminal Justice Reference Service (NCJRS)
P.O. Box 6000
Rockville, MD 20849-6000
Phone: (800) 851-3420
E-mail: askncjrs@ncjrs.org
http://ncjrs.org

National Enforcement Investigations Center (NEIC)
Bldg. 53, Box 25227
DFC Denver, CO 80225
Phone: (303) 236-5111
http://es.epa.gov/oeca/oceft/neic/lab1.html

National Law Enforcement and Corrections Technology Center (NLECTC)
P.O. Box 1160
Rockville, MD 20849-1160
Phone: (800) 248-2742
E-mail: asknlectc@nlelctc.org
http://www.nlectc.org

Occupational Safety and Health Administration (OSHA)
Office of Information and Consumer Affairs
200 Constitution Ave., Rm. 3647
Washington, DC 20210
Phone: (202) 693-1999
http://www.osha.gov

Office of Justice Programs (OJP)
810 Seventh St. NW
Washington, DC 20531
Phone: (202) 307-0703
E-mail: askocpa@ojp.usdoj.gov
http://www.ojp.usdoj.gov

Professional Associations

The following list includes some of the professional associations that contributed articles to (or were featured in) this book. They are classified by occupation.

Arson and Explosives Investigation

National Center for Forensic Science (NCFS)
University of Central Florida
P.O. Box 162367
Orlando, FL 32816-2367
Phone: (407) 823-6469
Fax: (407) 823-3162
E-mail:
natlctr@pegasus.cc.ucf.edu
http://ncfs.ucf.edu

Crime Laboratory Accreditation

American Society of Crime Laboratory Directors (ASCLD)
3200 34th St. S.
St. Petersburg, FL 33711
Phone: (813) 341-4409
Fax: (813) 341-4547
E-mail: webmaster@ascld.org
http://www.ascld.org/

Expert Witnesses

National Forensic Center
17 Temple Terrace
Lawrenceville, NJ 08648
Phone: (800) 526-5177
E-mail:
forenexpts@worldnet.att.net
http://www.ExpertIndex.com

Law Enforcement Assistance in Child Recovery

National Center for Missing and Exploited Children (NCMEC)
2101 Wilson Blvd., Ste. 550
Arlington, VA 22201-3077
Phone: (703) 235-3900; hotline:
(800) 843-5678
http://www.missingkids.org

Research and Education

The Forensic Sciences Foundation, Inc.
P.O. Box 669
Colorado Springs, CO 80901-0669
Phone: (719) 636-1100
Fax: (719) 636-1993
E-mail: Membship@aafs.org
http://www.aafs.org

National Association of Medical Examiners (NAME)
1402 S. Grand Blvd.
St. Louis, MO 63104
Phone: (314) 577-8298
Fax: (314) 268-5124
E-mail: randazdd@SLU.EDU
http://www.thename.org

Forensic Scientists

The following list features some of the forensic scientists who contributed articles to this book. They are classified by forensic science subspecialty.

Anthropology

John A Giacobbe
Stantec Consulting, Inc.
1440 W. Lobster Trap Dr.
Gilbert, AZ 85233
Phone: (602) 707-4716
Fax: (602) 431-9562
E-mail: jgiacobbe@stantec.com

Carrie M. Weiler
King County Medical
Examiner's Office
325 Ninth Ave.
Seattle, WA 98104
Phone: (206) 731-3235
Fax: (206) 731-8555
E-mail: cmweiler@eskimo.com
http://www.metrokc.gov/health/

Arson Investigation

Tony Cafe
T.C. Forensic Pty Ltd.
P.O. Box 8
Lansvale NSW Australia 2166
Phone: (02) 9725 6356
Fax: (02) 9724 9145
E-mail: tcforen@ozemail.com.au
http://www.ozemail.co.au/
~tcforen

Criminal Profiling

Brent Turvey, M.S.
Knowledge Solutions, LLC
1271 Washington Ave., #274
San Leandro, CA 94577-3646
Phone: (510) 483-6739
E-mail: bturvey@corpus-delicti.com.
http://www.corpus-delicti.com

Document Examination

Emily J. Will
P.O. Box 58552
Raleigh, NC 27658
Phone: (919) 556-7414
E-mail: qdewill@mindspring.com
http://www.webmasters.net/qde

Engineering

John Mustard, Centre of Forensic Sciences
University of Toronto at Mississauga, Erindale College
3359 Mississauga Rd.
Mississauga, ON, Canada L5L 1C6
Phone: (905) 828-3726
http://www.erin.utoronto.ca/academic/FSC

Entomology

Jason H. Byrd, Ph.D.
Dept. of Entomology and Nematology
P.O. Box 110620, Bldg. 970
University of Florida
Gainesville, FL 32611
Phone: (352) 392-1901 ext. 205
E-mail: jhby@gnv.ifas.ufl.edu
http://csssrvr.entem.ufl.edu/~pmc

Evidence Collection and Preservation

George Schiro, Forensic Scientist
Louisiana State Police Crime Laboratory
P.O. Box 66614
Baton Rouge, LA 70896
Phone: (504) 925-7791
http://police2.ucr.edu

Firearms Identification

Jeffrey Scott Doyle, Firearms Examiner
Jefferson Regional Forensic Laboratory
3600 Chamberlain Lane, Ste. 410
Louisville, KY 40241
Phone: (502) 426-8240
http://www.geocities.com/~jsdoyle

Graphics

Michael Bloomenfeld
Legal Arts Multimedia, LLC
444 High St., Ste. 244
Palo Alto, CA 94301
Phone: (888) 883-1101
E-mail: design@legalarts.com
http://www.legalarts.com

Nursing

Arlene Kent-Wilkinson R.N., M.N.
Forensic Nurse Educator/Consultant
116 Martindale Close NE
Calgary, Alberta, T3J 2V3
Canada
Phone: (403) 293-1598
Fax: (403) 285-1760
E-mail: kentwila@cadvision.com
http://www.mtroyal.ab.ca/programs/centrehs/forensic/

Virginia A. Lynch, M.S.N., R.N., FAAFS
International Association of Forensic Nurses
644 Brewer Dr.
Fort Collins, CO 80524
Phone: (609) 848-8356
http://members.aol.com/COCFCI/Vart.html

Odontology

Bruce R. Rothwell, D.M.D., M.S.D.
Chairman, Dept. of Restorative Dentistry
D-770 Health Sciences, University of Washington
Seattle, WA 98195
Phone: (206) 543-7496
E-mail: rothwell@u.washington.edu
http://www.washington.edu/home/staffdir.cgi

Palynology

Dr. Terry J. Hutter, Palynological Specialist
TH Geological Services, Inc.
P.O. Box 40
Sand Springs, OK 74063
Phone: (918) 245-1427
E-mail: tjhutter@ionet.net
http://www.geoscience.net/Forensic_Palynology.html

Pathology

Michael S. Pollanen, Ph.D.
Forensic Pathology Unit
Office of the Chief Coroner of Ontario
26 Grenville St.
Toronto, ON, Canada M7A 2G9
Phone: (416) 314-4100
Fax: (416) 314-0888

Photography

Lt. James O. Pex
Oregon State Police Forensic
Laboratory
3334 S. 4th
Coos Bay, OR 97420
Phone: (541) 269-2967
Fax: (541) 267-2007
E-mail: jim.pex@state.or.us

Psychiatry

Harold J. Bursztajn, M.D.
Associate Clinical Professor
Harvard Medical School
Cambridge, MA 02138
Phone: (617) 492-8366
E-mail:
burszt@warren.med.harvard.edu
http://www.forensic-psych.com/
newhome.html

Other Internet Sources

The following Internet addresses provide information on
forensic science topics, bibliogra-
phies, professional and educational institutions, and current
research.

http://galaxy.tradewave.com/gal-
axy/Medicine/Health-Occupa-
tions/Medicine/
Other-Specialties/Forensic-
Medicine.html

http://haven.ios.com/~nyrc/
homepage.html

http://plague.law.umkc.edu/
default.htm

http://pw2.netcom.com/~foren-
sic/weblinks.html

http://sis.nlm.nih.gov/toxtutr1/
index.htm

http://users.bart.nl/~geradts/
forensic.html

http://worldmall.com/erf/lec-
tures/env-23.htm

http://whyfiles.news.wisc.edu/
014forensic/index.html

http://www.smokefreekids.com/
medbooks/forensic.htm

http://www.soft-tox.org/forms/
toxlinks.htm

http://www.tncrimlaw.com/foren-
sic

http://www.uq.edu.au/asfd/
forlink.htm

http://www.vifp.monash.edu.au

Index

551

New York state
death investigation system, 30, 33
DNA evidence, 469
New York University
forensic odontology, 206
scientific evidence, 453
next of kin
death scene investigations, 97-98
forensic pathologists, 128
Niezgoda, Stephen, 377
911 emergency calls, domestic violence cases, 63-64
ninhydrin, 322-324
ninhydrin, defined, 533
North Carolina
death investigation system, 30, 33
DNA evidence, 469
Raleigh Police Department, 335
North Carolina State University, computational linguistics, 337
North Dakota
death investigation system, 30, 33
DNA evidence, 469
Northern Mariana Islands, death investigation system, 3134
Northwestern University, forensic odontology, 206
Northwest Territories, death investigation system, 31, 34
Nova Scotia, death investigation system, 31, 34
nuclear magnetic resonance spectroscopy, fire investigations, 84
nurses, forensic, 13, 26, 147-174
Nurses Association, American, 159
Nurses Networking on Violence Against Women, 159
Nursing, American Academy of, 159

O

oblique lighting technique, crime scene investigation, 48, 58
Occupational Safety and Health Administration
Office of Information and Consumer Affairs, 544
regulatory agency, 200

odor signatures, 347, 350
ODV, Inc., 365
Office of Law Enforcement Technology Commercialization (OLETC)
computer-aided criminal identification, 298
facial recognition technologies, 299
Justice, National Institute of (NIJ), 297
Ohio
death investigation system, 30, 33
DNA evidence, 469
Oklahoma
death investigation system, 30, 33
DNA evidence, 469
Omenn, Gilbert S., 453, 454
Ontario
Office of the Chief Coroner, 345
Ontario, death investigation system, 31, 34
OPO. *see* Organ Procurement Organizations (OPO)
orbit, defined, 533
Oregon
death investigation system, 30, 33
DNA evidence, 469
State Police Forensic Laboratory, 77, 548
organ donation, 163-166
organic toxins, 194-195
Organ Procurement Organizations (OPO)
anatomic gifts, 164, 166
osseous anomalies, defined, 533
osseous pathologies, defined, 533
ossification, defined, 533
osteometric board, defined, 534
osteon, defined, 534
osteophytic, defined, 534
oxidative phosphorylation, defined, 534

P

Pacific Northern National Laboratory (Hanford, WA), 367
paint, crime scene investigations, 56
palynology, forensic, 217-220

Q

R

S

South Dakota
  death investigation system, 30, 33
  DNA evidence, 469
spalling, defined, 536
special masters, defined, 536
spectrophotometers, evidence collection, 73
spectroscopy, 84, 384
  see also electromagnetic spectrum
  see also Fourier transform infrared spectroscopy (FTIR)
  see also gas chromatography/mass spectrometry (GC/MS)
  see also mass spectrometry
speech scientists, 13
Spencer, Timothy Wilson, 467
spontaneous combustion, 81
spousal abuse, evidence collection, 76
stabilizers, defined, 415
standard of care, expert testimony, 497-504
Standards and Technology, National Institute of
  Chemical Science and Technology Laboratory, 427
  Office of Law Enforcement Standards, 380
Stanley, Edward A., 219
Stantec Consulting, Inc., 545
state laws
  autopsy requirements, 36
  death investigations, 27-28
  death investigation systems, 30-34
  DNA databanking, 375
  DNA evidence, 469
  forensic psychiatry, 9
  malpractice evidence, 144
  standards of care, 500
  see also individual states
Statistics Canada, 29
Stehlin, Isadora B., 386
strangulation
  ligature, 109-110
  manual, 108-109
stress, domestic violence cases, 67
striated marks, described, 245
structure examinations
  fire scenes, 80-81
  forensic engineers, 6, 237

A Study of State Laws, Death Investigation Systems, Practices and Their Impact on Those Affected by Sudden Infant Death Syndrome, 27-28
substance abuse testing, 403-406
sudden deaths, medical examiners, 17
suffocation, defined, 107
suicides
  children, 393
  rapid anoxial death, 107
  statistics, 39
supracilliary arches, defined, 536
Supreme Court decisions
  Daubert v. *Merrell Dow Pharmaceuticals,* 326-329, 451, 454-455, 458-460, 468, 486n17, 506
  described, 527
  Goddard v. *Dupree,* 143
  Oncale v. *Sundowner Offshore Services, Inc., et al.,* 133
  Tank v. *Chronister,* 144
  see also court decisions
suspects
  childhood deaths, 395-396
  condom trace evidence, 434
  criminalists, 4
  criminal profiling, 273-281
suspicious deaths
  forensic nursing, 153
  statistics, 35-41
Svensson, Arne, 59
symphysial, defined, 536
systemic toxins, 193-195

T

T. C. Forensic Pty Ltd., 545
T. H. Geological Services, Inc., 547
Taber's Cyclopedic Medical Dictionary, 148
Tardieu's spots
  death scene investigations, 96
  defined, 536
target organs
  defined, 195, 536
  xenobiotics, 196
target tissues, defined, 195, 536
Taylor, Katherine, 189

Contagious & Non-Contagious Infectious Diseases Sourcebook

Basic Information about Contagious Diseases like Measles, Polio, Hepatitis B, and Infectious Mononucleosis, and Non-Contagious Infectious Diseases like Tetanus and Toxic Shock Syndrome, and Diseases Occurring as Secondary Infections Such as Shingles and Reye Syndrome, Along with Vaccination, Prevention, and Treatment Information, and a Section Describing Emerging Infectious Disease Threats

Edited by Karen Bellenir and Peter D. Dresser. 566 pages. 1996. 0-7808-0075-3. $78.

Death & Dying Sourcebook

Basic Information for the Layperson about End-of-Life Care and Related Ethical and Legal Issues, Including Chief Causes of Death, Autopsies, Pain Management for the Terminally Ill, Life Support Systems, Coma, Euthanasia, Assisted Suicide, Hospice Programs, Living Wills, Near-Death Experiences, Counseling, Mourning, Organ Donation, Cryogenics and Physician Training and Liability, Along with Statistical Data, a Glossary, and Listings of Sources for Additional Help and Information

Edited by Annemarie Muth. 600 pages. 1999. 0-7808-0230-6. $78.

Diabetes Sourcebook, 1st Edition

Basic Information about Insulin-Dependent and Noninsulin-Dependent Diabetes Mellitus, Gestational Diabetes, and Diabetic Complications, Symptoms, Treatment, and Research Results, Including Statistics on Prevalence, Morbidity, and Mortality, Along with Source Listings for Further Help and Information

Edited by Karen Bellenir and Peter D. Dresser. 827 pages. 1994. 1-55888-751-2. $78.

"…very informative and understandable for the layperson without being simplistic. It provides a comprehensive overview for laypersons who want a general understanding of the disease or who want to focus on various aspects of the disease." — *Bulletin of the MLA, Jan '96*

Diabetes Sourcebook, 2nd Edition

Basic Consumer Health Information about Type 1 Diabetes (Insulin-Dependent or Juvenile-Onset Diabetes), Type 2 (Noninsulin-Dependent or Adult-Onset Diabetes), Gestational Diabetes, and Related Disorders, Including Diabetes Prevalence Data, Management Issues, the Role of Diet and Exercise in Controlling Diabetes, Insulin and Other Diabetes Medicines, and Complications of Diabetes Such as Eye Diseases, Periodontal Disease, Amputation, and End-Stage Renal Disease; Along with Reports on Current Research Initiatives, a Glossary, and Resource Listings for Further Help and Information

Edited by Karen Bellenir. 725 pages. 1998. 0-7808-0224-1. $78.

Diet & Nutrition Sourcebook, 1st Edition

Basic Information about Nutrition, Including the Dietary Guidelines for Americans, the Food Guide Pyramid, and Their Applications in Daily Diet, Nutritional Advice for Specific Age Groups, Current Nutritional Issues and Controversies, the New Food Label and How to Use It to Promote Healthy Eating, and Recent Developments in Nutritional Research

Edited by Dan R. Harris. 662 pages. 1996. 0-7808-0084-2. $78.

"Useful reference as a food and nutrition sourcebook for the general consumer."
— *Booklist Health Sciences Supplement, Oct '97*

"Recommended for public libraries and medical libraries that receive general information requests on nutrition. It is readable and will appeal to those interested in learning more about healthy dietary practices."
— *Medical Reference Services Quarterly, Fall '97*

"With dozens of questionable diet books on the market, it is so refreshing to find a reliable and factual reference book. Recommended to aspiring professionals, librarians, and others seeking and giving reliable dietary advice. An excellent compilation." — *Choice, Feb '97*

Diet & Nutrition Sourcebook, 2nd Edition

Basic Consumer Health Information about Dietary Guidelines, Recommended Daily Intake Values, Vitamins, Minerals, Fiber, Fat, Weight Control, Dietary Supplements, and Food Additives; Along with Special Sections on Nutrition Needs throughout Life and Nutrition for People with Such Specific Medical Concerns as Allergies, High Blood Cholesterol, Hypertension, Diabetes, Celiac Disease, Seizure Disorders, Phenylketonuria (PKU), Cancer, and Eating Disorders, and Including Reports on Current Nutrition Research and Source Listings for Additional Help and Information

Edited by Karen Bellenir. 600 pages. 1999. 0-7808-0228-4. $78.

Domestic Violence Sourcebook

Basic Information about the Physical, Emotional and Sexual Abuse of Partners, Children, and Elders, Including Information about Hotlines, Safe Houses, Safety Plans, Resources for Support and Assistance, Community Initiatives, and Reports on Current Directions in Research and Treatment; Along with a Glossary, Sources for Further Reading, and Listings of Governmental and Non-Governmental Organizations

Edited by Helene Henderson. 600 pages. 1999. 0-7808-0235-7. $78.

Ear, Nose & Throat Disorders Sourcebook

Basic Information about Disorders of the Ears, Nose, Sinus Cavities, Pharynx, and Larynx, Including Ear Infections, Tinnitus, Vestibular Disorders, Allergic and Non-Allergic Rhinitis, Sore Throats, Tonsillitis, and Cancers That Affect the Ears, Nose, Sinuses, and Throat, Along with Reports on Current Research Initiatives, a Glossary of Related Medical Terms, and a Directory of Sources for Further Help and Information

Edited by Karen Bellenir and Linda M. Shin. 592 pages. 1998. 0-7808-0206-3. $78.

Endocrine & Metabolic Disorders Sourcebook

Basic Information for the Layperson about Pancreatic and Insulin-Related Disorders Such as Pancreatitis, Diabetes, and Hypoglycemia; Adrenal Gland Disorders Such as Cushing's Syndrome, Addison's Disease, and Congenital Adrenal Hyperplasia; Pituitary Gland Disorders Such as Growth Hormone Deficiency, Acromegaly, and Pituitary Tumors; Thyroid Disorders Such as Hypothyroidism, Graves' Disease, Hashimoto's Disease, and Goiter; Hyperparathyroidism; and Other Diseases and Syndromes of Hormone Imbalance or Metabolic Dysfunction, Along with Reports on Current Research Initiatives

Edited by Linda M. Shin. 632 pages. 1998. 0-7808-0207-1. $78.

Environmentally Induced Disorders Sourcebook

Basic Information about Diseases and Syndromes Linked to Exposure to Pollutants and Other Substances in Outdoor and Indoor Environments Such as Lead, Asbestos, Formaldehyde, Mercury, Emissions, Noise, and More

Edited by Allan R. Cook. 620 pages. 1997. 0-7808-0083-4. $78.

". . . a good survey of numerous environmentally induced physical disorders . . . a useful addition to anyone's library."
— Doody's Health Science Book Reviews, Jan '98

". . . provide[s] introductory information from the best authorities around. Since this volume covers topics that potentially affect everyone, it will surely be one of the most frequently consulted volumes in the *Health Reference Series*."   — Rettig on Reference, Nov '97

"Recommended reference source."
— Booklist, Oct '97

Ethical Issues in Medicine Sourcebook

Basic Information about Controversial Treatment Issues, Genetic Research, Reproductive Technologies, and End-of-Life Decisions, Including Topics Such as Cloning, Abortion, Fertility Management, Organ Transplantation, Health Care Rationing, Advance Directives, Living Wills, Physician-Assisted Suicide, Euthanasia, and More; Along with a Glossary and Resources for Additional Information

Edited by Helene Henderson. 600 pages. 1999. 0-7808-0237-3. $78.

Fitness & Exercise Sourcebook

Basic Information on Fitness and Exercise, Including Fitness Activities for Specific Age Groups, Exercise for People with Specific Medical Conditions, How to Begin a Fitness Program in Running, Walking, Swimming, Cycling, and Other Athletic Activities, and Recent Research in Fitness and Exercise

Edited by Dan R. Harris. 663 pages. 1996. 0-7808-0186-5. $78.

"A good resource for general readers."
— Choice, Nov '97

"The perennial popularity of the topic . . . make this an appealing selection for public libraries."
— Rettig on Reference, Jun/Jul '97

Food & Animal Borne Diseases Sourcebook

Basic Information about Diseases That Can Be Spread to Humans through the Ingestion of Contaminated Food or Water or by Contact with Infected Animals and Insects, Such as Botulism, E. Coli, Hepatitis A, Trichinosis, Lyme Disease, and Rabies, Along with Information Regarding Prevention and Treatment Methods, and a Special Section for International Travelers Describing Diseases Such as Cholera, Malaria, Travelers' Diarrhea, and Yellow Fever, and Offering Recommendations for Avoiding Illness

Edited by Karen Bellenir and Peter D. Dresser. 535 pages. 1995. 0-7808-0033-8. $78.

"Targeting general readers and providing them with a single, comprehensive source of information on selected topics, this book continues, with the excellent caliber of its predecessors, to catalog topical information on health matters of general interest. Readable and thorough, this valuable resource is highly recommended for all libraries."
— Academic Library Book Review, Summer '96

"A comprehensive collection of authoritative information."   — Emergency Medical Services, Oct '95

Continues next page

Gastrointestinal Diseases & Disorders Sourcebook

Basic Information about Gastroesophageal Reflux Disease (Heartburn), Ulcers, Diverticulosis, Irritable Bowel Syndrome, Crohn's Disease, Ulcerative Colitis, Diarrhea, Constipation, Lactose Intolerance, Hemorrhoids, Hepatitis, Cirrhosis, and Other Digestive Problems, Featuring Statistics, Descriptions of Symptoms, and Current Treatment Methods of Interest for Persons Living with Upper and Lower Gastrointestinal Maladies

Edited by Linda M. Ross. 413 pages. 1996. 0-7808-0078-8. $78.

". . . very readable form. The successful editorial work that brought this material together into a useful and understandable reference makes accessible to all readers information that can help them more effectively understand and obtain help for digestive tract problems." — *Choice, Feb '97*

Genetic Disorders Sourcebook

Basic Information about Heritable Diseases and Disorders Such as Down Syndrome, PKU, Hemophilia, Von Willebrand Disease, Gaucher Disease, Tay-Sachs Disease, and Sickle-Cell Disease, Along with Information about Genetic Screening, Gene Therapy, Home Care, and Including Source Listings for Further Help and Information on More Than 300 Disorders

Edited by Karen Bellenir. 642 pages. 1996. 0-7808-0034-6. $78.

"Provides essential medical information to both the general public and those diagnosed with a serious or fatal genetic disease or disorder." — *Choice, Jan '97*

"Geared toward the lay public. It would be well placed in all public libraries and in those hospital and medical libraries in which access to genetic references is limited." — *Doody's Health Sciences Book Review, Oct '96*

Head Trauma Sourcebook

Basic Information for the Layperson about Open-Head and Closed-Head Injuries, Treatment Advances, Recovery, and Rehabilitation, Along with Reports on Current Research Initiatives

Edited by Karen Bellenir. 414 pages. 1997. 0-7808-0208-X. $78.

Health Insurance Sourcebook

Basic Information about Managed Care Organizations, Traditional Fee-for-Service Insurance, Insurance Portability and Pre-Existing Conditions Clauses, Medicare, Medicaid, Social Security, and Military Health Care, Along with Information about Insurance Fraud

Edited by Wendy Wilcox. 530 pages. 1997. 0-7808-0222-5. $78.

"The layout of the book is particularly helpful as it provides easy access to reference material. A most useful addition to the vast amount of information about health insurance. The use of data from U.S. government agencies is most commendable. Useful in a library or learning center for healthcare professional students." — *Doody's Health Sciences Book Reviews, Nov '97*

Healthy Aging Sourcebook

Basic Consumer Health Information about Maintaining Health through the Aging Process, Including Advice on Nutrition, Exercise, and Sleep, Along with Help in Making Decisions about Midlife Issues and Retirement, Practical and Informed Choices in Health Consumerism, and Data Concerning the Theories of Aging, Aging Now, and Aging in the Future, Including a Glossary and Practical Resource Directory

Edited by Jenifer Swanson. 500 pages. 1999. 0-7808-0390-6. $78.

Immune System Disorders Sourcebook

Basic Information about Lupus, Multiple Sclerosis, Guillain-Barré Syndrome, Chronic Granulomatous Disease, and More, Along with Statistical and Demographic Data and Reports on Current Research Initiatives

Edited by Allan R. Cook. 608 pages. 1997. 0-7808-0209-8. $78.

Kidney & Urinary Tract Diseases & Disorders Sourcebook

Basic Information about Kidney Stones, Urinary Incontinence, Bladder Disease, End Stage Renal Disease, Dialysis, and More, Along with Statistical and Demographic Data and Reports on Current Research Initiatives

Edited by Linda M. Ross. 602 pages. 1997. 0-7808-0079-6. $78.

Learning Disabilities Sourcebook

Basic Information about Disorders Such as Dyslexia, Visual and Auditory Processing Deficits, Attention Deficit/Hyperactivity Disorder, and Autism, Along with Statistical and Demographic Data, Reports on Current Research Initiatives, an Explanation of the Assessment Process, and a Special Section for Adults with Learning Disabilities

Edited by Linda M. Shin. 579 pages. 1998. 0-7808-0210-1. $78.

Medical Tests Sourcebook

Basic Consumer Health Information about Medical Tests, Including Periodic Health Exams, General Screening Tests, X-ray and Radiology Tests, Electrical Tests, Tests of Body Fluids and Tissues, Scope Tests, Lung Tests, Gene Tests, Pregnancy Tests, Newborn Screening Tests, Sexually Transmitted Disease Tests, and Computer Aided Diagnoses; Along with a Section on Paying for Medical Tests, a Glossary, and Resource Listings

Edited by Joyce B. Shannon. 600 pages. 1999. 0-7808-0243-8. $78.

Men's Health Concerns Sourcebook

Basic Information about Health Issues That Affect Men, Featuring Facts about the Top Causes of Death in Men, Including Heart Disease, Stroke, Cancers, Prostate Disorders, Chronic Obstructive Pulmonary Disease, Pneumonia and Influenza, Human Immunodeficiency Virus and Acquired Immune Deficiency Syndrome, Diabetes Mellitus, Stress, Suicide, Accidents and Homicides; and Facts about Common Concerns for Men, Including Impotence, Contraception, Circumcision, Sleep Disorders, Snoring, Hair Loss, Diet, Nutrition, Exercise, Kidney and Urological Disorders, and Backaches

Edited by Allan R. Cook. 760 pages. 1998. 0-7808-0212-8. $78.

Mental Health Disorders Sourcebook

Basic Information about Schizophrenia, Depression, Bipolar Disorder, Panic Disorder, Obsessive-Compulsive Disorder, Phobias and Other Anxiety Disorders, Paranoia and Other Personality Disorders, Eating Disorders, and Sleep Disorders, Along with Information about Treatment and Therapies

Edited by Karen Bellenir. 548 pages. 1995. 0-7808-0040-0. $78.

"This is an excellent new book . . . written in easy-to-understand language."
— *Booklist Health Science Supplement, Oct '97*

". . . useful for public and academic libraries and consumer health collections."
— *Medical Reference Services Quarterly, Spring '97*

"The great strengths of the book are its readability and its inclusion of places to find more information. Especially recommended." — *RQ, Winter '96*

". . . a good resource for a consumer health library."
— *Bulletin of the MLA, Oct '96*

"The information is data-based and couched in brief, concise language that avoids jargon. . . . a useful reference source." — *Readings, Sept '96*

"The text is well organized and adequately written for its target audience." — *Choice, Jun '96*

". . . provides information on a wide range of mental disorders, presented in nontechnical language."
— *Exceptional Child Education Resources, Spring '96*

"Recommended for public and academic libraries."
— *Reference Book Review, '96*

Ophthalmic Disorders Sourcebook

Basic Information about Glaucoma, Cataracts, Macular Degeneration, Strabismus, Refractive Disorders, and More, Along with Statistical and Demographic Data and Reports on Current Research Initiatives

Edited by Linda M. Ross. 631 pages. 1996. 0-7808-0081-8. $78.

Oral Health Sourcebook

Basic Information about Diseases and Conditions Affecting Oral Health, Including Cavities, Gum Disease, Dry Mouth, Oral Cancers, Fever Blisters, Canker Sores, Oral Thrush, Bad Breath, Temporomandibular Disorders, and other Craniofacial Syndromes, Along with Statistical Data on the Oral Health of Americans, Oral Hygiene, Emergency First Aid, Information on Treatment Procedures and Methods of Replacing Lost Teeth

Edited by Allan R. Cook. 558 pages. 1997. 0-7808-0082-6. $78.

"Recommended reference source." — *Booklist, Dec '97*

Pain Sourcebook

Basic Information about Specific Forms of Acute and Chronic Pain, Including Headaches, Back Pain, Muscular Pain, Neuralgia, Surgical Pain, and Cancer Pain, Along with Pain Relief Options Such as Analgesics, Narcotics, Nerve Blocks, Transcutaneous Nerve Stimulation, and Alternative Forms of Pain Control, Including Biofeedback, Imaging, Behavior Modification, and Relaxation Techniques

Edited by Allan R. Cook. 667 pages. 1997. 0-7808-0213-6. $78.

"The information is basic in terms of scholarship and is appropriate for general readers. Written in journalistic style . . . intended for non-professionals. Quite thorough in its coverage of different pain conditions and summarizes the latest clinical information regarding pain treatment." — *Choice, Jun '98*

"Recommended reference source."
— *Booklist, Mar '98*

Continues next page

Physical & Mental Issues in Aging Sourcebook

Basic Consumer Health Information on Physical and Mental Disorders Associated with the Aging Process, Including Concerns about Cardiovascular Disease, Pulmonary Disease, Oral Health, Digestive Disorders, Musculoskeletal and Skin Disorders, Metabolic Changes, Sexual and Reproductive Issues, and Changes in Vision, Hearing, and Other Senses; Along with Data about Longevity and Causes of Death, Information on Acute and Chronic Pain, Descriptions of Mental Concerns, a Glossary of Terms, and Resource Listings for Additional Help

Edited by Heather E. Aldred. 625 pages. 1999. 0-7808-0233-0. $78.

Pregnancy & Birth Sourcebook

Basic Information about Planning for Pregnancy, Maternal Health, Fetal Growth and Development, Labor and Delivery, Postpartum and Perinatal Care, Pregnancy in Mothers with Special Concerns, and Disorders of Pregnancy, Including Genetic Counseling, Nutrition and Exercise, Obstetrical Tests, Pregnancy Discomfort, Multiple Births, Cesarean Sections, Medical Testing of Newborns, Breastfeeding, Gestational Diabetes, and Ectopic Pregnancy

Edited by Heather E. Aldred. 737 pages. 1997. 0-7808-0216-0. $78.

"... for the layperson. A well-organized handbook. Recommended for college libraries ... general readers."
— *Choice, Apr '98*

"Recommended reference source."
— *Booklist, Mar '98*

"This resource is recommended for public libraries to have on hand."
— *American Reference Books Annual, '98*

Public Health Sourcebook

Basic Information about Government Health Agencies, Including National Health Statistics and Trends, Healthy People 2000 Program Goals and Objectives, the Centers for Disease Control and Prevention, the Food and Drug Administration, and the National Institutes of Health, Along with Full Contact Information for Each Agency

Edited by Wendy Wilcox. 698 pages. 1998. 0-7808-0220-9. $78.

Rehabilitation Sourcebook

Basic Information for the Layperson about Physical Medicine (Physiatry) and Rehabilitative Therapies, Including Physical, Occupational, Recreational, Speech, and Vocational Therapy; Along with Descriptions of Devices and Equipment Such as Orthotics, Gait Aids, Prostheses, and Adaptive Systems Used during Rehabilitation and for Activities of Daily Living, and Featuring a Glossary and Source Listings for Further Help and Information

Edited by Theresa K. Murray. 600 pages. 1999. 0-7808-0236-5. $78.

Respiratory Diseases & Disorders Sourcebook

Basic Information about Respiratory Diseases and Disorders, Including Asthma, Cystic Fibrosis, Pneumonia, the Common Cold, Influenza, and Others, Featuring Facts about the Respiratory System, Statistical and Demographic Data, Treatments, Self-Help Management Suggestions, and Current Research Initiatives

Edited by Allan R. Cook and Peter D. Dresser. 771 pages. 1995. 0-7808-0037-0. $78.

"Designed for the layperson and for patients and their families coping with respiratory illness. . . . an extensive array of information on diagnosis, treatment, management, and prevention of respiratory illnesses for the general reader."
— *Choice, Jun '96*

"A highly recommended text for all collections. It is a comforting reminder of the power of knowledge that good books carry between their covers."
— *Academic Library Book Review, Spring '96*

"This sourcebook offers a comprehensive collection of authoritative information presented in a nontechnical, humanitarian style for patients, families, and caregivers."
— *Association of Operating Room Nurses, Sept/Oct '95*

Sexually Transmitted Diseases Sourcebook

Basic Information about Herpes, Chlamydia, Gonorrhea, Hepatitis, Nongonoccocal Urethritis, Pelvic Inflammatory Disease, Syphilis, AIDS, and More, Along with Current Data on Treatments and Preventions

Edited by Linda M. Ross. 550 pages. 1997. 0-7808-0217-9. $78.

Index